WORKING

WITH

FAMILIES

IN THE

ERA

OF

HIV/AIDS

D1301237

WORKING

WITH

FAMILIES

IN THE

ERA

OF

HIV/AIDS

Edited by

WILLO PEQUEGNAT

JOSÉ SZAPOCZNIK

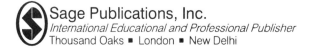

Sage Publications, Inc.
International Educational and Professional Publisher
Thousand Oaks ▪ London ▪ New Delhi

For information:

 Sage Publications, Inc.
2455 Teller Road
Thousand Oaks, California 91320
E-mail: order@sagepub.com

Sage Publications Ltd.
6 Bonhill Street
London EC2A 4PU
United Kingdom

Sage Publications India Pvt. Ltd.
M-32 Market
Greater Kailash I
New Delhi 110 048 India

Printed in the United States of America

Library of Congress Cataloging-in-Publication Data

Main entry under title:

Working with families in the era of HIV/AIDS /edited by
    Willo Pequegnat, José Szapocnik
        p.   cm.
    Includes bibliographical references and index.
    ISBN 0-7619-2216-4 (cloth: acid-free paper)
    ISBN 0-7619-2217-2 (pbk.: acid-free paper)
        1. AIDS (Disease)—Prevention. 2. HIV infections—Prevention.
    3. AIDS (Disease)—Patients—Family relationships. 4. HIV-positive persons—
    Family relationships. 5. Family—Health and Hygiene. 6. Parents of AIDS
    patients—Services for. 7. Children of AIDS patients—Services for.
    I. Pequegnat, Willo. II. Szapocznik, José
    RA644.A25.W659 2000   00-008360
    362.1′969792—dc21

00   01   02   03   10   9   8   7   6   5   4   3   2   1

Acquiring Editor:	Jim Brace-Thompson
Editorial Assistant:	Anna Howland
Production Editor:	Elly Korn
Editorial Assistant:	Victoria Cheng
Typesetter/Designer:	Marion Warren
Indexer:	Teri Greenberg
Cover Designer:	Candice Harman

Contents

Part I   Overview of Family and HIV/AIDS

Foreword

The AIDS epidemic has presented researchers, public health officials, and health and mental health professionals with constant challenges for two decades. With the introduction of new medical treatments, persons with AIDS (PWAs) are living longer, and HIV has become, for many, a chronic illness requiring long-term medical and home care. A great deal of the responsibility and burden of that care is on family members.

One challenge faced by medical and family practitioners has been to expand our definition of family to include nontraditional support systems, including extended family, nonblood kin, foster families, friends, partners, and families of choice. This book is unique in its emphasis on families as the focus of prevention and intervention and the wisdom of its authors in understanding the diversity and complexity of the families, partners, and other supportive persons who are affected by HIV/AIDS.

Drawing on the work of some of the most respected prevention researchers in the country, this book provides much-needed direction for the development of prevention programs for families at risk and interventions for HIV-infected and HIV-affected families. It focuses on populations experiencing alarming rates of increase in HIV/AIDS: African Americans, adolescents and young adults of color, and women. A number of chapters in this book have provided careful guidelines for the development of prevention programs involving parents in safe-sex education with their children and adolescents.

Many tools are provided for the practitioner as well as the researcher, and this book is unusual in offering both perspectives. Each chapter provides clear descriptions of the interventions and their different phases. The excellent use of case vignettes throughout brings the material alive.

Another contribution of this work is the emphasis on a high standard of cultural sensitivity in each research and clinical intervention. All of the researchers herein demonstrate a firsthand knowledge of the families with whom they work and their realities as well as their cultural strengths. The authors frequently emphasize the inclusion of community members in the design of the prevention programs. Many of these studies implement their interventions directly in the communities and, in some cases, the homes of their clients.

Researchers and program directors in community agencies often struggle with the process of training facilitators and practitioners. This book is unique in that an entire chapter (and sections of many others) is devoted to the issue of recruitment, personal characteristics, technical skills, training, and evaluation of facilitators who implement family interventions in community settings. The need for ongoing supervision to enhance the work of the facilitators and the overall quality of the intervention is also stressed.

An often forgotten group has been the children and adolescents orphaned by the AIDS epidemic. A number of chapters in this book lead the reader through a series of interventions that begin to answer the question of a child who will soon lose a parent to death due to AIDS—"Who will care for me?" These authors have designed interventions that address many facets of this problem, including the parenting challenges faced by a terminally ill mother or father, helping children and adolescents to live with and cope with a parent's chronic illness, helping adolescents deal with the often unrealistic expectations placed on them, disclosure to children and other family members, permanency planning for future custody of the children prior to a parent's death, and legal issues associated with custody decisions. They also address the needs of the surviving children and caregivers for bereavement counseling, help with the formation of a new family, social services, and other health and mental health needs.

The editors and authors of this book have brought together scientific knowledge, sound research methodology, clinical skill, and human compassion in a rare combination to produce this excellent volume. It will provide direction as we enter the 21st century in designing and implementing programs for families who are at risk for, living with, or affected by HIV and AIDS. It provides a road map for all of us who are committed to this work.

—Nancy Boyd-Franklin
Rutgers University

Prologue

As we marshal a national effort to prevent HIV infection, assist HIV-infected persons to live better lives, and help those dying of AIDS plan for an orderly transition for their children after their own deaths, we are once again struck by the pivotal roles that families play in these efforts. This book is the product of a national effort launched by the National Institute of Mental Health (NIMH) in 1990 to understand HIV and AIDS in the context of at-risk and affected families, as well as to encourage a program of research on family strategies in the prevention and adaptation to HIV and AIDS.

The purpose of this book is to encourage professionals to become involved in family-oriented services to prevent the spread of HIV and its consequences and to provide examples of strategies for mobilizing family resources in the prevention and adaptation to HIV and AIDS. The members of the NIMH Consortium on Families and HIV/AIDS have prepared these chapters, building on their research and practice experience. Together, some of the nation's most capable behavioral prevention and treatment scientists have developed these prevention programs based on sound scientific principles and are currently testing them in rigorous, controlled trials in communities across the country. Although these interventions have not yet been demonstrated to be effective, they have received rigorous peer review by independent scientists conducted under the auspices of the NIMH and were considered worthy of research support.

COMMUNITY COLLABORATION

One reason to be confident that these interventions will be successfully adopted in public health agencies and clinics is because they have been developed in close collaboration with research participants or with the communities where they are being implemented. Because of this collaborative approach, the interventions are community friendly and culturally appropriate. Without community involvement in the design, implementation, and evaluation of these projects, these potentially effective HIV prevention and treatment programs would not have been possible.

FOCUS OF BOOK

This book focuses on populations where HIV infection is now quickly spreading, and yet relatively little is known about family interventions with these populations. The prevention programs address the spectrum of programs to prevent the spread of HIV and its consequences. These HIV prevention programs are intended to promote greater responsibility in general and thus encourage healthier lifestyles with respect to drug use and sexual behavior among family members. Although not exclusively, the book focuses heavily on women and adolescents, and a large proportion of the programs presented in this book were designed for African American populations and address the prevention of the spread of HIV/AIDS and its consequences. With that caveat, however, it should be noted that these interventions also can be adapted for use with other cultural groups, other chronic diseases, sexually transmitted diseases (STDs), and multiple family configurations.

Family members may be left without resources as the health of the head of the household declines. Children may experience abandonment when their primary caretaker (mother, father, or both) is infected and eventually dies. Cultural background may influence who cares for these children (e.g., family members, foster parents, etc.). Increasingly, multigenerational losses may occur, which are devastating to the immediate and extended family.

OUTSIDE THE SCOPE OF THIS BOOK

So many different populations have been infected and affected by HIV/AIDS that it is not possible in one book to always include every population. Although this book focuses on some of the populations that have been heavily affected by the epidemic, it is also limited in that it does not report interventions with three groups and their families that have been heavily affected by HIV: (a) gay men, (b) intravenous drug users, and (c) hemophiliacs. To highlight the relevance of prevention in this program for all families, we will briefly review some research that highlights the significance of families in these three groups. The earliest group afflicted by the epidemic, homosexual men, has had to cope with conflicts that arise between members of their families of origin and their nontraditional families of choice. Gay men may rely on friends and lovers for many of the support functions typically provided by relatives for heterosexuals, yet these "nontraditional family members" may have no automatic legal status as heterosexual families do (Hays, Chauncey, & Tobey, 1990). Although gay friends have played an important role in promoting low-risk sexual activities, relatives of homosexual men, like their heterosexual counterparts, have played critical roles in providing care during illness episodes. Hays, Catania, McKusick, and Coates (1990), for example, found that whereas less than half of the HIV+ gay men who were not diagnosed with AIDS sought help from relatives for HIV-related concerns, once diagnosed with AIDS, more than 90% sought and obtained help from relatives. Thus, for homosexual men, the role of family members may change over the developmental course of an individual's HIV illness. As homosexuality has become increasingly accepted in society at large, gay men have developed closer and more open relationships with their families of origin, and there has been an increased understanding between families of origin and families of choice.

Drug users are another group that has been greatly infected and affected by the HIV epidemic (Szapocznik & Coatsworth, 1999). Although not designed for families coping with drug addiction, nearly all of the prevention programs discussed in this book consider drug use a risk factor for risky sexual behavior. Frequently, prevention programs in high-risk neighborhoods are likely to include families in which one or more of the responsible adults are active drug users, presenting additional challenges to prevention efforts with their children. For programs working with already infected family members, many became infected either through their own drug use or through sex with drug users. Here again, there are additional challenges because the individual's drug use might have caused a loss of family support, requiring targeted family work to repair and reintegrate the HIV+ individual and his or her family. Therefore, although not designed specifically for use with drug abusers, the interventions presented in this book can readily be adopted to include family members who are current or past drug users.

Another family group that has received special attention are hemophiliacs and their families (Klein, Forehand, Armistead, & Wierson, 1994). Between 60% and 75% of all hemophiliacs who used blood component therapy prior to May 1985 have contracted HIV infection. Individuals and family members must then cope with two chronic illnesses.

BRIDGING RESEARCH AND PRACTICE

We hope that this book, presenting the interventions designed and currently being tested by some of America's best prevention scientists, will be extremely useful to service providers in public health agencies and community-based organizations that are mounting primary and secondary prevention programs. This book is focused primarily on African American heterosexual families experiencing the challenges of HIV/AIDS. However, it is our hope to encourage more family work with families of all persons infected or affected by HIV/AIDS and other devastating diseases. Therefore, we encourage providers to consider adapting these interventions for work with other groups and other chronic illnesses.

ACKNOWLEDGMENTS

The drawing that appears on the cover of this book was developed by Katherine West, who is the graphic artist at the National Institute of Mental Health. She developed this logo for the annual NIMH Research Conference on the Role of Families in Preventing and Adapting to HIV/AIDS.

—Willo Pequegnat
—José Szapocznik

REFERENCES

Hays, R. B., Catania, J. A., McKusick, L., & Coates, T. J. (1990). Help seeking for AIDS-related concerns: A comparison of gay men of various HIV diagnoses. *American Journal of Community Psychology, 18,* 743-755.

Hays, R. B., Chauncey, S., & Tobey, L. (1990). The social support networks of gay men with AIDS. *Journal of Community Psychology, 18,* 374-385.

Klein, K., Forehand, R., Armistead, L., & Wierson, M. (1994). The contributions of social support and coping methods to stress resiliency in couples facing hemophilia and HIV. *Advances in Behavior Research and Therapy, 16,* 253-275.

Szapocznik, J., & Coatsworth, J. D. (1999). An ecodevelopmental framework for organizing the influences on drug abuse: An ecodevelopmental model for risk and prevention. In M. Glantz & C. R. Hartel (Eds.), *Drug abuse: Origins and interventions* (pp. 331-366). Washington, DC: American Psychological Association.

PART I

Overview of
Family and HIV/AIDS

Chapter 1

The Role of Families in Preventing and Adapting to HIV/AIDS

Issues and Answers

Willo Pequegnat

National Institute of Mental Health

José Szapocznik

University of Miami

Although the role of families in caring for its sick members is as old as humankind, only in recent years have researchers, health professionals, and family practitioners recognized the important role of the family in disease prevention and health promotion (Anderson & Bury, 1988; Cohen & Wills, 1985; Kazak, 1989). With enhanced treatments, HIV infection is now becoming a long-term chronic illness affecting hundreds of thousands of families. As a serious chronic illness, HIV infection is creating pressure on health care and social and mental health service providers to design comprehensive systems for families. For each of the more than 688,200 persons in the United States with AIDS, there are parents, siblings, aunts and uncles, and friends and partners in the family constellation who are affected (Centers for Disease Control and Prevention [CDC], 1998b). The family is de facto and often de jure caretakers when one of its members is ill or in trouble (Pequegnat & Bray, 1997).

AUTHORS' NOTE: The second author was partially supported in writing this chapter by NIMH Grant R37 MH55796. Requests for further information on this chapter should be sent to Dr. Willo Pequegnat, Associate Director, Primary Prevention, Translational, and International Research, Center for Mental Health Research on AIDS, National Institute of Mental Health, 6001 Executive Boulevard, Room 6205, MSC 9619, Bethesda, MD 20892 (Express Mail: Rockville, MD 20852); e-mail: Wpequegn@nih.gov.

In the United States today, 2 people younger than age 25 become HIV infected every hour, whereas in the world this number is estimated to be 450. This means that a generation of families may not be able to fulfill their potential. Fortunately, the AIDS mortality rate in the United States has been reduced in recent years with the advent of life-saving medications. Perinatal transmissions have been essentially eliminated in the United States, and cost-effective strategies are being explored in developing countries. However, for those infected who are fortunate enough to receive medical care, medication regimes can be so rigorous that doctors will not always recommend the most complex regimens for fear that patients will fail to adhere with dire consequence: the emergence of drug-resistant strains.

AIDS is changing the demographics of families not only in the United States but in other countries as well (Ankrah, 1991; Bor, 1990; Bor & Elford, 1994). The generation that should be parenting the next generation and participating actively in the workforce is experiencing the highest infection rates because AIDS has most severely affected persons between the ages of 25 to 44. AIDS differs from other diseases in an important way: It infects persons when they potentially have a long life span ahead of them. Africa best illustrates the devastation of AIDS for families and economies when people in their most productive years are struck down. In some African villages, there are primarily grandparents and children because the parent generation has died of AIDS. Remarkably, all the gains made in the past 30 years in life span have been wiped out by HIV disease in many sub-Saharan countries where the life expectancy has again fallen to 40 years old. In countries with a long history of AIDS, a new phenomenon of child-headed households is emerging (Foster, 1998). This provides a picture of the devastation that could occur in the AIDS urban epicenters in the United States if prevention programs are not pursued vigorously.

The epidemiology of AIDS has made it difficult to use traditional family models in studying and providing care to infected and affected groups. Families coping with HIV infection, unlike the standard American family of television sitcoms, are often nontraditional. Family networks include extended family members, nonblood relations, foster parents, and friends and partners chosen for familial roles. Offering services to families therefore requires a thoughtful consideration of the many configurations and types of families in modern America. When affected by HIV/AIDS, families from all walks of life may need our services.

The programs presented in this book are highlighted in the appropriate sections of this chapter to place the work of the National Institute of Mental Health (NIMH) Consortium on Families and HIV/AIDS in context. There are a range of perspectives in the chapters, from those that focus on the role of parents in preventing HIV infection in their children (DiIorio et al., 2000 [this volume];

Jemmott et al., 2000 [this volume]; Krauss et al., 2000 [this volume]; McKay et al., 2000 [this volume]) to seropositive mothers who must work out permanency planning for their adolescents to ensure a better future for their youth, including good mental health outcomes (Bauman, Draimin, Hudis, & Levine, 2000 [this volume]; Rotheram-Borus & Lightfoot, 2000 [this volume]). In urban epicenters of infection, there are adequate medical and social services for seropositive women; Mitrani, Szapocznik, and Robinson-Batista's (2000 [this volume]) program to help women adapt to HIV/AIDS focuses on interventions to improve family relations and other natural support systems and improve relations between natural supports and formal services. In contrast, in rural areas where there are few social services and seropositive women experience severe isolation, Wingood and DiClemente's (2000 [this volume]) prevention program focuses on helping these women develop a family-like social support system of seropositive women like themselves. Although many of the programs proposed are built on behavioral theory, mostly social cognitive theoretical orientation, some that work with HIV-affected families directly use systemic family principles (Mitrani et al., 2000; Rapkin, Weston, Murphy, Bennett, & Munoz, 2000 [this volume]).

This chapter is organized into six major sections: (a) epidemiology of HIV infection in family members, (b) definition of family, (c) families as a framework for prevention and adaptation to HIV, (d) role of families in preventing the spread of HIV, (e) role of family in adapting to and dying of HIV, and (f) conclusions.

EPIDEMIOLOGY OF HIV INFECTION IN FAMILY MEMBERS

Poverty, substance abuse, and community violence are disproportionately present in the lives of inner-city children (Bell & Jenkins, 1993; Garbarino, Kostelny, & Dubrow, 1991). In addition, the incidence of HIV and AIDS infection has risen dramatically in poor, primarily minority neighborhoods (Boyd-Franklin, Aleman, & Lewis, 1995). Because many significant stressors co-occur in these poor communities, it is not surprising that being reared within an inner-city environment has been associated with exposure to a wide range of health and psychological risks (Eng & Butler, 1997).

As the third decade of the AIDS epidemic approaches, several trends in the number of reported AIDS cases have emerged—trends that are likely to affect the nature of the epidemic for years to come. Of special significance is the growing number of adolescents and young adults infected with HIV, particularly women and people of color. In fact, inner-city African Americans represent 50% of all new HIV cases diagnosed with AIDS (Boyd-Franklin et al., 1995; CDC,

1998b). By the end of 1998, almost 700,000 AIDS cases had been reported in the United States, and of these, almost 100,000 were among adolescents and young adults ages 13 to 24 (CDC, 1998b).

Adolescents

African American youth are disproportionately represented among adolescent cases of HIV infection. The number of adolescents infected is doubling every 14 months (CDC, 1998c). The primary risk factor for contracting HIV among adolescents is unprotected sexual intercourse. Reflecting the level of sexual risk in the nation, each year approximately 12 million new sexually transmitted disease (STD) cases are reported, of which 3 million are individuals younger than age 20, with minorities overrepresented (CDC, 1998b; IOM, 1997). Although African American adolescents are overrepresented in current HIV cases, current risk for adolescent Hispanics is also high because of the poor rates of reported condom use at last intercourse: 48% for Hispanics as compared to 64% of African Americans (CDC, 1998a).

With 60% of 12th graders from a national sample reporting having had sexual intercourse (CDC, 1998c), a fairly substantial proportion of adolescents are at potential risk for contracting HIV. Because school connectedness is linked to later onset of sexual intercourse, most likely the 60% estimate among 12th graders represents a considerable underestimation of the actual rate of sexual intercourse among 17-year-old youth who have dropped out of school. Although each emerging cohort of adolescents has been aware of the need to use condoms for protection against HIV and other STDs, less than 50% of adolescents use condoms consistently (Jemmott, Jemmott, & Fong, 1998).

Women

During the past decade, the percentage of AIDS cases among women has grown from 9% in 1985 to 16% at the end of 1998, with a significant number of these infections due to heterosexual transmission (CDC, 1998b). Although representing 12% of the U.S. population, African American men account for 35% of AIDS cases among males in the 13 to 24 age group, and African American women account for 51% of cases among women in the same age group (CDC, 1998b). For that reason, most prevention programs in this book are focused on African American women and their families.

As Wingood and DiClemente (2000) and others have suggested, HIV infection is increasing in women, and they are often at risk because of the behavior of their partners (Ginzburg, Trainor, & Reis, 1990; Grinstead, Kegeles, Binson, & Eversley, 1993). Because of the imbalance in status and power, interventions have focused on issues of empowerment, skills training, and effective sexual negotiation (Amaro, 1995; El-Bassel & Schilling, 1992). More recent approaches have worked with couples directly to improve couple communication and understanding (e.g., Mitrani et al., 2000).

There is strong evidence that there is more efficient transmission of HIV from men to women. One of the facilitators of transmission may be the presence of an STD that increases vulnerability to HIV infection (Wyatt & Chin, 1999; Wyatt, Moe, & Guthrie, 1999). Because there are frequently no symptoms for STDs in women, they may not seek treatment. Consequently, women who engage in fewer risky acts than men may still be at greater risk of becoming infected (Pequegnat & Stover, 1999). Another aspect of HIV places women at higher risk of disease progression. Women, even with a lower viral load than men, appear to have a poorer disease course. Women experience more HIV-associated problems, progress to an AIDS diagnosis more quickly, and die from the disease sooner than men.

Few studies have examined the unique stressors that affect women living with HIV. Semple et al. (1993) identified the major stressors in 31 predominantly Caucasian women living with HIV. The main HIV-related stressors were being informed of their HIV serostatus (27.8%), having chronic financial strain (11.1%), terminating an exclusive relationship as a result of learning their HIV serostatus (11.1%), having a child develop behavioral problems subsequent to learning their serostatus (11.1%), and coping with the death of a friend from AIDS (11.1%). Other studies report additional gender-specific stressors for women with HIV, such as the caretaking responsibilities for a seropositive child, the decision to continue or terminate a pregnancy, the shame and stigmatization about having HIV, the isolation of not knowing other women with HIV, the lack of physicians who are knowledgeable about the medical and gynecological conditions common among women with HIV, and the lack of HIV support groups (Rehner, 1994; Selwyn, O'Connor, & Schottenfeld, 1995). In a recent study, African American poor urban women reported poverty and the problems associated with poverty as their greatest problems, regardless of HIV status (Smith et al., 2000). These burdens are made worse by the absence of supportive family relationships to assist women in effectively coping with these stresses, often not being prescribed the latest therapies, and barriers that poor women and women of color experience in accessing health care.

Children and Adolescents as Orphans
and Abandoned Children

In New York City, where two of the interventions associated with children in this book were conducted, at one time it had been estimated that 75,000 adolescent children would have been orphaned by HIV/AIDS by the year 2000 (Levine & Stein, 1994). However, with the advent of medications in the United States, these numbers may be much lower. Internationally, 1 in every 3 children orphaned by HIV/AIDS is younger than age 5, and increasing numbers of abandoned children live in bands in urban cities in Africa. The chronic illness and death of a parent are uniquely stressful life events (Christ, Siegel, & Sperber, 1994; Rutter, 1966), perhaps the most difficult experience a youth can face. In the Western world, about 5% of children experience the death of a parent before age 15 (Silverman & Worden, 1992; Weller, Weller, Fristad, & Bowes, 1991). However, as can be expected, in U.S. urban HIV/AIDS epicenters, this number is considerably higher.

Children of mothers with HIV/AIDS may receive services while their parents are alive. However, because they are not designated as recipients of services, the responsibility of any existing social service system may be terminated when the parent dies; often there is no safety net for them. Because few of the children are HIV infected, they will not qualify for the same level of services the parent had obtained. If the parent has made no permanency plans for them, they may need to fend for themselves. If they end up in foster care, there are limited or no income supports, no bereavement assistance, and no support options for higher education. Although the evidence is clear that a secure placement with supportive and loving caregivers can be cost-effective, custody planning is labor intensive and time-consuming and requires resources. However, the cost for not providing for proper permanency planning may be even greater in terms of school failure, early sexual debut, substance abuse, delinquency, and other behaviors that may ultimately cost society more and result in a squandered life.

DEFINITION OF FAMILY

The so-called "ideal nuclear family" only accounts for 7% of the total number of households in the United States (Levine, 1994). In recognition of this reality, the NIMH Center for Mental Health Research on AIDS (formerly the NIMH Office of AIDS) has adopted the definition of a "network of mutual commitment" to connote the range of organizational structures that are the reality of families today (Pequegnat & Bray, 1997). (NIMH has developed a logo that captures the diversity of modern families; see Figure 1.1.) Thus, persons who fulfill the roles traditionally specified by genetics and legal terms are acknowledged as family members (Mellins, Ehrhardt, Newman, & Conrad, 1996). The members of these nontraditional families may be more similar in shared values and interests than traditional extended family members because they select each other more often than is the case for members of biological families. Intergenerational families that include grandmothers parenting their grandchildren is only one configuration that is meeting the challenge of the global orphan problem (Williamson, 1994). A model that has elegantly served the needs of gay men is the differentiation between family of origin and family of choice (Lovejoy, 1989). Although

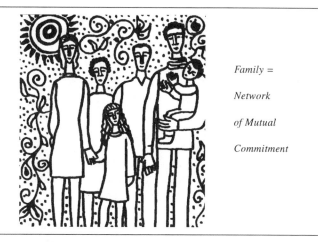

Family =

Network

of Mutual

Commitment

Figure 1.1. NIMH Logo

gay men in the 1990s may have "come out" to their parents and siblings and may consequently rely on their family of origin's support more than has been the case historically, many familial needs have been and continue to be filled by families of choice, composed of partners and extended family and friendship networks. Social networks, such as those of intravenous drug users, share intimate social experiences and paraphernalia in shooting galleries or on the streets. These social networks at times perform many familial roles even when substance abusers are in close touch with their families (Bekir, McLellan, Childress, & Gariti, 1993; Page, 1990). Although not generally known, 26 out of 28 reports attest to the regularity with which most drug addicts maintain contact with one or more of their parents or parent surrogates (Stanton & Shadish, 1997).

FAMILY CONFIGURATIONS

The following are some family configurations that are common in families infected and affected by HIV/AIDS and are based on real families, but the names are fictitious. Ruby had several children before she became infected in her 30s; when she died, her two uninfected and one infected children were left to be cared for by her mother—the children's grandmother. The grandmother already had her daughter-in-law and her two children fathered by the grandmother's son in her household. The daughter-in-law and the grandchildren have been living with the grandmother since her son was incarcerated and received a 7- to 10-year prison sentence. A second family is a mixed serostatus couple—such as John and David—who have a close circle of friends who play multiple familial roles. A third family can be a seropositive single mother, Jean, who lives with her children, some of whom are seropositive and others seronegative, and her current boyfriend—Raphael—who is not the father of any of the children. The fourth family is a seropositive woman and her boyfriend—Juanita and Sam—who are trying to decide if they are going to have a baby and, if so, whether Juanita will take the full AZT regimen to prevent vertical transmission. A fifth family can be members of a social network of injection drug users in an urban area—such as Frank and Jim—who participate in a relatively stable social network that injects together in shooting galleries and other gathering places known only to them; they play both the instrumental and social support roles of extended family members to others in their social network. Finally, there is the family in the chapter by Rapkin et al. (2000) in which an HIV+ man in a homosexual relationship is providing the social support to the grandmother of his partner's brother's girlfriend's baby.

FAMILIES AS A FRAMEWORK FOR PREVENTION AND ADAPTATION PROGRAMS

Historically, Western scientists and service providers have had an individualistic perspective (Szapocznik, 1994), but those among them with a family systems perspective balance the interests of individuals, on one hand, with the collective well-being of the family, on the other (Boyd-Franklin, 1989). In tackling problems related to preventing HIV infection and adapting to HIV/AIDS within families, it is important to understand HIV-related behaviors in the social context in which they are learned and reinforced (cf. Perrino, Gonzalez, Soldevillo, Pontin, & Szapocznik, in press; Szapocznik & Coatsworth, 1999; Szapocznik & Kurtines, 1993). Noncontextual, fragmented approaches may complicate the problem and create a sense of hopelessness on the part of individuals, families, peers, and health care workers rather than promoting family efficacy and more effective family resource use.

Impact of Which Family Member Is Seropositive

Although families most affected by the AIDS epidemic have problems in common, they are likely to face very distinct issues based on the lifestyle and premorbid vulnerability of the infected family member. The challenges faced by the family member can be quite dissimilar depending on, for example, whether the person is a gay man, an older woman, a pregnant adolescent, or an infant. A double crisis can occur when the family discovers unsuspected homosexuality, bisexuality, infidelity, or drug use at the same time that they learn of an HIV+

status. The family member must then cope with lifestyle as well as chronic health problems and death and dying issues. Social isolation may result from the stigma associated with HIV infection, a possible high-risk lifestyle, real or perceived rejection by family and friends, desire to remain anonymous, and not knowing how or with whom to talk about concerns and to whom to disclose their serostatus (Roffman, Gillmore, Gilchrist, Mathias, & Krueger, 1990).

Family Composition and Roles

In addition to the differences due to who in the family is infected, the problems families face and the ways that they cope are largely influenced by family composition. For example, women are more likely to be single parents, whereas gay men may be more likely to consider friendship networks as family. The current "family system" of living with a person with AIDS (PWA) may or may not include significant partners, parents, grandparents, children, siblings, in-laws, other relatives, close friends, and even neighbors and unrelated members of the PWA's household (Mellins et al., 1996). Critical differences among families are associated with family culture and with family members' ages and genders, the makeup of their households, their lifestyles and patterns of contact, and length of tenure in the house. The distribution of family roles and responsibilities— such as raising children, bringing in an income, and assisting the PWA—can also play a large part in shaping the kinds of problems families face, as well as options for coping with those problems. While providing support to the seropositive family member, families are also trying to prevent further infection among its members.

ROLE OF FAMILY IN PREVENTING
THE SPREAD OF HIV

As HIV infection has spread among heterosexuals, researchers have focused on risk reduction activities among families and social networks. Families are considered by many to be the single most influential force in the life of children and adolescents (Szapocznik & Coatsworth, 1999). HIV prevention family programs have typically taken the form of education about HIV/AIDS and interventions aimed at developing parental competencies that can influence adolescents' behaviors. Increased attention has been given to examining how families serve to promote or encourage adolescents to adopt responsible behavior that decreases high-risk behaviors (Brooks-Gunn & Paikoff, 1993). It has been suggested that negative family life experiences are risk factors for high-risk behaviors among adolescents. In contrast, parental monitoring of adolescent activities delays initiation of sexual behavior (Romer et al., 1994; Stanton et al., 1993; St. Lawrence, 1993). Other researchers have explored the impact of socioculturally related factors and family system functioning on issues relevant to the perception of HIV/STD risk and risk reduction among poor, urban, and ethnic families, particularly African Americans and Hispanics (Boyd-Franklin, 1989; Szapocznik & Kurtines, 1993). Due to economic and social conditions, these subgroups of families have been identified as the most at risk of acquiring HIV infection.

The increasing numbers of sexually active adolescents and their failure to use condoms consistently, along with the upward trend in HIV infection among adolescents, have renewed public health efforts to provide information on protective sexual practices to adolescents. Consistent with the public health model, most sex education programs are individually directed toward adolescents themselves and are provided through convenient venues such as school and community agencies. Some students may understand and use the information delivered this way, but others may not be ready to appreciate its significance, and still others may not be ready or predisposed to adopt recommended behaviors. Repeated exposure to sexual health messages presented in a variety of forums during the formative years can help ensure that information is available when youth are ready to receive it.

One option for matching readiness of youth with availability of information is to provide parents with information and skills (including training on developmentally appropriate ways of relating and communicating about sex) to guide their adolescents in making responsible decisions regarding sexual behavior. The assumption here is that information provided to parents will, in turn, be presented to their adolescents, and skills developed in parents will permit them to present and reinforce information in developmentally appropriate ways about sexual risk behavior throughout the teen years. Moreover, parents can do a lot more than present information about sex. Parents communicate values, model appropriate behavior, encourage bonding to family and school, encourage children to form a long-term view of their behavior, and monitor the behavior of their children and their friends. Consequently, alert parents can have considerable information about what is occurring in the life of an adolescent at any one time and can adapt their interventions to the life conditions and the potential risks facing their adolescent. Because families are the most proximal and fundamental social system influencing human development (Bronfenbrenner, 1986), they are a strategic point of entry for effective and lasting behavioral change— that is the objective of the interventions described in this book.

Research has overwhelmingly demonstrated the role that families play in healthy development (Christopherson, Miller, & Norton, 1994; Leland & Barth, 1993). The quality of parent-child relations is also an important predictor of sexual risk behaviors. Adolescents who report low levels of parental support (Biglan et al., 1990) or more emotional distance from their families are more likely to engage in sexual behaviors at a younger age (Whitebeck, Conger, &

Kao, 1993). Remarkably, children's perceptions of their relationships with their parents at ages 7 to 11 predict age of first sexual intercourse 11 years later (Miller, Norton, Curtis, Hill, & Schvaneveldt, 1998). Level of mother's coercive behavior and "love withdrawal" predict earlier age of first intercourse for women (Miller et al., 1998). Positive family factors have also proven protective of sexual risk behaviors (Leland & Barth, 1993). In particular, adolescents' beliefs that they have a close relationship with their parents are protective against early sexual intercourse. Paikoff and colleagues found that there is greater risk of early sexual debut with earlier pubertal maturation if there is family conflict (Paikoff et al., in press).

Although the overall quality of the parent-child relationship is important in preventing risky sexual behaviors in teens, parent-child communication is a critical determinant of their risky sexual behaviors. The lack of open and comfortable discussion about sexuality, even in the most relevant relationships, is a major concern for adolescent HIV prevention (IOM, 1997). In general, parents and children do not speak sufficiently about sexuality (Hutchinson & Cooney, 1998), and, as a result, adolescents overestimate their mothers' level of approval of their sexual behavior, whereas mothers underestimate the amount of sexual activity of their teens (Jaccard, Dittus, & Gordon, 1998). Parent-child communication about sex decreases HIV risk behaviors (Leland & Barth, 1993; Stanton et al., 1993). Youth reporting parent-child discussions about sex are more likely to delay sexual activity (Fox, 1981; Darling & Hicks, 1982; Stanton et al., 1993). Mother-adolescent discussions regarding condom use prior to first sexual intercourse increase the chances of adolescents using condoms during first sexual intercourse and subsequent encounters (Christ, Raszka, & Dillon, 1998; Christopherson et al., 1994; Miller et al., 1998).

Given the important role that parents can play in promoting the sexual health of their adolescents, particularly as it relates to HIV prevention, several parent-oriented interventions have been developed by members of the NIMH Consortium on Families and HIV/AIDS and are presented in this book (DiIorio et al., 2000; Jemmott et al., 2000; Krauss et al., 2000; McKay et al., 2000). Krauss has developed a prevention program for mothers and fathers to use with preadolescent children to help parents become experts in their children's eyes (Krauss et al., 2000). In this way, parents can teach and model for their children knowledge, attitudes, and behaviors about HIV/AIDS and safer sexual practices. These efforts are aimed at fostering family involvement in the sexual health of adolescents, including delay of sexual intercourse, acquisition of information about HIV/AIDS, and enactment of HIV risk reduction practices. Parents participate in four 3-hour group training sessions, given once a week. These sessions cover HIV knowledge and HIV safety skills; child development; parent-child communication; communication about sex, drugs, and HIV; recognition of risky situations and how to avoid them; negotiation skills to handle risky situations; and sensitive and safe interactions with persons with HIV. The initial parent training is followed by a parent-child session in which each parent and child meet alone with a facilitator, the parent chooses activities to perform with the child, and the child has an opportunity to ask any unanswered questions. The parent group meets again after 3 months to discuss real-life situations that have occurred.

Parents play a pivotal role in guiding adolescents' sexual behavior during transition years in which situations of "sexual possibilities" are likely to increase (McKay et al., 2000). A sexual possibility is an opportunity for young people to engage in risky behavior because they are not closely supervised. The intervention developed by Paikoff (1995) combines both parent-only groups and child-only groups with multiple-family groups. It is meant to promote comfort and communication about information and values related to puberty, early sexual behavior, and HIV/AIDS. Work in this realm has borrowed heavily from Bronfenbrenner's (1986) social ecological theory, which considers parents as the most fundamental social context influencing children's development into adaptive or maladaptive adolescents (i.e., children who manage more or less constructively their social relationships). This work recognizes that the sexual behavior of adolescents must be approached as part of the social development of the youth and that parents have a crucial role to play in guiding and shaping the social and sexual development of their children. It should be noted that within this movement there are two streams: One of these builds on the evidence that parents or parent figures lose influence as children reach adolescence, and the other builds on the evidence that parents or parent figures continue to have considerable influence on their children, even as children grow into adolescence, but that as youth mature and grow in their search for autonomy, it takes considerable skill to harness this influence in such a way that it can continue to guide youth even after they enter into a world in which peer norms—perceived and real—gain significant influence. Clearly, the work of Paikoff et al. (in press; see McKay et al., 2000) is representative of the latter approach.

DiIorio and her colleagues (2000) have developed a prevention program for mothers and their adolescents (11 to 14 years old). The long-term objectives of this approach are to foster family involvement in the sexual health of adolescents, including delay of sexual intercourse, acquisition of information about HIV/AIDS, and the enactment of HIV risk reduction practices. Mothers and adolescents meet every 2 weeks over 3 months for a total of seven sessions. All sessions are designed to be interactive with the use of games, videos, role-plays, and skits to demonstrate and practice skills learned in the session. There are also take-home activities in which each participant can set a personal goal to be accomplished before the next session.

Interventions with parents, particularly mothers, may be critically important to reduce HIV risk-associated sexual behaviors of African American male adolescents. Jemmott and her colleagues (2000) have therefore developed an intervention that is designed so that mothers can teach their sons about sex to decrease risky behavior among this very at-risk population. This program helps mothers examine their personal values related to sexuality and provides them with factual information to share with their sons. Activities are intended to increase mothers' understanding about developmental challenges and social stressors that their sons are experiencing and to improve their parental communication skills.

ROLE OF FAMILY IN ADAPTING TO AND DYING OF HIV

Although AIDS until recently was almost universally a fatal disease, with adequate treatment it is increasingly becoming a chronic disease. When adherence to treatment is a challenge, when symptoms persist, when the infected individual is psychologically or physically debilitated by the illness, or when there are other complicating factors such as substance abuse, mental illness, or other severe chronic conditions, families continue to be under considerable stress, and their commitment to the patient continues to be challenged. Many issues within families can be addressed in preventive interventions, such as the following:

1. disclosure of disease status and symptoms;
2. disclosure and stigma about revealing within the family the route of infection (homosexuality, drug use);
3. overcoming obstacles in the past relationship between the seropositive person and her or his family;
4. developmental issues and changing roles (e.g., an adult who for many years was independent needs to be reintegrated into family for care, the teenager of a dying parent trying to move toward emancipation, a drug-addicted mother in recovery who needs to regain a role as mother and daughter within her family, etc.);
5. stress and coping abilities of the seropositive individual and family; and
6. adaptation to disease, infectiousness, and the dread of a "death" sentence.

There are also issues of the family in relation to its social environment, such as social stigma if extended family, friends, and neighbors find out about the HIV status; relationship between family of origin, on one hand, and family of choice and friends, on the other; and relationship between the various aspects of family and the health care system.

Multiple problems create obstacles and challenges for families attempting to cope with AIDS, including geographical distance; competing demands for family members' time, energy, or other resources (Stoller & Pugliesi, 1989); lack of knowledge about how to be helpful (Good, Good, Schaffer, & Lind, 1990; Starrett, Bresler, Decker, Waters, & Rogers, 1990); and a history of negative interactions (Shinn, Lehmann, & Wong, 1984; Fiore, Becker, & Coppel, 1983; Fobair et al., 1986). As illness advances, some family members withdraw due to physical or emotional exhaustion or overidentification with the patient (Carl, 1986; Dunkel-Schetter & Wortman, 1982; Flaskerud, 1989; Namir, Wolcott, & Fawzy, 1989). Family members may also be reticent to discuss problems with the PWA, for fear of making the PWA sicker by worrying him or her. By the same token, PWAs may be reluctant to become a burden to their family members (Hays, Catania, McKusick, & Coates, 1990). The problems of coping with illness are compounded by the stigma of AIDS. PWAs and their families may experience rejection from friends, loss of jobs, and harassment (Bor, Miller, & Goldman, 1993). Concerns about disclosure may cause parents affected by AIDS considerable difficulty in seeking support, disclosing to their children, and making permanency plans for children who will be orphaned at their death (Smith & Rapkin, 1995, 1996).

Families affected by AIDS face multiple health care and psychosocial problems throughout the illness trajectory. Problems include complex medical management and caregiving issues, disruption of family roles and routines, and concerns about the family's future as illness progresses. The course of illness and the efficacy of treatment are both unpredictable at the level of an individual, making it impossible for families to know precisely when and with what problems they will need to cope. Often families have not resolved issues associated with the PWA's exposure to HIV, including homosexuality, bisexuality, substance use, and infidelity prior to finding themselves in a caretaking role.

Family members may have caretaking concerns that include helplessness associated with being overwhelmed by the needs of their ill family member for time, energy, or money, and they may feel that they do not possess the abilities needed to be good caregivers. Major adjustments in the family's lifestyle may need to occur if the ill family member lives at home. Siblings and spouses may have additional concerns such as having their needs ignored as the family attends to the sick member. There may be anger in low-income families where everyone is expected to contribute to the household but the seropositive person is unable because of fatigue and unpredictable health.

Several studies conducted prior to the advent of the newest medications have provided an initial taxonomy of the problems experienced by families affected by symptomatic AIDS cases (Pequegnat & Bray, 1997). These stressors are still relevant when the seropositive family member is unable to tolerate treatment, is unresponsive to such treatment, or has other conditions that make medication adherence difficult (e.g., substance abuse, mental illness) and consequently continue to manifest severe physical symptomatology:

1. concerns about recurring acute illness episodes;
2. difficulty in adhering to a complex medical regimen;

3. isolation from other family members and friends, contributing to the deterioration of partner and family relationships;
4. emotions associated with illness (e.g., depression, confusion, loneliness, fear, and suicidal ideation);
5. guilt about having infected others;
6. difficulty in maintaining a predictable routine;
7. anxiety about financial problems;
8. complicated task of relating to multiple health and mental health providers;
9. lack of good medical care and counseling;
10. lack of available and affordable housing and related services because of their known health status;
11. possible need to address problems of substance abuse and change in lifestyle;
12. lack of respite from providing care and inadequate or unavailable alternative child care;
13. need to plan for bereavement and future of the survivors; and
14. handling the stigma of a disease with moral overtones.

Obviously, AIDS places an enormous strain on family systems. Families are called on to respond and manage an unpredictable illness while managing other chronic and acute stressors, often with little or no specialized training, guidance, or support. Given the scope and uncertainty of the challenges they face, families affected by AIDS need flexible coping skills that can be applied to a variety of circumstances. It is interesting to note that the patterns of reliance on family seem to differ according to population or site. In a study of the use of public health service in the New York City greater metropolitan area, Crystal and Kersting (1998) found that asymptomatic persons tend to rely on social support from their families, but as the disease progressed, public health services are used more for more complex health complications. In contrast, a study in San Francisco revealed that seropositive gay men tended to rely on their families of choice and extended support network, but as the disease progressed, they tended to rely more on their family of origin (Hays et al., 1990). These differences may be explained by proximity to family. In New York, a larger heterosexual population tended to live closer to their families. As the disease progressed, the family may have become exhausted or burdened with having to care for more than one seropositive family member. In San Francisco, on the other hand, the population was more largely homosexual with parents not living in the area. As the disease progressed, the family of choice or the extended family of choice may have become exhausted, and in fact romantic partners may have also become ill and died, at which time the seropositive person tended to seek the support of their families, who often lived out of town and had not been taxed up to that point with the stress of day-to-day care.

Coping with AIDS is exacerbated when more than one family member in a household, or even in the close extended family, is HIV infected, including children. Indeed, many families have already experienced significant losses due to AIDS. PWAs and their families are subject to considerable distress associated with these demands and concerns. Of course, problems related to AIDS co-occur with other issues facing the family. Given high levels of poverty, substance use, unemployment, and poor health care, at any given time, AIDS-related problems may not even be the most pressing for these families (Smith et al., 2000). In addition to the stressors experienced by all families, AIDS-affected families have additional challenges that require family solutions, such as caretaking for the ill family members and reassigning roles filled by the seropositive person prior to the illness. Rapkin et al. (2000) have developed an intervention to enhance AIDS-affected families' abilities to problem solve. The Family Health Project (Rapkin et al., 2000) teaches families problem-solving skills. Problem solving is broken down into its component elements, and families are encouraged to follow these steps: (a) create a comfortable climate for problem solving, (b) identify the problem, (c) brainstorm, (d) weigh the consequences of various alternatives, (e) think through together the implementation of possible solutions, (f) set goals, and (g) evaluate solution outcomes.

Taking another tack, Szpaocznik and colleagues (see Mitrani et al., 2000) have designed an intervention to improve the quality of the social relations and supports of African American seropositive women. In their work, this team found that one out of every two seropositive African American women who reported problems with their families had a recent history (less than 3 years) of drug addiction or abuse. Not surprisingly, however, for all the women—those who had been drug abusers and those who had not—the usual problems in living confronted by inner-city minority families were prevalent: poverty, parenting issues, day care, family conflict, marital infidelity, and violence in the neighborhood causing the loss of lives of close friends and family members, among others. For these women, family therapy to assist in the integration to the family of origin was needed because frequently, family members felt that they had been betrayed in prior episodes of sobriety that ended in relapse. An approach focusing on changing the quality of relationships, building family trust, increasing mutual support, and reducing blaming and personal attacks (family negativity) was successful in helping the seropositive women regain a valued role with their families. Often family work targeted restoring the woman to a parenting role with her young children, whose guardianship she had frequently lost to her mother because of addiction and neglect. A broadly social ecological perspective also helps to rebuild a supportive network around the woman and her family that includes the family's relation to kin and other neighborhood supports, faith community, and HIV support groups, among others.

Although Szapocznik and colleagues' prevention program reintegrates women into their social support system, a program that helps seropositive women build social support networks to enhance and prolong their lives is the WiLLOW program (Wingood & DiClemente, 2000). The WiLLOW program creates HIV support networks for women in semirural areas, where these women feel isolated through stigma and low rates of disclosure. There are several compelling clinical and public health reasons to design a secondary prevention program for women living with HIV aimed at building supportive social networks, increasing coping skills, and reducing stress, risky sexual behaviors, and STDs. First, an effective program could reduce the risk of disease progression among women living with HIV that may result from women's exposure to other strains of HIV or sexually transmitted diseases during unprotected sex. Second, an effective program could promote quality of life among women living with HIV that may result from reducing stressors, enhancing coping skills, and building stronger social networks that, it is hoped, will translate into a more healthy life and less need for expensive health care. Third, an effective program could reduce risk of HIV transmission to seronegative sexual partners. Finally, an effective program could reduce risk of HIV transmission to unborn children.

Children and Adolescents as Orphans and Abandoned Children

Based on the literature on childhood bereavement, it is anticipated that children and adolescents who are orphaned will experience long-term difficulties in adjustment as a result of losing a parent (see Sandler et al., 1992, for a review). Losing a parent in adolescence is of particular concern because it may affect developmental processes of self-concept and identity formation, interpersonal relations, schoolwork, family involvement, and psychological well-being. At the individual level, bereavement can impede a youth's successful completion of these developmental tasks and interfere with a successful transition to adulthood (Balk, 1991). The negative impact on adolescents whose parents live with HIV/ AIDS may be even greater than would be suggested by the bereavement literature because these families typically experience additional AIDS-specific stressors, including stigma (Herek & Capitanio, 1993), protracted illness that may disrupt childhood, internal and familial conflict over disclosure (to whom? when? how much?), and, because HIV/AIDS is associated with poverty, a lack of buffering resources such as a second parent in the home and involvement in substance use subcultures, which may adversely affect pre-AIDS family coping.

At the family social ecological level, having a parent incapacitated by AIDS and later losing that parent to AIDS have ecodevelopmental consequences (cf. Szapocznik & Coatsworth, 1999). When families are functioning in an adaptive way, parents are typically the family leaders, and when they are ill or die, that family leadership and connectedness may be lost unless provision has been made to have it taken over by someone else. Parents connect the child to the extended family. Parents also have critical roles to play in providing guidance, nurturance, and support. Moreover, they can be involved in collaborative relations with teachers to help a child achieve in school and may exert sufficient influence to guide youth toward prosocial peers and away from antisocial peers. When a parent becomes ill or dies, these important ecodevelopmental functions are lost or at best imperiled.

The literature on childhood parental loss has focused mainly on post-death factors and has tended to neglect pre-death factors. Parents who are dying of AIDS are often burdened by poverty, inadequate medical care, and a host of other interrelated social problems. Many of these chronic stressors and those that occur in poor communities have been found to affect children's mental health (Achenbach, Howell, Quay, & Conners, 1991; Florenzano, 1991; Garbarino et al., 1991; Jaenicke et al., 1987; Masten, Best, & Garmezy, 1990; Quinton, 1989; Wallerstein & Kelly, 1980).

The parent's terminal illness itself is a chronic stressor that may create psychological risk for children (Garmezy & Rutter, 1988; Rutter, 1979). Garmezy and Rutter (1988) found that repeated stressors (e.g., multiple hospital admissions of an ill parent) were more likely to be related to psychological disturbance in children in the context of chronic psychosocial adversity. The effects were not cumulative but geometric: Children were 4 times more likely to demonstrate psychiatric disorder when exposed to two stressors and 10 times more likely when exposed to more than five stressors. Because children of parents with AIDS may have many potent risk factors for psychological disturbance before parental death, they may be especially vulnerable to psychological disorder after the death.

To address these problems with children and adolescents orphaned by HIV/AIDS, two prevention programs that were developed with a community-based organization are presented. Although AIDS orphans are an appropriate target for preventive efforts, few systematic attempts have been made to intervene. Bauman et al. (2000) have developed Project Care, which is a preventive intervention designed to improve the psychological functioning of children who survive the death of a parent from AIDS. This intervention has four specific goals: (a) facilitating disclosure decisions and heightening communication between the ill parents and their children and future caregivers, (b) enhancing the stability and security of the child's future through development of an appropriate and feasible custody plan prior to the parent's death, (c) working with the caregiver and child after parental death to ease the transition to the new family, and (d) providing access to concrete resources and social support. This is accomplished by a carefully crafted home-based program that is delivered in two parts: (a) after parental diagnosis with AIDS (or late-stage HIV disease) and (b) after parent death. Family specialists meet with the family approximately every 2 weeks to access the resources that are required (e.g., lawyers, social workers, etc.) to move the family along the permanency planning continuum and to accomplish disclosure and transition goals. A range of psychoeducational materials is used to address healthy eating, stress management, and relaxation.

Another program designed to help parents make decisions regarding disclosure and custody as well as to increase a family's ability to maintain positive daily routines while the PWA is ill has been developed by Rotheram-Borus and Lightfoot (2000). The coping skills of a family to handle the challenges of HIV disease are extremely important in their adjustment to HIV and normalizing life. The ultimate goal of this prevention program is the long-term adjustment of the adolescent children after their parent has died. This program is designed to address issues of social identity, roles, rules, and behaviors of these youth. There are different phases of the intervention: coping skills intervention, illness phase, and adjustment phase, which occurs after the parent has died.

CONCLUSIONS

AIDS has presented families with a whole constellation of new prevention and adaptation challenges. The prevention programs presented in this book provide service providers with an array of options for working with families around these issues. Family-oriented prevention programs can greatly enhance the quality of life of families infected and affected by HIV. They also provide programs that can enhance the social service options of service agencies and may ultimately prove to be cost-effective by keeping family members from becoming infected and by keeping those who are infected out of the expensive public health care system.

REFERENCES

Achenbach, T., Howell, C., Quay, H., & Conners, C. (1991). National survey of competencies and problems among 4-16 year olds: Parents' reports for normative and clinical samples. *Monograph of the Society for Research in Child Development, 56*(3), 1-131.

Amaro, H. (1995). Love, sex, and power: Considering women's realities in HIV prevention. *American Psychologist, 50,* 437-447.

Anderson, R., & Bury, M. (1988). *Living with chronic illness: The experience of patients and their families.* London: Unwin Hyman.

Ankrah, E. M. (1991). The impact of AIDS on the social, economic, health and welfare systems. In G. B. Rossi, E. Beth-Giraldo, L. Chieco-Bianchi, F. Dianzani, G. Giraldo, & P. Verani (Eds.), *Science challenging AIDS* (pp. 175-187). Basel, Switzerland: Karger.

Balk, D. E. (1991). Death and adolescent bereavement: Current research and future directions. *Journal of Adolescent Research, 6*(1), 7-27.

Bauman, L. J., Draimin, B., Levine, C., & Hudis, J. (2000). Who will care for me? Planning the future care and custody of children orphaned by HIV/AIDS. In W. Pequegnat & J. Szapocznik (Eds.), *Working with families in the era of HIV/AIDS* (pp. 155-188). Thousand Oaks, CA: Sage.

Bekir, P., McLellan, T., Childress, A. R., & Gariti, P. (1993). Role reversals in families of substance misusers: A transgenerational phenomenon. *International Journal of Addiction, 28*(7), 613-630.

Bell, C., & Jenkins, E. J. (1993). Community violence and children on Chicago's South Side. *Psychiatry: Interpersonal and Biological Processes, 56,* 46-54.

Biglan, A., Metzler, C. W., Wirt, R., Ary, D., Noell, J., Ochs, L., French, C., & Hood, D. (1990).
    Social and behavioral factors associated with high-risk sexual behavior among adolescents.
    Journal of Behavioral Medicine, 13, 245-261.
Bor, R. (1990). The family and HIV/AIDS. *AIDS Care, 2*(4), 409-412.
Bor, R., & Elford, J. (1994). *The family and HIV.* New York: Cassell.
Bor, R., Miller, R., & Goldman, E. (1993). HIV/AIDS and the family: A review of research in the
    first decade. *Journal of Family Therapy, 15,* 187-204.
Boyd-Franklin, N. (1989). *Black families in therapy: A multisystems approach.* New York:
    Guilford.
Boyd-Franklin, N., Aleman, J.-G., & Lewis, L. Y. (1995). Cultural sensitivity and competence: Afri-
    can American, Latino, and Haitian families with HIV/AIDS. In N. Boyd-Franklin, G. L. Steiner,
    & M. G. Boland (Eds.), *Children, families and HIV/AIDS: Psychosocial and therapeutic issues*
    (pp. 115-126). New York: Guilford.
Bronfenbrenner, U. (1986). Ecology of family as a context for human development research. *Ameri-
    can Psychologist, 32,* 513-531.
Brooks-Gunn, J. & Parkoff, R. L. (1993). Sex is a gamble, kissing is a game: Adolescent sexuality,
    contraception, and pregnancy. In S. Millstein, A. C. Petersen, & E. Nightengale (Eds.), *Promo-
    tion of healthy behavior during adolescence* (pp. 180-208). New York: Oxford Press.
Carl, D. (1986). Acquired immune deficiency syndrome: A preliminary examination of the effects
    on gay couples and coupling. *Journal of Marital and Family Therapy, 12*(3), 241-247.
Centers for Disease Control and Prevention (CDC). (1998a). *Prevention and treatment of sexually
    transmitted diseases as an HIV prevention strategy—November 1998.* Atlanta, GA: Author.
Centers for Disease Control and Prevention (CDC). (1998b). *Year-end 1998* (HIV/AIDS Surveil-
    lance Reports). Atlanta, GA: Author.
Centers for Disease Control and Prevention (CDC). (1998c). *Youth risk behavior survey 1997* (CD-
    ROM). Atlanta, GA: Author.
Christ, G. H., Siegel, K., & Sperber, D. (1994). Impact of parental terminal cancer on adolescents.
    American Journal of Orthopsychiatry, 64(4), 604-613.
Christ, J. J., Raszka, W. V., & Dillon, C. A. (1998). Prioritizing education abut condom use among
    sexually active female adolescents. *Adolescence, 33*(132), 735-744.
Christopherson, C. R. (1994). Pubertal development, parent-teen communication, and sexual values
    as predictors of adolescent sexual intentions and sexually related behaviors. *Dissertation Ab-
    stracts International Section A: Humanities and Social Sciences 54*(12A), 4599.
Cohen, S., & Wills, T. A. (1985). Social support, stress and the buffering hypothesis. *Psychological
    Bulletin, 98,* 310-357.
Crystal, S., & Kersting, R. C. (1998). Stress, social support, and distress in a statewide population of
    persons with AIDS in New Jersey. *Social Work in Health Care, 28*(1), 41-60.
Darling, C. A., & Hicks, M. W. (1982). Parental influence on adolescent sexuality: Implications for
    parents as educators. *Journal of Youth and Adolescent, 11,* 231-245.
DiIorio, C., Resnicow, K., Denzmore, P., Rogers-Tillman, G., Wang, D. T., Dudley, W. N., Lipana,
    J., & Van Marter, D. F. (2000). Keepin' it R.E.A.L.! A mother-adolescent HIV prevention pro-
    gram. In W. Pequegnat & J. Szapocznik (Eds.), *Working with families in the era of HIV/AIDS*
    (pp. 113-132). Thousand Oaks, CA: Sage.
Dunkel-Schetter, C. A., & Wortman, C. B. (1982). The interpersonal dynamics of cancer: Problems
    in social relationships and their impact on the patient. In H. S. Friedman & M. R. DiMateo (Eds.),
    Interpersonal issues in health care (pp. 69-100). New York: Academic Press.
El-Bassel, N., & Schilling, R. (1992). Fifteen-month followup of women methadone patients taught
    skills to reduce heterosexual HIV transmission. *Public Health Reports, 107,* 500-504.
Fiore, J., Becker, J., & Coppel, P. B. (1983). Social network interactions: A buffer or stress? *Ameri-
    can Journal of Community Psychology, 11,* 423-439.

Flaskerud, J. H. (1989). Psychosocial and neuropsychiatric aspects. In J. H. Flaskerud (Ed.), *AIDS/ infection: A reference guide for nursing professionals* (pp. 145-168). Philadelphia, PA: W. B. Saunders.

Florenzano, R. (1991). Chronic mental illness in adolescence: A global overview. *Pediatrician, 18*(2), 142-149.

Fobair, P., Hoppe, R. T., Bloom, J., Cox, R., Varghese, A., and Spiegel, D. (1986). Psychosocial problems among survivors of Hodgkin's disease. *Journal of Clinical Oncology, 4*(5), 805-814.

Foster, G. (1998, July). *Child-headed households in the era of parental deaths from AIDS.* Invited plenary address to the NIMH Conference on the Role of Families in Preventing and Adapting to HIV/AIDS, Washington, DC.

Fox, J. L. (1981). The family's role in adolescent sexual behavior. In T. Ooms (Ed.), *Teenage pregnancy in a family context* (pp. 73-130). Philadelphia, PA: Temple University Press.

Garbarino, J. E., Kostelny, K., & Dubrow, N. (1991). What children can tell us about living in danger. *American Psychologist, 46,* 376-382.

Garmezy, N., & Rutter, M. (1988). *Stress, coping, and development in children.* Baltimore, MD: Johns Hopkins University Press.

Ginzburg, H. M., Trainor, J., & Reis, E. (1990). A review of epidemiologic trends in HIV infection of women and children. *Pediatric AIDS and HIV Infection: Fetus to Adolescent, 1,* 11-15.

Good, M. D., Good, B. J., Schaffer, C., & Lind, S. E. (1990). American oncology and the discourse on hope. *Culture, Medicine, and Psychiatry, 12,* 59-79.

Grinstead, O. A., Kegeles, B., Binson, E., & Eversley, R. (1993). Women's sexual risk for HIV: The National AIDS Behavioral Surveys. *Family Planning Perspectives, 6,* 252-257.

Hays, R. B., Catania, J. A., McKusick, L., & Coates, T. J. (1990). Help seeking for AIDS-related concerns: A comparison of gay men of various HIV diagnoses. *American Journal of Community Psychology, 18,* 743-755.

Herek, G. M., & Capitanio, J. P. (1993). Public reactions to AIDS in the United States: A second decade of stigma. *American Journal of Public Health, 83,* 574-577.

Hutchinson, K. M., & Cooney, T. M. (1998). Patterns of parent teen sexual risk communication: Implications for intervention. *Family Relations: Interdisciplinary Journal of Applied Family Studies, 47*(2), 185-194.

Eng, T. R., & Butler, N. T. (Eds.) (1997). *The hidden epidemic: Confronting sexually transmitted diseases.* Washington, DC: National Academy Press.

Jaccard, J., Dittus, P. J., & Gordon, V. V. (1998). Parent-adolescent congruency in reports of adolescents' sexual behavior and in communication about sexual behavior. *Child Development, 69*(1), 247-261.

Jaenicke, C., Hammen, C., Zupan, B., Hiroto, D., Gordon, D., Adrian, C., & Burge, D. (1987). Cognitive vulnerability in children at risk for depression. *Journal of Abnormal Child Psychology, 15*(4), 559-572.

Jemmott, J. B., III, Jemmott, L. S., & Fong, G. T. (1998). Abstinence and safer sex HIV riskreduction interventions for African American adolescents: A randomized controlled trial. *Journal of the American Medical Association, 279,* 1529-1536.

Jemmott, L. S., Outlaw, F., Jemmott, J. B., III, Brown, E. J., Howard, M., & Hopkins, B. H. (2000). Strengthening the bond: The mother-son health promotion project. In W. Pequegnat & J. Szapocznik (Eds.), *Working with families in the era of HIV/AIDS* (pp. 133-151). Thousand Oaks, CA: Sage.

Kazak, A. E. (1989). Families of chronically ill children: A systems and social-ecological model of adaptation and challenge. *Journal of Consulting and Clinical Psychology, 57,* 25-30.

Krauss, B. J., Godfrey, C., Yee, D., Goldsamt, L., Tiffany, J., Almeyda, L., Davis, W. R., Bula, E., Reardon, D., Jones, Y., DeJesus, J., Pride, J., Garcia, E., Pierre-Louis, M., Rivera, C., Troche, E., Daniels, T., O'Day, J., & Velez, R. (2000). Saving our children from a silent epidemic: The PATH program for parents and preadolescents. In W. Pequegnat & J. Szapocznik (Eds.), *Working with families in the era of HIV/AIDS* (pp. 89-112). Thousand Oaks, CA: Sage.

Leland, N. L., & Barth, R. P. (1993). Characteristics of adolescents who have attempted to avoid HIV and who have communicated with their parents about sex. *Journal of Adolescent Research, 8,* 58-76.

Levine, C. (1994). AIDS and the changing concept of the family. In R. Bor & J. Elford (Eds.), *The family and HIV* (pp. 3-22). London: Cassell.

Levine, C., & Stein, G. (1994). *Orphans of the HIV epidemic: Unmet needs in six U.S. cities.* New York: The Orphans Project.

Lovejoy, N. C. (1989). AIDS: Impact on the gay man's homosexual and heterosexual families. *Marriage and Family Review, 14,* 285-316.

Masten, J. A., Best, F., & Garmezy, N. (1990). Resilience and development: Contributions from children who overcome adversity. *Development and Psychopathology, 2,* 425-444.

McKay, M. M., Baptiste, D., Coleman, D., Madison, S., Paikoff, R., & Scott, R. (2000). Preventing HIV risk exposure in urban communities: The CHAMP Family Program. In W. Pequegnat & J. Szapocznik (Eds.), *Working with families in the era of HIV/AIDS* (pp. 67-87). Thousand Oaks, CA: Sage.

Mellins, C. A., Ehrhardt, A. A., Newman, L., & Conard, M. (1996). Selective kin: Defining the caregivers and families of children with HIV disease. In L. S. Jemmott & A. O'Leary (Eds.), *Women and AIDS: Coping and care* (pp. 123-149). New York: Plenum.

Miller, B. C., Nortin, M. C., Curtis, T., Hill, E. J., & Schvaneveldt, P. (1998). The timing of sexual intercourse among adolescents: Family, peer and other antecedents. *Youth and Society, 29*(3), 390.

Mitrani, V. B., Szapocznik, J., & Robinson Batista, C. (2000). Structural ecosystems therapy with HIV+ African American women. In W. Pequegnat & J. Szapocznik (Eds.), *Working with families in the era of HIV/AIDS* (pp. 243-279). Thousand Oaks, CA: Sage.

Namir, S., Wolcott, D. L., & Fawzy, F. I. (1989). Social support and HIV spectrum disease: Clinical research perspectives. *Psychiatric Medicine, 7,* 97-105.

Page, J. B. (1990). Shooting scenarios and risk of HIV infection. *American Behavioral Scientist, 33,* 478-490.

Paikoff, R. L. (1995). Early heterosexual debut: Situations of sexual possibilities during the transition to adolescence. *American Journal of Orthopsychiatry, 65*(3), 389-401.

Pequegnat, W., & Bray, J. (1997). Families and HIV/AIDS: Introduction to the special sections. *Journal of Family Psychology, 11*(1), 3-10.

Pequegnat, W., & Stover, E. (1999). Considering women's contextual and cultural issues in HIV/ST prevention research. *Cultural Diversity and Ethnic Minority Psychology, 5*(3), 287-291.

Perrino, T., Gonzalez, A., Soldevillo, A., Pontin, H., & Szapocznik, J. (in press). The role of families in adolescent HIV prevention: A review. *Clinical Child and Family Psychology Review.*

Quinton, D. (1989). Adult consequences of early parental loss. *British Medical Journal, 299*(6701), 694-695.

Rapkin, B., Bennett, J. A., Murphy, P., & Muñoz, M. (2000). The Family Health Project: Strengthening problem solving in families affected by AIDS to mobilize systems of support and care. In W. Pequegnat & J. Szapocznik (Eds.), *Working with families in the era of HIV/AIDS* (pp. 213-242). Thousand Oaks, CA: Sage.

Rehner, T. A. (1994). *Depression in Alabama women with HIV.* Ph.D. dissertation, School of Social Work in the Graduate School, University of Alabama.

Roffman, R., Gillmore, M., Gilchrist, L., Mathias, S. A., & Krueger, L. (1990). Continuing unsafe sex: Assessing need for AIDS-prevention counseling. *Public Health Reports, 105,* 202-208.

Romer, D., Black, M., Ricardo, I., Feigelman, S., Kaljee, L., Galbraith, J., Nesbit, R., Hornick, R. C., & Stanton, B. (1994). Social influences on sexual behavior of youth at risk for HIV exposure. *American Journal of Public Health, 84,* 977-985.

Rotheram-Borus, M. J., & Lightfoot, M. (2000). Helping adolescents and parents with AIDS to cope effectively with daily life. In W. Pequegnat & J. Szapocznik (Eds.), *Working with families in the era of HIV/AIDS* (pp. 189-211). Thousand Oaks, CA: Sage.

Rutter, M. (1966). *Children of sick parents: An environmental and psychiatric study.* London: Oxford University Press.

Sandler, I. N., West, S. G., Baca, L., Pillow, D. R., Gersten, J. C., Rogosch, F., Virdin, L., Beals, J., Reynolds, K. D., Kallgren, C., Tein, J.-Y., Kriege, G., Cole, E., & Ramirez, R. (1992). Linking empirically based theory and evaluation: The family bereavement program. *American Journal of Community Psychology, 20*(4), 491-521.

Selwyn, P. A., O'Connor, P. G., & Schottenfeld, R. A. (1995). Female drug users with HIV infection: Issues for medical care and substance use treatment. In H. Minkoff, J. A. DeHovitz, & A. Duerr (Eds.), *HIV infection in women* (pp. 241-262). New York: Raven.

Semple, S. J., Patterson, T. L., Temoshok, L. R., McCutchan, J. A., Straits-Troster, K. A., Chandler, J. L., & Grant, I. (1993). Identification of psychobiological stressors among HIV-positive women. *Women & Health, 20,* 15-36.

Shinn, M., Lehmann, S., & Wong, N. W. (1984). Social interaction and social support. *Journal of Social Issues, 40*(4), 5-76.

Silverman, P. R., & Worden, J. W. (1992). Children's reactions in the early months after the death of a parent. *American Journal of Orthopsychiatry, 62*(1), 93-104.

Smith, L., Feaster, D. J., Prado, G., Kamin, M., Blaney, N., & Szapocznik, J. (2000). *The effect of HIV status on the psychosocial functioning of African American recent mothers.* Manuscript submitted for publication.

Smith, M. Y., & Rapkin, B. D. (1995). Unmet needs for help among persons with AIDS. *AIDS Care, 7*(3), 353-363.

Smith, M. Y., & Rapkin, B. D. (1996). Social support and barriers to family involvement in caregiving for persons with AIDS: Implications for patient education. *Patient Education and Counseling, 27,* 85-94.

St. Lawrence, J. S. (1993). African-American adolescents' knowledge, health-related attitudes, sexual behavior, and contraceptive decision: Implications for the prevention of adolescent HIV infection. *Journal of Consulting and Clinical Psychology, 61,* 104-112.

Stanton, B., Romer, D., Ricardo, I., Black, M., Feigelman, S., & Galbraith, J. (1993). Early initiation of sex and its lack of association with risk behaviors among adolescent African Americans. *Pediatrics, 92,* 13-19.

Stanton, M. D., & Shadish, W. R. (1997). Outcome, attrition, and family-couples treatment for drug abuse: A meta analysis and review of the controlled, comparative studies. *Psychological Bulletin, 122*(2), 170-191.

Starrett, R. A., Bresler, C., Decker, J. T., Waters, G. T., & Rogers, D. (1990). The role of environmental awareness and support networks in Hispanic elderly persons' use of formal social services. *Journal of Community Psychology, 18,* 218-227.

Stoller, E. P., & Pugliesi, K. L. (1989). Other roles of caregivers: Competing responsibilities or supportive resources? *Journal of Gerontology, 44,* 31-38.

Szapocznik, J. (1994, August). *Hispanic families' contributions to a psychology for all people.* Invited address presented at the 102nd annual meeting of the American Psychological Association, Los Angeles.

Szapocznik, J., & Coatsworth, J. D. (1999). An ecodevelopmental framework for organizing the influences on drug abuse: An ecodevelopmental model for risk and prevention. In M. Glantz & C. R. Hartel (Eds.), *Drug abuse: Origins and interventions* (pp. 331-366). Washington, DC: American Psychological Association.

Szapocznik, J., & Kurtines, W. M. (1993). Family psychology and cultural diversity: Opportunities for the theory, research and application. *American Psychologist, 48*(4), 400-407.

Wallerstein, J., & Kelly, J. (1980). *Surviving the breakup.* New York: Basic Books.

Weller, R. A., Weller, E. B., Fristad, M. A., & Bowes, J. M. (1991). Depression in recently bereaved prepubertal children. *American Journal of Psychiatry, 148*(11), 1536-1540.

Whitebeck, L. B., Conger, R. D., & Kao, M. (1993). The influence of parental support, depressed affect, and peers on the sexual behavior of adolescent girls. *Journal of Family Issues, 14,* 261-278.

Williamson, J. (1994). *Action for children affected by AIDS: Programme profiles and lessons learned.* New York: World Health Organization and UNICEF.

Wingood, G. M., & DiClemente, R. J. (2000). The WiLLOW program: Mobilizing social networks of women living with HIV to enhance coping and reduce sexual risk behaviors. In W. Pequegnat & J. Szapocznik (Eds.), *Working with families in the era of HIV/AIDS* (pp. 281-298). Thousand Oaks, CA: Sage.

Wyatt, G. E., & Chin, D. (1999). HIV and ethnic minority women, families, and communities. *Cultural Diversity and Ethnic Minority Psychology, 5*(3), 179-182.

Wyatt, G. E., Moe, A., & Guthrie, D. (1999). The gynecological, reproductive, and sexual health of HIV-positive women. *Cultural Diversity and Ethnic Minority Psychology, 5*(3), 183-196.

Chapter 2

Assessment and Evaluation of HIV/AIDS Families

Applications to Prevention and Care

James H. Bray   Ernest Frugé

Baylor College of Medicine

Sylvia and her partner have come to the clinic for 6 weeks. They originally came because Sylvia did not feel that Jimmy understood how difficult it was to be seropositive and care for three children. In the process, the therapist determined that Sylvia and Jimmy are unable to successfully problem solve because when a difference of opinion arises, they revert to attacking each other. Sylvia declared that she now feels that Jimmy understands her, and she feels no need to come back for additional therapy. Although Sylvia now feels supported, Sylvia and Jimmy do not yet have the skills to problem solve on their own. The therapist is concerned that when Sylvia's father comes back to live with the couple, their inability to problem solve their differences about how to manage the father's intrusions into the couple's lives will cause a deterioration in the couple's relationship.

Sylvia's report of her perceived needs is somewhat different from the therapist's assessment of the problems confronting the couple. Although the therapist perceives the issues of empathy and support that brought Sylvia to seek services, the therapist also perceives that the couple's conflict resolution skills are

AUTHORS' NOTE: The first author's contribution to this chapter was partially supported by National Institute of Alcohol Abuse and Alcoholism Grant RO1 AA/DA 08864. Correspondence concerning this chapter should be addressed to James H. Bray, Ph.D., Department of Family and Community Medicine, Baylor College of Medicine, 5510 Greenbriar, Houston, TX 77005; e-mail: JBRAY@BCM.TMC.EDU.

maladaptive. In addition, the therapist is concerned because an external stressor will soon challenge the couple's problem-solving skills: Sylvia's father's intrusions into the couple's relationship. This discrepancy between individual self-reports and observed behaviors represents an important theme in the family assessment and the family intervention fields.

Accurate assessment of family relationships and functioning is an important issue in evaluating and treating families. This truism for all families is also true for families in which one or more family members have HIV/AIDS. Formal assessment is always a challenge for service providers because of the press of time to develop and execute a treatment plan. However, in family interventions, just as in individual psychotherapy, the success of a treatment plan often depends on accurate assessment of the nature of the problem and the potential for solutions (Szapocznik & Kurtines, 1993).

The purpose of this chapter is to make available to providers some of the experience that has been developed in research and evaluation of families. On one hand, information on family assessment issues and strategies will improve providers' abilities to quickly determine the nature of problems in families. On the other hand, findings from research on family evaluation will alert providers to "blind spots" that can mislead providers as they work with families. This can enhance their conduct of family interventions in general and with families with HIV/AIDS in particular.

This chapter is organized along the following topics: (a) What is a family in the HIV/AIDS arena? What are strategies for identifying the family? Who should be included in the assessment? (b) What are important characteristics of family functioning? (c) What are important factors that influence our observations of family functioning? (d) What are the issues in assessing families? (e) What is the clinical application of family assessment?

WHAT IS A FAMILY IN THE HIV/AIDS ARENA?

The composition of modern American families is quite diverse and includes traditional two-parent families with children, single-parent families, stepfamilies, extended kin families, quasi-kin families, and a host of other configurations (Bray, 1993; Levine, 1994). In the case of individuals suffering from HIV/AIDS, family compositions may be even more unique—in many cases, with nonbiological relationships as their functional core. In recognition of this fact, the National Institute of Mental Health (NIMH) defined *family* as a network of mutual commitment (Pequegnat & Bray, 1997). Thus, persons who fulfill relationship roles heretofore traditionally specified by biological or legal relationships are now considered family members for the purpose of supporting patients and understanding their social contexts (Mellins, Ehrhardt, Newman, & Conrad, 1996).

Families formed by mutual commitment are quite common for gay men and injection drug users (Pequegnat & Bray, 1997) and are increasingly common in heterosexual family relations. Networks of gay men have developed families of choice, in addition to their families of origin (Lovejoy, 1989). Likewise, injection drug users may have intimate social networks who perform family functions but may still be in close contact with their biological family members (Page, 1990). The mostly heterosexual HIV+ individuals participating in the family interventions described in this volume were all part of a family. The targets of these interventions range from mother-child dyads to families transitioning from parental illness and death due to AIDS through foster care placement of a child orphaned to HIV/AIDS.

Which type of family member performs what type of role can change with time and circumstances, particularly during the course of a chronic, debilitating, and life-threatening illness. When the burdens of caregiving become more extreme, patients, institutions, or the government often call on biological kin. For example, grandmothers and other kin are often left to parent children in multigenerational families because of the deaths of mothers from AIDS.

The diversity of family compositions presents unique challenges for service providers. Some of the challenges include (a) how to define families and determine which individuals should be included in services, (b) where to draw the boundaries that define "the family" in any particular case, and (c) how to handle the fluidity of some families in which family composition changes over time (e.g., due to death, beginning or ending of romantic involvements, or as a result of interventions that change the boundaries of families to include additional supports or to separate disruptive or detrimental influences such as drug-abusing family members).

PROCEDURE FOR IDENTIFYING THE FAMILY

Pequegnat et al. (2000) describe a procedure to identify the family. The first step in the family identification protocol is to construct a genogram with the HIV+ client. The genogram is a method used to obtain a visual representation of several generations of the family of the target individual. With minority families, the authors recommend including four generations in the genogram, as well as biological and nonbiological relations that are "like family." In this family tree, the nature of relationships (strong, weak, conflicted, severed) is indicated by thick, thin, jagged, or broken lines, respectively, and the roles are indicated. After the genogram is completed, additional information is obtained on the length of time individuals have lived in the household of the target individual. Furthermore, the nature of contributions by individuals who live and do not live in the family, such as who cares for the children, who does household tasks, and who provides emotional and financial support, is also assessed. The reason for such an elaborate procedure is that although in some cultures individuals are unlikely to reveal individuals with whom they have conflictive relations within their intimate family, in other cultures individuals are likely to be overly inclusive of who they report as a family member. From a service provision perspective, it is important to identify all individuals who have an ongoing functional relation (positive or negative) as well as to identify individuals who are potential yet untapped sources of support.

The NIMH definition of *family* as a "network of mutual commitment" (Pequegnat & Bray, 1997) is a case in point. This definition may certainly facilitate a more realistic picture of the caregiving context of the person with AIDS. However, the basic definition includes such a broad spectrum of potential family members that consistent definitions of family may be difficult. One possible guideline is to relate the definition of family makeup to the goals of the treatment plan. For example, if the outcome of interest is developing a competent caregiving system for the person with HIV, then the members of the family invited to preventive and treatment interventions might include only those family members who directly care (or potentially could care) for that person. On the other hand, if the treatment goals include the children of persons with HIV, then the boundaries of the family could be extended to those involved in the care of the children as well as those who can facilitate or impede this important family function.

Regardless of the particular definition, the constellation of family membership is dynamic and changes over time. Changes in the composition of families are a common finding in service provisions to HIV-involved families. Because of the changing and progressive nature of the disease and, in some cases, unstable relationship systems, it is highly probable that family composition may change over the course of either short- or long-term treatment. In addition, some prevention and treatment programs may result in changes in family composition, such as when an abusive or drug-abusing family member is removed from the family.

IMPORTANT CHARACTERISTICS
OF FAMILY FUNCTIONING

Efforts to capture the complexity and subtlety of family relationships, their natural processes, and the influences of family members on family life over time have led to a variety of assessment strategies. Such diversity of perspectives is useful in reflecting the uniqueness of each family and the rich tapestry of family dynamics. However, four types of family characteristics are frequently assessed in research and evaluation of families. Because these characteristics have been so frequently measured in family research (Bray, 1995a; Fisher, 1976; Grotevant, 1989), we suggest that they may be useful for providers as well. These include (a) family composition, (b) family process, (c) family affect, and (d) family organization. Family complexity and diversity interact among all four of these factors.

Family Composition

Family composition refers to family membership (e.g., couple only, couple with children, single-parent family), structure of the family (e.g., nuclear family, divorced family, stepfamily), and factors such as ethnic group (e.g., African American, Hispanic). Family composition is a key marker for other aspects of family functioning.

Family Process

Family process factors include behaviors and interactions and transactions among family members that characterize essential elements or patterns of behavioral exchanges between or among family members and the function or outcomes associated with these exchanges. Process measures attempt to reflect core features of transactional behavior such as conflict, differentiation, communication, problem solving, and control. Family process is distinguished from content. Family process is the transactions between family members without regard to content. For example, when Sylvia says to Jimmy, "You never help me take out the garbage," the content is "garbage" and "chores." However, the process of "You never help me" could easily apply to any content area other than garbage. In this regard, process also refers to the message or metacommunication, "I feel unsupported by you."

Process can sometimes also refer to the nature of the transactional patterns. For example, if Jimmy says to Sylvia, "I would like to make love with you now," and Sylvia responds by saying, "You never take out the garbage," the function of "You never take out the garbage" may be to avoid discussion or action on Jimmy's request to make love. Consequently, exactly the same words (content), depending on their context, could have very different functions (process). In this case, what is reflected may be part of a pattern in which an emotionally laden request receives a response that changes the topic of conversation.

Family Affect

Family affect refers to the nature of the emotional expression among family members. The emotional tone and volume of interactions are important aspects of the context of family processes and greatly affect how family members experience or interpret communications. Measures of expressed emotion between family members, particularly negative emotion, offer some of the most reliable predictors of outcome in studies of chronic problems such as schizophrenia, mood disorders, and alcoholism. Similarly, considerable research has found that negative affect is prominent in families with acting-out and antisocial adolescents.

Actually, a broad range of affective qualities must be considered in determining the character of family relations. These range from loving, supportive, and nurturing affect to negative, hostile, and sarcastic. In addition, the level or volume of affective tone is also important and may range from families in which there is little affect, or affect is overcontrolled, to families in which the volume of either positive or negative affect is very high. Negative affect at high volume is usually disruptive of family life. Hence, there is widespread acceptance that negative affect is undesirable, and interventions to correct it are needed. In addition, very high levels of affectivity in general can in some families be problematic but need not be problematic in every case.

Family Organization

Family organization factors refer to rules and roles within the family and expectations for behavior that contribute to family functioning. These factors include aspects such as (a) boundaries, (b) decision hierarchy, and (c) the distribution of labor and emotional support functions. Because issues around boundaries are very useful to understand in families affected by HIV/AIDS, we present an expanded discussion on this topic. Boundaries refer to the emotional and psychological closeness or distance between family members and between the family and the external world (Szapocznik & Kurtines, 1993). In general, boundaries need to be permeable to permit interaction across them, but the nature of which boundaries are appropriate may differ with the developmental stage of the family (see below on context). Families with an infant, for example, naturally have strong boundaries around the mother and infant. As the infant grows, the boundary between mother and infant becomes more flexible, and eventually, when the child and siblings are developmentally in a similar stage, the boundaries among siblings may be stronger than the boundary around the mother and child.

Another interesting boundary issue occurs in the relation of nuclear and extended family or kin networks. In some cultures, boundaries around the nuclear family are quite rigid, whereas in other cultures, boundaries between the nuclear family and their extended or kinship network are quite fluid. As indicated below (under context), culture is an important defining feature of families—it will prescribe the nature of the family interactions that are acceptable. What is acceptable may change considerably from family to family and from culture to culture.

FAMILY DIVERSITY AND COMPLEXITY

Family diversity and complexity are responsible for important variations within and across the factors presented earlier. For example, family process may be quite different for different family compositions in different ethnic groups at different developmental stages, and these differences may result in important differences in individual functioning for family members in different family roles (cf. Bray, 1995a; Fine, 1993; Szapocznik & Kurtines, 1993). For example, hypothesized relationships among these factors may not hold in different family structures, such as single-parent families or stepfamilies (Hetherington & Clingempeel, 1992). Families are also dynamic rather than static systems. Relationships between factors noted at one point may change in form over time. Thus, as families develop and family members move into different family roles (i.e., infant grows and begins school; children leave the home), the nature of family composition, process, affect, and organization will all be affected by these important developmental transitions.

FACTORS THAT INFLUENCE OBSERVATIONS
OF FAMILY FUNCTIONING

Context plays a critical role in influencing families. The contexts in which families are observed may dramatically affect how families behave. Consequently, we may see very different family relationships and interactions depending on the context in which the family is observed and what the family is asked to do (i.e., discussing a family problem vs. planning a family vacation). For example, in a clinic, a family may be on their best behavior, but in their own dining room, they may interact in a more typical way. Several chapters in this volume deliver their interventions in different settings and contexts. For instance, Bauman, Draimin, Hudis, and Levine (2000 [this volume]) and Mitrani, Szapocznik, and Robinson Batista (2000 [this volume]) use home-based interventions, whereas Jemmott et al. (2000 [this volume]) deliver interventions in housing projects.

Another example of the context of family is consideration of how the stage of a family's life cycle may influence the behavior of a family. Family life cycle theory teaches us that most families progress through a definable set of stages, each characterized by an interrelated set of developmental tasks and dynamics (e.g., caring for young children). Life cycle theory suggests that the ways families adapt to both predictable and unpredictable challenges and changes are greatly influenced by the life cycle stage of the family (Carter & McGoldrick, 1988).

Yet a third example of context is the consideration of the broader cultural and ethnic attributes that may specifically define and influence family life cycle stages and the characteristic behaviors of certain groups of families. Thus, the appraisal of family functioning, particularly the definition of *normality*, should be considered in the context of the specific life cycle stages as well as in context of cultural and ethnic dimensions.

Most of the current models of family relationships and functioning are based on White middle-class families that do not necessarily reflect variations that may be typical for families from different cultural and ethnic backgrounds and those suffering with an HIV family member (Bray, 1995a). Indeed, most family measures, with a few exceptions (e.g., Szapocznik & Kurtines, 1993), are based on these models and have not been validated with families from diverse ethnic backgrounds (Baer & Bray, 1999; Bray, 1995b; Hampson, Beavers, & Hulgus, 1990; Morris, 1990). Researchers and clinicians are cautioned to keep this limitation in mind when using measures and instruments developed on one ethnic group to assess the health and dysfunction of families from other ethnic and cultural backgrounds. The readers are referred to the recent issue of the journal *Family Relations* on family diversity for further information (Fine, 1993).

However, standardized family measures can still be useful in providing information about the family at several different points using the same assessment ruler. So-called "objective measures" can then be interpreted in the broader context of what is known about the life and culture of the family. Hence, although many measures have not been used with a particular cultural group, the practitioner can nevertheless use the measure across a sample of ethnically specific families and establish her or his own sense of how families compare with each other on a particular measure. This "don't throw the baby out with the bath water" approach is intended to encourage practitioners to not fully discount family measures that have been used with their population. Rather, learn how these measures can be helpful in your practice setting and what they tell you about the specific cultural group served in your practice setting.

ISSUES IN ASSESSING FAMILIES

In choosing a family assessment strategy, service providers should first determine which aspects of family functioning are most likely to be relevant to the goals of prevention and treatment that are of most interest. This consideration involves several dimensions: (a) the members of the family who are being evaluated, (b) the methods of the assessment that have been selected, and (c) the methods of examining the family system by using all these sources of information (Dakof, 1996). It is also important in assessing interpersonal interactions to distinguish between properties of the relationship (e.g., conflict, cohesion) from feelings or attitudes (e.g., anger, positivity-negativity) that individuals have about the relationship (Thompson & Walker, 1982). As previously stated, deciding on whom to include in the assessment of the family system is a major issue in the HIV/AIDS arena.

Wisdom has emerged from family research that can be very useful for clinical applications. For example, family research measures are often based on self-report data from individual family members describing their own perceptions of the family, rather than reports from multiple family members or direct observations of families in interaction (Bray, 1995a, 1995b; Fisher, Kokes, Ransom, Phillips, & Rudd, 1985). Most surveys and assessments of individual family members use this type of information, with the assumption that self-report information represents valid and complete information on family functioning.

Family research reveals that information obtained from an individual may or may not accurately reflect the functioning of the entire family (Fisher et al., 1985; Ransom, Fisher, Phillips, Kokes, & Weiss, 1990). Several studies have found statistically significant and clinically important differences among family members' reports of family functioning (Cole & McPherson, 1993; Cook & Goldstein, 1993). For instance, research on the breakup of relationships indicates that there are frequently significant differences reported by the partners in satisfaction with the relationship and why it is ending. The examination of the differences in perceptions between individual family members can be useful for prevention and treatment efforts; logic and clinical practice suggest that bridging these differences in perception can have therapeutic value for improving the quality of relationships (Bray, 1995a).

Although the assessment of an individual's perceptions is suitable for evaluating certain aspects of the family system (e.g., differentiation within the family of origin), these assessments are not truly measures of the family system as a whole. Information obtained from individuals within a family can be transformed into relational measures by various means that are beyond the scope of this chapter (Bray, 1995a, 1995b; Cole & McPherson, 1993; Fisher et al., 1985; Kolevzon, Green, Fortune, & Vosler, 1988; Ransom et al., 1990). Suffice it to say that family-level measures can be developed from averaged or weighted responses of individual family members. This provides an overall evaluation of the family that may be helpful if it provides information about how distressed this family is in comparison to other families with whom the practitioner has successfully worked (Olson, 1977). As mentioned earlier, the self-reports of individual family members can also simply be compared to other members of the family to see how much agreement there may be on issues that are likely to be important in the prevention or treatment programs.

An alternative approach would be to directly observe how family members interact and try to solve a problem when there are likely to be diverse points of view. The interactions that occur around a task may reveal the typical positive and negative patterns of family interaction. Fisher et al. (1985) termed this category of measurement *transactional assessment*. Transactional assessment involves some type of direct observation of family members in a predefined standard task or structured interaction. Transactional assessments reflect interactions at a system level, rather than a simple sum or averaging of individual points of view. These assessments can measure the interactions of all the participating members of the family or focus on several individuals who seem to dominate the discussion and decision-making process within the family.

In contrast to self-report measures, these directly observed transactional assessments also represent an outsider's view of the family. These assessments involve a trained professional making judgments about family interactions. However, family members can also make ratings and observations about family interactions, as exemplified by Gottman's work on marital relationships (Gottman & Levenson, 1992).

There is unresolved controversy about the necessity to assess the entire family in both the research and clinical literatures (Bray, 1995b; Carlson, 1989). Occasionally, examining the interactions of various family dyads (e.g., a couple within the family) and triads (e.g., two parents and a child) may be more useful than examining the family as a whole (Bray, 1995a; Cole & Jordan, 1989; Gable, Belsky, & Crnic, 1992; Kashy & Kenny, 1990; Kenny & LaVoie, 1984). Sometimes, information from smaller family subgroups can lead to more focused treatment plans. Changing the behavior of a few members of a family will ultimately lead to shifts in the entire family (Szapocznik & Kurtines, 1993). This marks a shift from viewing and discussing the family exclusively as a coherent whole. In recognizing that many critical aspects of family functioning are reflected in specific processes and interactions between particular family members (e.g., the couple), the arena of family assessment and intervention has become more differentiated—recognizing that sometimes individual perceptions are most useful, but other times contrasts in individual perceptions, measures of full family functioning, or measures of the functioning of family subsystems may be most useful.

Without a consensus on what constitutes a "gold standard" in family measurement (Bray, 1995a), researchers and clinicians usually rely on more than one method for assessing family process (how the family behaves when it is together) and outcomes (whether the family successfully achieves the goals that it has articulated). The two most common measurement methods in family assessment are the use of self-report instruments and behavioral observations of family interactions (Bray, 1995b). It is important to understand that the information obtained by these methods does not always agree with each other (Cole & McPherson, 1993; Cook & Goldstein, 1993; Kolevzon et al., 1988; Markman & Notarius, 1987).

SELF-REPORT METHODS

Self-reports of family functioning are probably the most common means of assessing family relations and processes in research contexts (Bray, 1995b), and there are hundreds of published self-report measures of family functioning. The intervention programs described in this book used family measures that are applicable to the HIV/AIDS arena. Self-report measures include perceptions of the family by individual family members, ratings by family members of other family members' behavior or relationships, and self-reports of affect and emotions while engaging in certain behaviors (Bray, 1995b). It is beyond the scope of this chapter to review them in any detail, and the reader is referred to excellent books by Fredman and Sherman (1987), Grotevant and Carlson (1989), and Touliatos, Perlmutter, and Straus (1990) for reviews of many of the family measures. A review of self-report measures used and recommended by the NIMH Consortium on Families and HIV/AIDS represented in this book is found in Pequegnat et al. (2000).

There are many benefits to self-report instruments of family functioning (Bray, 1995b). Foremost, self-reports are usually economical, are easy to collect in a clinical setting, and can be administered in repeated sessions to document changes within the family. Self-report measures thus can be a convenient gauge for changes in outcomes as a result of a preventive or treatment intervention. To measure changes over time, however, the clinician must be careful to select measures that reflect the kinds of changes that are likely to occur in the prevention or treatment program rather than a measure of stable family or individual characteristics. It is also wise to select more specific measures of family functioning with reasonable theoretical or empirical linkages to the prevention or treatment interventions being evaluated, in addition to global reports on family functioning. For example, an intervention that is trying to restore a woman to a responsible role in the family should assess not only her individual perceptions but also her actual behaviors within the family to determine if the woman, in fact, has been restored to a responsible role in the family.

A good example of a self-report scale of family functioning that has demonstrated reliability and better-than-average association with other indicators of family coping with medical illness is the Family Environment Scale, developed by Rudolf Moos and his colleagues (Phipps & Mulhern, 1995).

OBSERVATIONAL METHODS

Observations of families can range from qualitative measures, such as narrative descriptions of family relations, to very quantitative approaches such as the specific coding of interactional sequences (e.g., microanalytic coding; Carlson & Grotevant, 1987; Ransom et al., 1990). Observational measures attempt to measure the real-time patterning of family interactions that are of interest to family clinicians.

There are three dimensions of standardized observations: (a) what is observed (i.e., what task family members are asked to perform), (b) where it is observed (i.e., home, office), and (c) how it is observed (i.e., the coding system employed; Bray, 1995b). To facilitate comparisons between families, it is desirable to establish a specific task to be performed by each family (e.g., plan a menu). The form of the task chosen often reflects common problematic situations in average family life (e.g., discussing how to solve a discipline problem with a child). Alternatively, the specific task may be carefully designed to stimulate dimensions of interaction that are thought to be particularly relevant to the problem being investigated (e.g., discussing who is going to have custody of a child after the mother dies from AIDS).

What Is Observed?

Problem-solving tasks in which family members are asked to identify a common problem, discuss it, and attempt to develop a solution to the problem (Markman & Notarius, 1987) are widely used. These tasks are engaging and often revealing of typical patterns of family interactions. This type of task can elicit discord, creativity, and a family's usual style or pattern of conflict resolution. Problems selected may be identified as internal to the family or couple versus external. There are also standardized games, such as the Simulated Family Activity Measurement (SIMFAM; Straus & Tallman, 1971), which can be used as the catalyst for a problem-solving task. Other types of tasks include providing emotional support or encouragement for a family member, planning pleasant events (e.g., a family trip or vacation), describing qualities of the family, making up stories to standardized pictures (e.g., the Thematic Apperception Test), putting together puzzles or games, and talking about what happened during the day (Grotevant & Carlson, 1989).

Each type of task tends to elicit different types of family interactions. For instance, the task of discussing differences in individual views asks family members to defend their position on certain ideas and values and can reflect issues of power, group pressure, and autonomy, whereas the planning tasks may be more likely to elicit positive interactions and role relationships. In all family assessments, it is important to sample various content domains to ensure that one obtains a picture of how the family functions across a variety of meaningful domains.

Where Does the Observation Take Place?

Direct observation of family interaction is often set in a clinic due to financial and logistical constraints. Direct observations, however, can also be set in more natural settings such as the home (e.g., dinner table conversations) or school (e.g., classroom). Recent research indicates that families show little reactivity to observation per se (Jacob, Tennenbaum, Seilhamer, Bargiel, & Sharon, 1994) and to exposure to standardized tasks, although different types of behavior may be exhibited in different settings. Thus, the setting used for observation should be selected for the purpose of the assessment and chosen to maximize the chances for a relevant sample of behavior. For example, if parent management strategies for child behavior problems are the target, then a home observation setting may be particularly useful. The use of more naturalistic and longer-term observational approaches may also be required in the case of behavior that occurs rarely, such as temper tantrums or abusive behaviors.

How Are Families Observed?

Family interactions can be used to obtain global ratings (e.g., positive to negative quality of interaction), on one hand, or highly specific frequency counts of a particular behavior (e.g., how many times did a parent criticize a child), on the other (Bray, 1995b). The latter type of observation can be very useful for identifying linked patterns of behaviors (Gottman, 1994; Markman & Notarius, 1987). For example, what follows a parental criticism of a child? Is a critical parental behavior followed by adolescent compliance or rebellious behavior? Actually, it may vary by family. In some families, parental criticism of an adolescent may result in an adolescent compliant response, but in another family it may result in an adolescent rebellious response. The reader is referred to Grotevant and Carlson (1989) and Markman and Notarius (1987) for reviews of various behavioral observation systems and to Pequegnat et al. (2000) for observational methods currently in use in HIV-related family studies.

CLINICAL APPLICATION OF FAMILY ASSESSMENTS

Even though there are good family measures, family-oriented practitioners are not likely to use standardized or formal family assessments in their practices (Boughner, Hayes, Bubenzer, & West, 1994; Bray, 1995b; Floyd, Weinand, & Cimmarusti, 1989). Yet, there are many reasons for clinicians to use formal, standardized methods for assessing families (Bray, 1995b). Evaluations conducted before prevention or treatment intervention begins can provide a rich source of information about the family and can be used to develop initial hypotheses about problem areas, causes of problems, and potential areas of strengths. Assessment also ensures that a broad range of routine information is collected to make certain that important areas are not overlooked. By using a battery of self-report methods, a substantial amount of information can be ascertained with minimal clinician time. In addition, given that most clients and family members initially view the presenting problem as within an individual, completing family assessment instruments begins to redefine the problem as a family systems issue, which can start the therapeutic process.

Most of the available family measures and methods have been developed for research contexts and have not been specifically applied to clinical practice. Consequently, many instruments do not provide either the instructions or clinically relevant norms and comparisons necessary for use in practice settings. These factors may explain the recent survey finding that most family practitioners do not necessarily view formal family assessment as an important part of clinical practice (Boughner et al., 1994). Few researchers have developed manuals to assist practitioners to use their methods as part of routine clinical practice. One exception is the work of Szapocznik and Kurtines (1993), who provide a detailed guide to the use of observational measures as part of family therapy practice with behavior problem adolescents.

Using a standard battery of instruments also facilitates comparisons between a family's current functioning and published normative data. Given the limitations of family assessment, it is probably wise to view the normative data as suggestive rather than as defining pathology. Likewise, clinicians and researchers need to be cognizant of different norms for various family structures (e.g., nuclear, single parent, stepparent) and ethnic backgrounds (Bray, 1995b). In addition, initial assessments can be compared to posttreatment assessments to document intervention-related changes. With the changes in health care reimbursement and the demand for the demonstration of treatment efficacy, formal assessments that document positive change are becoming a central part of the therapeutic process. Clinicians who are able to empirically demonstrate treatment effectiveness are likely to be in greater demand in the near future. The use of measures will make it easier for clinicians to compare families and gain insights that may be applicable to future client families.

It is clear that more attention is needed to develop methods that can capture the complex phenomena of family relationships found in this arena. A number of new and promising methods are currently being developed in other areas of family research that may provide clinicians with innovative ways of assessing family relationships and outcomes. These types of innovations will facilitate the further development of effective family prevention and treatment interventions to prevent and adapt to HIV/AIDS.

REFERENCES

Baer, P. E., & Bray, J. H. (1999). Adolescent individuation and alcohol usage. *Journal of Studies on Alcohol, 13,* 52-62.

Bauman, L., Draimin, B., Levine, C., & Hudis, J. (2000). Who will care for me? Planning the future care and custody of children orphaned by HIV/AIDS. In W. Pequegnat & J. Szapocznik (Eds.), *Working with families in the era of HIV/AIDS* (pp. 155-188). Thousand Oaks, CA: Sage.

Boughner, S. R., Hayes, S. F., Bubenzer, D. L., & West, J. D. (1994). Use of standardized assessment instruments by marital and family therapists: A survey. *Journal of Marital and Family Therapy, 20,* 69-75.

Bray, J. H. (1993). Families in demographic perspective: Implications for family counseling. *The Family Journal, 1,* 94-96.

Bray, J. H. (1995a). Assessment of family health and distress: An intergenerational-systems perspective. In J. C. Conoley & E. Werth (Eds.), *Family assessment* (pp. 67-102). Lincoln, NE: Buros Institute of Mental Measurement.

Bray, J. H. (1995b). Family assessment: Current issues in evaluating families. *Family Relations, 44,* 469-477.

Carlson, C. I. (1989). Criteria for family assessment in research and intervention contexts. *Journal of Family Psychology, 3,* 158-176.

Carlson, C. I., & Grotevant, H. D. (1987). A comparative review of family rating scales: Guidelines for clinicians and researchers. *Journal of Family Psychology, 1,* 23-47.

Carter, E. A., & McGoldrick, M. (Eds.). (1988). *The changing family life cycle* (2nd ed.). New York: Gardner.

Cole, D. A., & Jordan, A. E. (1989). Assessment of cohesion and adaptability in component family dyads: A question of convergent and discriminant validity. *Journal of Counseling Psychology, 36,* 456-463.

Cole, D. A., & McPherson, A. E. (1993). Relation of family subsystems to adolescent depression: Implementing a new family assessment strategy. *Journal of Family Psychology, 7,* 119-133.

Cook, W. L., & Goldstein, M. J. (1993). Multiple perspectives on family relationships: A latent variables model. *Child Development, 64,* 1377-1388.

Dakof, G. A. (1996). Meaning and measurement of family: Comment on Gorman-Smith et al. (1996). *Journal of Family Psychology, 10,* 142-146.

Fine, M. A. (Ed.). (1993). Family diversity (Special issue). *Family Relations, 42*(3).

Fisher, L. (1976). Dimensions of family assessment: A critical review. *Journal of Marriage and Family Counseling, 2,* 367-382.

Fisher, L., Kokes, R. F., Ransom, D. C., Phillips, S. L., & Rudd, P. (1985). Alternative strategies for creating "relational" family data. *Family Process, 24,* 213-224.

Floyd, F. J., Weinand, J. W., & Cimmarusti, R. A. (1989). Clinical family assessment: Applying structured measurement procedures in treatment settings. *Journal of Marital and Family Therapy, 15,* 271-288.

Fredman, N., & Sherman, R. (1987). *Handbook of measurements for marriage and family therapy.* New York: Brunner/Mazel.

Gable, S., Belsky, J., & Crnic, K. (1992). Marriage, parenting, and child development: Progress and prospects. *Journal of Family Psychology, 5,* 276-294.

Gottman, J. M. (1994). *What predicts divorce?* Hillsdale, NJ: Lawrence Erlbaum.

Gottman, J. M., & Levenson, R. W. (1992). Marital processes predictive of later dissolution: Behavior, physiology, and health. *Journal of Personality and Social Psychology, 63,* 221-233.

Grotevant, H. D. (1989). The role of theory in guiding family assessment. *Journal of Family Psychology, 3,* 104-117.

Grotevant, H. D., & Carlson, C. I. (1989). *Family assessment: A guide to methods and measures.* New York: Guilford.

Hampson, R. B., Beavers, W. R., & Hulgus, Y. (1990). Cross-ethnic family differences: Interactional assessment of White, Black, and Mexican-American families. *Journal of Marital and Family Therapy, 16,* 307-319.

Hetherington, E. M., & Clingempeel, W. G. (1992). Coping with marital transitions: A family systems perspective. *Monographs of the Society for Research in Child Development, 57*(2-3, Serial No. 227).

Jacob, T., Tennenbaum, D., Seilhamer, R. A., Bargiel, K., & Sharon, T. (1994). Reactivity effects during naturalistic observation of distressed and nondistressed families. *Journal of Family Psychology, 8,* 354-363.

Jemmott, L. S., Outlaw, F., Jemmott, J. B., III, Brown, E. J., Howard, M., & Hopkins, B. H. (2000). Strengthening the bond: The mother-son health promotion project. In W. Pequegnat & J. Szapocznik (Eds.), *Working with families in the era of HIV/AIDS* (pp. 133-151). Thousand Oaks, CA: Sage.

Kashy, D. A., & Kenny, D. A. (1990). Analysis of family research designs: A model of interdependence. *Communication Research, 17,* 462-482.

Kenny, D. A., & LaVoie, L. (1984). The social relations model. In L. Berkowitz (Ed.), *Advances in experimental social psychology* (Vol. 18, pp. 141-182). Orlando, FL: Academic Press.

Kolevzon, M. S., Green, R. G., Fortune, A. E., & Vosler, N. R. (1988). Evaluating family therapy: Divergent methods, divergent findings. *Journal of Marital and Family Therapy, 14,* 277-286.

Levine, C. (1994). AIDS and the changing concept of the family. In R. Bor & J. Elford (Eds.), *The family and HIV* (pp. 3-22). London: Cassell.

Lovejoy, N. C. (1989). AIDS: Impact on the gay man's homosexual and heterosexual families. *Marriage and Family Review, 14,* 285-316.

Markman, H. J., & Notarius, C. I. (1987). Coding marital and family interaction: Current status. In T. Jacob (Ed.), *Family interaction and psychopathology: Theories, methods, and findings* (pp. 329-390). New York: Plenum.

Mellins, C. A., Ehrhardt, A. A., Newman, L., & Conard, M. (1996). Selective kin: Defining the caregivers and families of children with HIV disease. In L. S. Jemmott & A. O'Leary (Eds.), *Women and AIDS: Coping and care* (pp. 123-149). New York: Plenum.

Mitrani, V. B., Szapocznik, J., & Robinson Batista, C. (2000). Structural ecosystems therapy with HIV+ African American women. In W. Pequegnat & J. Szapocznik (Eds.), *Working with families in the era of HIV/AIDS* (pp. 243-279). Thousand Oaks, CA: Sage.

Morris, T. M. (1990). Culturally sensitive family assessment: An evaluation of the family assessment device used with Hawaiian-American and Japanese-American families. *Family Process, 29,* 105-116.

Olson, D. H. (1977). Insiders' and outsiders' view of relationships: Research strategies. In G. Levinger & H. Raush (Eds.), *Close relationships* (pp. 115-135). Amherst: University of Massachusetts Press.

Page, J. B. (1990). Shooting scenarios and risk of HIV infection. *American Behavioral Scientist, 33,* 478-490.

Pequegnat, W., Bauman, L. J., Bray, J. H., DiClemente, R., DiIorio, C., Hoppe, S. K., Jemmott, L. S., Krauss, B., Miles, M., Paikoff, R., Rapkin, B., Rotheram-Borus, M. J., & Szapocznik, J. (in press). *Families and HIV/AIDS: Measurement relevant to family process. Aids and Behavior.*

Pequegnat, W., & Bray, J. H. (1997). Families and HIV/AIDS: Introduction to the special section. *Journal of Family Psychology, 11,* 3-10.

Phipps, S., & Mulhern, R. K. (1995). Family cohesion and expressiveness promote resilience to the stress of pediatric bone marrow transplant: A preliminary report. *Journal of Developmental & Behavioral Pediatrics, 16,* 257-263.

Ransom, D. C., Fisher, L., Phillips, S., Kokes, R. F., & Weiss, R. (1990). The logic of measurement in family research. In T. W. Draper & A. C. Marcus (Eds.), *Family variables: Conceptualization, measurement, and use* (pp. 48-66). Newbury Park: CA: Sage.

Straus, M. A., & Tallman, I. (1971). SIMFAM: A technique for observational measurement and experimental study of families. In J. Aldous (Ed.), *Family problem-solving* (pp. 381-438). Hinsdale, IL: Dryden.

Szapocznik, J., & Kurtines, W. M. (1993). Family psychology and cultural diversity: Opportunities for the theory, research and application. *American Psychologist, 48,* 400-407.

Thompson, L., & Walker, A. (1982). The dyad as the unit of analysis: Conceptual and methodological issues. *Journal of Marriage and the Family, 44,* 889-900.

Touliatos, J., Perlmutter, B. F., & Straus, M. A. (Eds.). (1990). *Handbook of family measurement techniques.* Newbury Park, CA: Sage.

Chapter 3

Training Facilitators to Deliver HIV Manual-Based Interventions to Families

Mary Jane Rotheram-Borus   Noelle R. Leonard

University of California, Los Angeles

Facilitators are being hired to deliver interventions to families to help parents protect their children from HIV. Which of the following applicants would you hire?

Tom is a 26-year-old HIV+ advocate who is very educated about HIV prevention. He becomes very emotional when talking about HIV and can use his own life as an example of making poor choices in high-risk situations. He graduated from college with a degree in social work, has training in substance abuse, and has good social skills. He does not have children in his life.

◇ ◇ ◇

AUTHORS' NOTE: This chapter was completed with the support of National Institute of Mental Health Grant 1ROI MH49958-04 to the first author. We thank the staff of the Family Center/MHRA and Housing Works, as well as Coleen Cantwell, Tri Cisek, Ernesto De Guzman, Jennifer Elliott, Earl Foss, Carlos Garcia, Nionne James, Kris Langabeer, Julie Lehane, Patrice Lewis, Javelle McElhaney, Sheldon McLeod, Sutherland Miller, Tanko Mohammed, Sanna Moore, Fred Muench, Wilfredo Rosado-Ordonez, Laura Rosen, Marion Riedel, Martha Saab, Karen Schlichting, Phyllis Sena, and Karen Wyche. For more information about this chapter, please contact Dr. Mary Jane Rotheram-Borus, Professor and Director, Clinical Research Center, UCLA Neuropsychiatric Institute, 10920 Wilshire Boulevard, Suite 350, Los Angeles, CA 90024-6521; e-mail: mjrotheram@npimain. medsch.ucla.edu.

Susan, a 50-year-old mother of three children, has returned to work after raising her children. She was initially uncomfortable about intervening to help parents and their children talk about sex but now believes she will be very effective in helping to increase parents' comfort level in discussing issues of sexuality.

Barbara, a 30-year-old Latino woman, has been teaching sixth graders in a middle school for the past 7 years. She is enthusiastic, smart, and warm with people. She has little experience with HIV but expresses interest in the topic. She is active in her community and believes that families are the solution to social problems.

What would be the most important questions to ask each of these candidates? On what basis would you decide whom to hire? Does personal investment in the topic area (e.g., being HIV+) increase or decrease a potential applicant's ability to execute a job? Does experience with children count? Does ethnic background of the families to receive the intervention influence who is hired? How would you compare the social skills of the three potential facilitators? Does the theoretical orientation of the candidates influence who should be selected? This chapter attempts to address some of these questions. There are no clear answers to each question, but there are methods of identifying the characteristics and skills that are most important for your specific intervention.

Each family intervention described in this volume is delivered by a facilitator or a team of cofacilitators using a manual that specifies the goals, activities, and time allocation for the intervention. Each intervention requires facilitators with different skills and levels of previous education and experience. However, a set of common personal characteristics and technical skills are prerequisites for every family intervention, HIV related or not. The goal of this chapter is to review the (a) interpersonal skills, (b) technical skills for conducting groups, (c) training required to implement manual-based interventions such as those described in this book, and (d) methods to supervise and evaluate the quality of the implementation of interventions.

CONTINUUM OF INTERVENTIONS

Before describing factors for interpersonal and technical skills, training, and supervision of facilitators, it is critical to distinguish interventions on the theoretical rationale and the degree of expertise needed for the delivery of different types of interventions. Family interventions to reduce risk for acquiring HIV, as

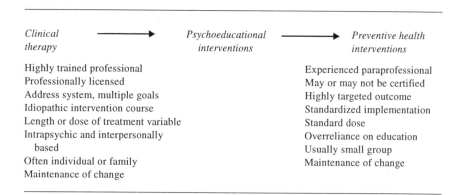

Figure 3.1. Types of Skills and Level of Competence Required by Facilitators

well as to help families cope with a family member who has HIV, can be placed on a continuum from clinical or therapeutic interventions to health education programs (see Figure 3.1). For example, the intervention of Szapocznik and colleagues (Mitrani, Szapocznik, & Robinson Batista, 2000 [this volume]) is a clinical intervention requiring significant analysis of a family's ecosystem and tailoring strategies for the specific family. In contrast, psychoeducational family groups of Wingood and DiClemente (2000 [this volume]) represent an intervention in which individuals consistently use the same sequencing of activities and allocate the same time, and the content of the information delivered and skills taught are similar for all clients. In the middle of the spectrum, Rotheram-Borus's intervention (Rotheram-Borus & Lightfoot, 2000 [this volume]) requires a high degree of skill, and the sequence of skills taught is consistent across clients in their order, timing, and content. However, the intervention is tailored for the specific problems of each participant. Figure 3.1 describes some of the variations in the types of skills and level of competence required of facilitators who implement interventions of differing levels of structure and predictability.

The persons who deliver interventions have been called facilitators, clinicians, leaders, counselors, therapists, or providers. Variations in titles used to describe each person at times reflect the underlying assumptions of those designing the intervention programs as well as the level of clinical expertise. At one end of the continuum, clinical interventions require facilitators who are typically identified as "clinicians" and who are often licensed. On the other end of the spectrum, facilitators are more likely to be identified as health educators and may only need some high school or college education. In this chapter, we use the title *facilitator* to describe any person who implements the prevention program.

PERSONAL CHARACTERISTICS OF FACILITATORS

There has been a debate on whether to focus on selecting facilitators with natural therapeutic skills or to intensively train facilitators once they are recruited (Bergin & Garfield, 1994). Actually, there are probably three components to successfully delivering a manual-based intervention: (a) interpersonal skills that would be difficult to train, (b) technical skills that can be trained but the facilitators should possess before being hired or selected to conduct the prevention programs in this book, and (c) knowledge of the manual-based intervention that can be trained on the job. For example, warmth, empathy, and genuineness are interpersonal skills of a person that are prerequisites for selection as an intervention facilitator (Bergin & Garfield, 1994). Even if there are significant variations in leadership style (Yalom, 1995), interpersonal skills are prerequisites. Facilitators who are effective stimulators of group interaction must also be warm, empathic, and genuine, or else their provocative statements may not stimulate reevaluation and behavior change by participants.

Warmth, empathy, and genuineness are characteristics that enable facilitators to provide an environment which participants are eager to return. However, as important as environment and attendance are, interpersonal skills are not sufficient for a facilitator to be effective. Facilitators' interpersonal skills must be coupled with important technical skills. Some skills are dependent on the theoretical orientation of the intervention model. For example, for those implementing a systems-focused intervention, facilitators must be able to perceive interaction patterns that recur over time (typically multiple times within a session). They must also be able to demonstrate the skills that the program attempts to enhance; at the very least, the facilitator must be able to model the skills that the intervention seeks to modify. For example, intervention programs attempting to modify social skills require that facilitators be able to demonstrate passive, assertive, and aggressive behaviors and be able to apply interpersonal behaviors appropriately in different situations when they are likely to be most effective (Rotheram-Borus, 1980).

At a minimum, facilitators must possess some modicum of the following technical skills to be effective:

- Articulate the theoretical model of the intervention through their behaviors, perceptions, and emotional responses. For example, within a behavioral paradigm, a facilitator should readily reinforce or validate desirable statements and behaviors ("It is wonderful how you are able to tell your child to engage in safer sexual behaviors because you love her and don't want anything bad to happen to her.").

- Establish a bond with participants by creating a supportive environment that permits trust and risk-revealing personal issues. For example, a participant might be able to reveal for the first time that he or she was abused as a child and felt guilty about it.
- Set realistic goals and anticipate gradual changes in behavior over time by using a series of successive approximations in expectations of others. This requires considerable patience and maturity, permitting the facilitator to perceive progress in very small increments. For example, if the goal is to ensure that adolescents use condoms during sexual intercourse, a first step might be to locate the pharmacy. A second step might be to speak about it with a (nonsexual) friend.
- Tolerate and manage the expression of strong emotions in multiple domains (e.g., hurt, anger, dependency, excitement, desire, rage). For example, some facilitators will not feel comfortable with the expression of negative affect such as anger, but others might not feel comfortable when a participant behaves in a needy and dependent fashion toward the facilitator. Being able to tolerate these expressions on the part of the participant is a first step in helping the participant grow in these areas.
- Perceive a rank-ordered set of strategies for changing the behavior, thoughts, or emotions of others; systematically be able to implement the strategies in a flexible style. It is easy to become overwhelmed with the many needs of some participants. The effective facilitator will need to establish priorities that enable him or her to focus, when needed, on one important issue at a time. "Let's concentrate on how we can keep your boyfriend from hitting you before we take up safer sex. Your safety is the most important thing."
- Use problem-solving skills to cope with emerging issues in a positive style. Nearly all interventions described in this book foster problem-solving skills— the facilitator needs to model effective problem-solving skills. "What are some of the ways Lily might be able to monitor her child's behavior?"
- Understand methods of coping with crisis situations within the intervention setting. It is critical, for example, that facilitators demonstrate appropriate responses to the expression of suicidal thoughts and threats of physical violence toward others in the intervention. These are extremely serious situations that can arise in nearly any contact with participants. "I am concerned about you, and I want you to talk with our crisis intervention counselor now."
- Articulate the differences between the participants and the facilitator (e.g., to set boundaries between the two). For example, it would not be unusual for a child whose parent is dying of AIDS to tell the facilitator, "I wish you could take me home." It is critical to respond in a caring fashion, yet effectively demarcate the reality and boundaries of the facilitator-participant relationship. "You are a wonderful child and your mother is working out a good plan for you."

• Respect and use the attributes of various ethnic groups, especially when clients are of a different ethnic group than the facilitator. Conversely, facilitators must be able to acknowledge and challenge cultural norms that are not health promoting. For example, some cultural norms can enhance risk for HIV. In some cultures, for example, machismo beliefs can condone older men seeking young virgins. In mainstream American culture, the belief in individual rights often supersedes the well-being of the group (Spiegel, 1982). For example, some HIV+ individuals may deliberately have unprotected sex with others, yet we lack the societal mechanism to support behavior change. Facilitators must be willing to confront social norms judged to promote ill health.

• Demonstrate expertise in specific areas or be trained prior to initiation of the specific intervention training. For example, facilitators must possess accurate information about HIV, positive attitudes toward HIV prevention that do not include homophobia or exclusion of acceptability of a range of prevention strategies (e.g., condom use is acceptable), and the ability to discuss sexuality, substance use, and other intimate topics.

• Be able to professionally endorse the critical aspects of the intervention and have the ability to become a representative of the intervention. This requires the facilitator to not have been overtrained in a modality or theoretical approach that is inconsistent with the current approach. Almost all interventions included in this book are based either on social learning theory (Bandura, 1977, 1986) or systems theory (Szapocznik & Kurtines, 1989). All of these interventions require the facilitators to be active problem solvers and to consider a broad range of ecological factors. Each facilitator is an active leader who must select a strategy that will be implemented to effect change in the family's ongoing behavior patterns. Each of the programs requires that facilitators learn, assimilate, and implement the intervention as outlined, both in practice and in philosophy. If a potential facilitator has received training in a particular orientation that is incompatible in some essential way, it may be difficult for a facilitator to have the flexibility to implement a manualized prevention program that is incompatible with essential aspects of his or her training. For example, facilitators whose experience and training have focused solely on individual psychoanalytic treatment will have a difficult time becoming active initiators, as required by most of our interventions. Psychoanalytic psychotherapists are more likely to be responsive as therapists rather than highly initiative (Ingram, 1991). It may also be difficult for psychoanalytically trained psychotherapists to shift from their intrapsychic approach to clients to a family process perspective, as needed by the interventions of Rapkin, Murphy, Bennett, and Munoz (2000 [this volume]) and Szapocznik and colleagues (see Mitrani et al., 2000). Moreover, psychoanalytically trained therapists are taught to show noncontingent positive regard, which would make it difficult for them to provide the contingent reinforcements required by Rotheram-Borus's interventions (Rotheram-Borus & Lightfoot,

2000). Intervention models differ in the amount of facilitator self-disclosure they encourage. Although in some humanistic models, disclosure is greatly discouraged, many of the interventions in this volume encourage a moderate amount of facilitator disclosure either as a mechanism for bonding or to model self-disclosing behavior.

This is not an exhaustive list of prerequisite technical skills for facilitators, but rather it is a list of minimum requirements for the interventions described in this volume in addition to interpersonal skills, such as warmth, empathy, and genuineness.

HIRING AND SELECTION

Although it is easy to outline the interpersonal and technical skills that are desirable among facilitators, it is much harder to identify these attributes in potential facilitators. Traditional hiring practices include reviewing previous employment history and recommendations and conducting a personal interview. It is advantageous if the potential facilitator possesses experience in the type of intervention being delivered, experience with the population being targeted (i.e., being a member of the target community), or exceptional interpersonal skills and training.

Performance evaluations of facilitators in simulated intervention situations also have been used and are highly recommended in selecting and hiring facilitators. For example, in the Group Assessment of Interpersonal Traits (Dooley, 1980), potential facilitators are invited to role-play as a counselor and counselee for 5 minutes each in a small group interview of six to eight potential facilitators. When each facilitator plays a counselor and counselee, the group observes the interaction. Ratings are made of the interpersonal skills and technical skills of the role-playing counselors and counselees by program staff. These ratings can then be used to assist in selecting facilitators to lead the intervention or in hiring new facilitators. If the potential facilitators rate each other, these ratings provide evidence of their evaluation clinical skills (i.e., whether the facilitators were good observers and raters of others' behaviors). If experienced staff and members of the participant population (e.g., mothers with AIDS, parents of adolescents) also observe the interactions, their ratings can be compared to the those of the potential facilitators.

Asking potential facilitators to conduct mock sessions from the proposed prevention program is another strategy for evaluating facilitators. Before the interview, potential facilitators can be sent a single session of the intervention and asked to role-play some section of the intervention with mock participants. The potential facilitators' interpersonal skills and technical skills can be observed in the mock intervention session. In the work of Szapocznik and colleagues (see

Mitrani et al., 2000), prospective facilitators are asked to conduct an interview with a representative family. The interview is videotaped and reviewed by supervisors and colleagues for style, comfort, and abilities in engaging families in conversation.

Although educational experience is not included in the list of prerequisites for being an intervention facilitator, it is anticipated that selection criteria may be previous intervention experience, a B.A. or M.A. in an appropriate discipline, and positive interpersonal skills. Some models, however, such as that of Jemmott and colleagues (Jemmott et al., 2000 [this volume]) and Paikoff and colleagues (McKay et al., 2000 [this volume]), use trained members of the participant community who are less likely to have college degrees.

Many community-based agencies do not have the luxury of hiring new staff members to conduct interventions. Although existing staff members usually possess many of the interpersonal and technical skills described in this chapter, especially those involving clinical skills such as establishing a relationship with clients and managing strong emotions, they may be unfamiliar with manual-based interventions, in which the goals of the sessions, specific exercises, and time allocation are carefully articulated and should be implemented with fidelity. All of the interventions presented in this volume are manual based. Manual-based interventions are intended to standardize delivery of an intervention and, as such, to maximize the impact of the manual-based intervention and minimize the impact of facilitator-specific styles and behaviors. For this reason, manual-based interventions are considered "standardized."

Existing staff members can be evaluated on their abilities and willingness to learn a new method of intervention delivery that may be much more directive and explicit than they currently provide. The training of existing staff should focus on capitalizing on their existing skills and knowledge of the population they serve while providing the new information and skills necessary for implementation of the manual-based intervention. These existing facilitators' knowledge of the intervention setting and the population can assist the agency in tailoring the intervention to their particular service site. In addition, because many community-based agencies are moving toward short-term interventions (in response to the demands of managed care insurers), the implementation of manualized interventions may be incorporated into the overall changing practices of the agency.

MANUAL-BASED TRAINING PROGRAMS

Intervention Manual

Each intervention described in this book has an intervention manual that outlines the activities and approaches that are to be adopted at each stage of the intervention. Because all of these manuals were developed and tested over time within a research context, they are intended to be very specific, clear, and easy to follow. They are written with the facilitator in mind, providing explicit direction and guidance. Many of the interventions have both a participant workbook and a facilitator guidebook to help facilitators achieve the objectives for each intervention session. The facilitators' guidebook contains a statement of goals to be accomplished, rationale, summary of the exercises, materials needed, time allowed for each exercise, and a word-for-word example of what the facilitator might say for each session exercise. In behavioral interventions, for example, each session of the manual is scripted as a model for the facilitator, but facilitators are encouraged to adapt the script to their own words and interpersonal style to help them tailor the material to the clients and present it easily. In addition, when facilitators are aware of which topics may arise soon, they can capture critical moments that occur in sessions and turn them into learning experiences.

The participant workbook contains information on the intervention topics for each session, self-assessment material, skills modeling, role-play scenes, exercises to be worked on with the facilitator, and tasks to be accomplished between sessions. The intent is to make the workbook and facilitator guidebook as simple and user-friendly as possible while encouraging both adherence to the intervention and quality control. Rapkin et al. (2000) and Rotheram-Borus and Lightfoot (2000) have detailed workbooks for the participating families. Table 3.1 shows an example from the latter program of the possible objectives for a single session—in this case, a small group session for parents living with AIDS. See Rapkin et al. [chap. 10, this volume] for an example of a page from that workbook.

Overview of the Training Process

The training process described here assumes that the facilitator who has been hired or selected already has excellent interpersonal skills, including warmth, empathy, genuineness, and good technical skills. Given these basic skills, training is needed to implement the manualized intervention. There are typically at least four phases of training: (a) providing a didactic review of intervention theory, (b) mastering the manual content, (c) observing and practicing how to conduct intervention sessions, and (d) conducting a complete intervention. On completion of the training program, facilitators will be "certified."

Phase 1: Didactic Review of Theory

The interventions in this book require that facilitators acquire information about the underlying model of change on which the intervention is based. The theory provides a cognitive road map or guide to the process of behavior change.

TABLE 3.1 Session 6: "Coping With Whether to Tell I Have AIDS" From the Teens and Adolescents Learning to Communicate (Project TALC) Intervention Manual

Objective 1	Mothers will learn about the concerns involved with disclosure.
Objective 2	Mothers will define disclosure decisions as problems.
Objective 3	Mothers will develop information about the problem.
Objective 4	Mothers will define why the outcomes they want relate to each problem.
Objective 5	Mothers will brainstorm alternative solutions for problems.
Rationale	Problem solving is a key coping strategy with ample evidence of its effectiveness. Although it can be used in many situations, in this workshop, it introduces and applies to the problem of disclosure. The problem process is explained and then used to work through the decision of whether to disclose one's AIDS status to a specific person. Because problem solving an issue, such as whether to disclose, takes more time than one session allows, this session stops with having generated action alternatives. The next session will deal with evaluating alternatives, making a selection, implementation, and evaluation.
Procedure 1	Introduce the participants, use a scene to introduce the topic of telling someone else about having AIDS, and check feelings about telling and what telling mothers have done. (15 minutes)
Procedure 2	Introduce the steps in problem solving and practice getting rid of attitudinal barriers to problem solving. (20 minutes)
Procedure 3	Practice defining the problem by focusing on a specific person the participant is considering telling and identify the information one would want to obtain. (20 minutes)
Procedure 4	Clarify the goals in telling a person. Introduce the topic through an illustrative script and practice figuring out the goals in telling the person what the mother is focused on. (15 minutes)
Procedure 5	Do a relaxation exercise. (10 minutes)
Procedure 6	Practice brainstorming a list of actions that could be taken regarding telling a specific person. (15 minutes)
Procedure 7	End with a lottery, between-sessions goal setting, a positive mantra, and showing appreciation to each other. (15 minutes)

This cognitive road map can anticipate critical moments that invariably occur during sessions and can guide the facilitator in making crucial choices for how to proceed. For example, when confronted by a very emotional participant who is crying, does the facilitator consider the behavioral shaping that may occur if the facilitator shows sympathy, warmth, and consideration toward the participant? Would the facilitator evaluate the crying as an ineffective coping strategy, possibly as a means to avoiding problem solving and refusing to take responsibility in the situation? On the other hand, the release of such strong emotion may be interpreted as a breakthrough and a signal of a basic organizational change in the participant's relationships. The training provides facilitators with a consistent set of behavioral guidelines to follow when confronted with the many critical moments of decision making throughout the intervention. In addition, intervention adherence improves when facilitators understand the "big picture," that is, what the intervention does to bring about change and the process by which it does.

Several of the intervention programs presented in this volume required the trainee to read a book or take a certain set of university-based classes prior to being eligible to be recruited as a facilitator. Programs that recruited community members as collaborators for the intervention design provided the theoretical framework to the trainees in interesting and fun workshops (Jemmott & Jemmott, 1994; McKay et al., 2000).

Phase 2: Mastering the Manual Content

Each intervention presented in this volume has a carefully developed manual, and some also have participant workbooks and facilitator guidebooks. Demonstration of mastery can proceed in several alternative ways. In Rotheram-Borus's intervention (Rotheram-Borus & Lightfoot, 2000), facilitators prepare small file cards (prompts or cues) containing the key activities for each session and the time frame for each activity. The manual contains model scripts for each activity; however, to master the content and be able to effectively deliver the intervention, facilitators must present it in their own language and style (i.e., they must own the material). Other programs do not require formal preparation of cards but test the trainees' knowledge on the content of each session's activities.

Phase 3: Observation and Practice
Conducting the Intervention Sessions

After acquiring a road map and an understanding of the goals, exercises, and process in each session, the facilitators experience an entire sequence of the intervention, typically in small groups or families that are "simulated" or in analog situations. The trainees role-play participants, and some trainees act as the facilitators. The senior trainers may first model the desirable intervention behavior for the trainees or may provide videotaped models of positive facilitation. Substantial feedback is given to trainees throughout this process. Some programs use these mock sessions as screening criteria to evaluate who might be an effective intervention facilitator.

Phase 4: Conduct a Complete Intervention

Finally, after mock training, the first sequence of intervention activities conducted by the facilitator with actual clients is closely monitored with videotape, through cofacilitation, or with live feedback by supervisors. Typically, the trainees are certified only after successfully demonstrating positive facilitator behaviors with clients in a real-world setting, and careful monitoring is conducted with quality assurance ratings. Only certified facilitators can independently deliver the intervention.

Depending on which prevention program is selected, other training issues may need to be considered. Prior to the initiation of the prevention program, an assessment should be done to ensure that the training is comprehensive to ensure the successful adoption of the program. For example, if the program is implemented in a storefront site in a dangerous community, staff may need to receive training in field safety methods. If the program requires close collaboration among facilitators or other staff members, the training should also have some modules on team building. Learning how to conduct and benefit from supervision might also be useful if there has been limited moderating of the conduct of sessions and there is likely to be some resistance.

ONGOING SUPERVISION OF PREVENTION PROGRAM

Rationale for Ongoing Supervision

We are mindful in this section that the quality and quantity of supervision that we recommend are likely to be more than what currently occurs in most practice settings. However, we want to be candid with providers: To accurately implement the interventions in this book, considerable supervision is needed on an ongoing basis.

Systematically supervising each session is critical to ensuring quality implementation of the prevention program. It has been well established in the psychotherapy literature that "drift" occurs when there is no anticipation of supervisory monitoring (Webb, 1966). Weisz and Weiss (1993) have demonstrated that clinical interventions for children that repeatedly have been shown to be effective in research settings are not replicated with positive outcomes in real-world settings. Successful research programs may not be successful in practice settings because facilitators' behaviors are rarely strictly monitored to ensure standardized delivery of the interventions. Practitioners must implement the model with fidelity to ensure that the intervention is as effective in the practice setting as it was in the research setting. The replication in the practice setting of research-based interventions may take far more training and adherence to research-developed models than both practitioners and researchers had recognized. However, it is better to deliver a successful program that will lead to desired behavior change on the part of the client, or this person will keep returning for treatment services for sexually transmitted diseases (STDs) or other health-related problems.

In the context of research, the quality of the intervention is ensured by audiotaping or videotaping each session for review by the facilitator, the facilitator's peer group, and the supervisor. This kind of session review allows for an examination of whether facilitators complete each exercise within the required time frame and with the quality outlined in the manual. Even in nonresearch contexts, ongoing supervision is essential to ensure fidelity to the intervention.

Supervision is a critical mechanism for monitoring quality and is an integral part of many programs described in this volume. Without it, an agency implementing any of these prevention programs may not be adhering to the intervention. Both group and individual supervision models are typically needed for delivering high-quality interventions and can contribute to maintaining the motivation of facilitators to deliver the prevention program. Group supervision sessions provide a context to build cohesion and motivation among facilitators, allow facilitators to learn from each other, problem solve difficult intervention situations, role-play difficult situations and choice points, and implement a cost-efficient intervention. Supplementing group supervision with individual sessions allows the facilitators to share and learn about highly uncomfortable situations and discuss personal deficiencies in a private setting. Supervisors should be mindful of conducting supervision in the broad model of the intervention—for example, setting a format and adhering to it (e.g., keeping to the agreed-on day, time, and length), providing positive reinforcement, role modeling, and using any other techniques specific to the intervention model the way facilitators should be conducting their group.

Enhancing Fidelity

To enhance fidelity to the intervention, each session must adhere to the content, theory, and guidelines of the manual, and this should be evaluated in supervision regularly. A set of written criteria, similar to a detailed employee performance evaluation, may assist in the supervision process. This list might include items such as the following: Does the facilitator consistently meet the objectives of sessions? Is the facilitator modeling desired behaviors? Does the facilitator use material brought up by the clients in a manner that brings the client back to the session's objectives? When responding to problematic behavior, does the facilitator make choices consistent with the theory? A list of these examples may help those initiating programs to develop their own methods of monitoring efficacy. To assess facilitator adherence to the intervention curricula and the quality of the implementation on an ongoing basis, programs can monitor fidelity with activities such as (a) rating of videotaped sessions, (b) facilitators' self-evaluation of sessions, and (c) participants' evaluation of sessions.

Rating of Videotaped Intervention Sessions

Every intervention session should be videotaped. For group supervision, randomly selected videotapes can be reviewed by the group of facilitators and their supervisor. From such tapes, the supervisor and facilitators can evaluate characteristics such as (a) the amount of time spent on the task, (b) frequency of social rewards, (c) time allocation for each activity, (d) completeness of conducting all activities outlined in the manual, (e) handling of crisis situations appropriately, and (f) the types of statements made by the facilitator (percentage of interpretations, reflective statements, rewards, etc.). The opportunity to have any facilitator's tape selected will enhance adherence to the model. The group's rating and discussion of the videotape also help to maintain adherence to the manualized intervention. Review of the tapes therefore becomes both a quality assurance process and a learning exercise.

Facilitators' Self-Evaluation of Session

After each session, the facilitator can complete a checklist of intervention topics and exercises covered, derived from the curriculum guide for that module. In addition to self-monitoring of content, it is important that facilitators evaluate themselves immediately after each session regarding issues such as how well the session went, client reactions to facilitator's feedback, interaction with their cofacilitator, and issues they want to address in supervision.

Participants' Ratings of Session

After each session, participants typically complete a brief checklist of topics covered derived from the workbook for that module. Participants will be assured that the facilitators will not have access to their ratings and that their ratings will not influence their relationship with the facilitators. The supervisors will have access to these ratings and will use them to help facilitators improve their work.

After each intervention, the participants will complete a questionnaire on facilitator clarity, interest, knowledgeability, relevance (to participant's personal situation), responsiveness (to expressed needs), feelings of trust, and accessibility. At a minimum, most interventions in this volume rely on the establishment of a sense of trust, warmth, and genuineness by the facilitators to provide a positive context for delivering the intervention.

Supervisor's Evaluation of Facilitator

The supervisor's observations and judgments about the skills and attributes of the facilitator are important. Supervisors are able to integrate information from multiple sources, such as from their observations of the facilitator's interpersonal style, judgment, and fidelity to the program. They may also incorporate client reactions as part of their overall evaluation. These ratings are likely to be most useful as summary judgments that integrate more information than other sources can.

Supervision is an important way in which these plans can be reviewed both before and after implementation. The following is an excellent example of when another opinion was critical in shifting the quality of the relationships of different members of the team working with an HIV+ woman.

AN EXAMPLE OF THE VALUE OF SUPERVISION

In structural ecosystems therapy (Mitrani et al., 2000; Szapocznik, Scopetta, Ceballos, & Santisteban, 1994), a crucial aspect of training and supervision involves helping the therapist avoid becoming entangled in the family's or other system's processes. Systems have well-established patterns of interaction that can be extremely powerful (especially in the case of families and complex or "political" service systems) and can pull the therapist into its system, often without his or her knowledge. In these cases, therapists often feel impotent and confused about how to move the case forward. The therapist's supervisor and clinical colleagues can help the therapist become aware of these situations and offer a road map for becoming disentangled from the system's pattern. Although these entanglements present roadblocks to therapeutic progress, they can also provide unique opportunities for assessing and developing interventions for difficult cases. In the process of being entangled in the system's processes, the therapist gains firsthand experience of its most problematic interactions and therefore gains a level of understanding of the experience of the individuals who interact with the system.

An example is the case of Katrina, who lived with her mother and brother in the mother's home. Katrina was a recovering cocaine abuser and had managed to put her life on a more positive track. She worked overtime cleaning offices and had a steady boyfriend, with whom she enjoyed spending her spare time. Katrina's mother had recently become very ill with kidney disease and required dialysis treatment and frequent monitoring at home. Katrina was highly stressed by her mother's caregiving needs and was angry because her brother did not provide any assistance. Katrina also had a grown daughter with whom she had a conflictive relationship, characterized by frequent periods in which they would not speak to one another due to some slight disagreement. In general, Katrina was irritable and antagonistic toward her family and would respond impatiently to her mother's requests for assistance.

Katrina was well known in her HIV clinic as an uncooperative patient. She would vary her medications (HIV and psychotropic) without consulting her nurse and then complain about the clinic's failure to treat her symptoms.

The therapist had great difficulty in establishing a working relationship with Katrina because of her oppositional, haughty, and demanding attitude. The therapist also was offended by Katrina's harsh treatment of her mother and her disparaging attitude toward her brother, who the therapist felt was justified in storming out of the house after Katrina asked him to "move your behind for a change."

In reviewing this case in supervision, the supervisor noted that there had been little contact in the month since the first session and that this sensitive and nurturant therapist expressed no empathy for Katrina. Although validating the therapist's dismay, the supervisor presented an alternative interpretation of Katrina's behavior as a symptom of her despair at the disruption to her tenuously balanced stability. This supervisory intervention helped the therapist to reengage Katrina with a more sympathetic approach. In the next session, Katrina responded well to the therapist's support and the opportunity to freely express her distress. She admitted that she sometimes acted impulsively and inappropriately toward her family and others and thanked the therapist for listening to her.

It was clear that the therapist's initial interaction with Katrina mirrored the interactions that Katrina had with others. Katrina felt her own pain so deeply that she failed to see the impact of her behavior on others and then blamed them for turning away from her. In a subsequent discussion of this case in supervision, the therapist related that she was now keenly aware that her own initial reaction to Katrina's off-putting behavior had contributed to their interaction. This helped the therapist develop a strategy for intervening in Katrina's relationship with her family and the clinic. Knowing how easily others could be pulled into Katrina's manner of interacting, the therapist was better prepared to engage Katrina's mother, brother, daughter, and nurse and lay the groundwork for transforming their interactions.

For example, to restructure Katrina's interaction with her nurse, the therapist called the nurse on the day before the next clinic appointment. The therapist related her sympathy for Katrina's stressful life circumstances and communicated that her own experience with Katrina was more productive once she lent a sympathetic ear. The therapist also expressed her admiration for Katrina's ability to juggle work, socializing, caregiving, and her own health care while maintaining her sobriety. Equally as important, the therapist validated the nurse's frustration regarding the difficulty of giving Katrina the individual attention she craved in a busy clinic session. This call served to "reframe" the nurse's view of Katrina and rendered her more receptive to the next appointment. The therapist also had prepared Katrina for the clinic visit by suggesting that she keep a record of her medications and symptoms for 3 days prior to the visit. One week later, the therapist learned from both the nurse and Katrina that the clinic visit had gone well and that Katrina had received a structured plan for varying her psychotropic medications as needed.

CHALLENGES OF IMPLEMENTATION

Even if facilitators arrive at the session with the requisite interpersonal skills, technical skills, and manual-based intervention skills, they still face a number of common challenges: (a) establishing group cohesion, (b) effectively using social influence, and (c) dealing with unanticipated problems from participants.

Establishing Group Cohesion

All facilitators possess a set of assumptions, beliefs, and behavioral plans about how to accomplish their goals. For example, building trust is a basic goal of most facilitators. Most interventions in this group are delivered in small groups. Therefore, group cohesion is typically conceptualized as a motivating force for members that substantially increases the probability of behavior change. When 6 to 10 persons are encouraging new behaviors, small group interventions—with strangers or families—are likely to be very efficient in shaping new behaviors and much more efficient than could be possible by one-on-one meetings between a facilitator and a client. It has been demonstrated that if group leaders use the word *we* several times during the sessions, encouraging the sense of a cohesive group, the sense of belonging, trust, and cohesion will be significantly higher. "We certainly did a good job on that role-play." "We seem to care for each other a great deal." Systematic encouragement of "groupness" is a positive leader behavior.

Effectively Using Social Influence

Facilitators can use social influence to encourage change among participants in small groups or families. Variations in social status exist among members of any group. The facilitator has the most power within the group and should recognize the increased influence that their positive and negative comments may have. However, clients may also exert significant power within a setting. For example, Rotheram-Borus (1980) had high school cheerleaders participate in intervention groups with ninth graders. The presence of the cheerleaders was a key social influence in encouraging mature behaviors by the younger children with behavior problems. These are only two examples of the strategic planning that all facilitators must make before confronting these issues in an intervention setting.

Unanticipated Problems From Participants

In general, the facilitator aims to ignore inappropriate behavior, redirect participants toward appropriate behavior, and reward even the slightest movement toward appropriate behavior. This manner of coping with difficult interpersonal situations has been outlined by Miller, Hunter, and Rotheram-Borus (1991). Prior to the initiation of any intervention, the manual and the design of the intervention must identify how the facilitator should handle each of the following issues: (a) disruptive behavior, (b) excessive talkativeness or reticence, (c) frequent arguments and conflicts among participants, (d) clinical crises (suicide threats and attempts), (e) revelation of sexual abuse or history of sexual abuse and physical battery, and (f) unexpectedly learning of HIV seropositivity of a member of the family or a spouse's homosexuality or infidelity. The sheer length of the list of potential problems is often sobering to new facilitators. However, if the facilitator has established group cohesion and can effectively use social influence, the group can be mobilized to address the problems of individual members.

SUMMARY OF TRAINING

All interventions presented in this volume depend on having skilled, committed, caring facilitators delivering them. Although it is feasible that interventions may emerge in the future that are not so facilitator dependent, the current state of family interventions depends on our ability to select and train effective leaders. This chapter reviews some of the key challenges in selecting and training such facilitators. As more innovative intervention models evolve, the challenges associated with delivering an intervention in a high-quality manner and with integrity (i.e., as it was designed to be delivered) will increase.

REFERENCES

Bandura, A. (1977). *Social learning theory.* Englewood Cliffs, NJ: Prentice Hall.
Bandura, A. (1986). *Social foundations of thought and action: A social cognitive theory.* Englewood Cliffs, NJ: Prentice Hall.

Bergin, A. E., & Garfield, S. L. (Eds.). (1994). *Handbook of psychotherapy and behavior change.* New York: John Wiley.

Dooley, C. D. (1980). Screening of paratherapists: Empirical status and research directions. *Professional Psychology, 11,* 242-251.

Ingram, D. H. (1991). Intimacy in the psychoanalytic relationship: A preliminary sketch. *American Journal of Psychoanalysis, 51,* 403-411.

Jemmott, J. B., III, & Jemmott, L. S. (1994). Interventions for adolescents in community settings. In R. J. DiClemente & J. L. Peterson (Eds.), *Preventing AIDS: Theories and methods of behavioral interventions* (pp. 141-174). New York: Plenum.

Jemmott, L. S., Outlaw, F., Jemmott, J. B., III, Brown, E. J., Howard, M., & Hopkins, B. H. (2000). Strengthening the bond: The mother-son health promotion project. In W. Pequegnat & J. Szapocznik (Eds.), *Working with families in the era of HIV* (pp. 133-151). Thousand Oaks, CA: Sage.

McKay, M. M., Baptiste, D., Coleman, D., Madison, S., Paikoff, R., & Scott, R. (2000). Preventing HIV risk exposure in urban communities: The CHAMP Family Program. In W. Pequegnat & J. Szapocznik (Eds.), *Working with families in the era of HIV* (pp. 67-87). Thousand Oaks, CA: Sage.

Miller, S., Hunter, J., & Rotheram-Borus, M. J. (1991). *Adolescents living safely: AIDS awareness, attitudes, and actions for gay, lesbian, and bisexual youths.* New York: HIV Center for Clinical and Behavioral Studies, Columbia University.

Mitrani, V. B., Szapocznik, J., & Robinson Batista, C. (2000). Structural ecosystems therapy with HIV+ African American women. In W. Pequegnat & J. Szapocznik (Eds.), *Working with families in the era of HIV* (pp. 243-279). Thousand Oaks, CA: Sage.

Rapkin, B., Bennett, J. A., Murphy, P., & Muñoz, M. (2000). The Family Health Project: Strengthening family problem solving in families affected by AIDS to mobilize systems of support and care. In W. Pequegnat & J. Szapocznik (Eds.), *Working with families in the era of HIV/ AIDS* (pp. 213-242). Thousand Oaks, CA: Sage.

Rotheram-Borus, M. J. (1980). Social skills training with elementary school and high school students. In D. Rathjen & J. Foreyt (Eds.), *Social skills throughout the lifespan* (pp. 69-112). New York: Pergamon.

Rotheram-Borus, M. J., & Lightfoot, M. (2000). Helping adolescents and parents with AIDS to cope effectively with daily life. In W. Pequegnat & J. Szapocznik (Eds.), *Working with families in the era of HIV/AIDS* (pp. 189-211). Thousand Oaks, CA: Sage.

Spiegel, J. (1982). An ecological model of ethnic families. In M. McGoldrick, J. Pearch, & J. Giordano (Eds.), *Ethnicity and family therapy* (pp. 31-51). New York: Guilford.

Szapocznik, J., & Kurtines, W. M. (1989). *Breakthroughs in family therapy with drug-abusing and problem youth.* New York: Springer.

Szapocznik, J., Scopetta, M. A., Ceballos, A., & Santisteban, D. (1994). Understanding, supporting and empowering families: From microanalysis to macrointervention. *The Family Psychologist, 43*(10), 23-26.

Webb, E. J. (1966). *Unobtrusive measures: Nonreactive research in the social sciences.* Chicago: Rand McNally.

Weisz, J. R., & Weiss, B. (1993). *Effects of psychotherapy with children and adolescents.* Newbury Park, CA: Sage.

Wingood, G. M., & DiClemente, R. J. (2000). The WiLLOW project: Mobilizing social networks of women living with HIV to enhance coping and reduce sexual risk behaviors. In W. Pequegnat & J. Szapocznik (Eds.), *Working with families in the era of HIV/AIDS* (pp. 281-298). Thousand Oaks, CA: Sage.

Yalom, I. D. (1995). *The theory and practice of group psychotherapy* (4th ed.). New York: Basic Books.

PART II

Prevention—Preventing the Spread of HIV Infection

Chapter 4

Preventing HIV Risk Exposure in Urban Communities

The CHAMP Family Program

Mary McKernan McKay

Doris Coleman

Roberta Paikoff

Donna Baptiste

Sybil Madison

Richard Scott

University of Illinois at Chicago

M s. P., an African American 38-year-old mother, is raising four children—Sandra, 9 years; DeAndre, 10 years; Kendra, 18 years; and Samual, 20 years—in an inner-city community in a large Midwestern city. Ms. P. is a committed parent who is exceptionally proud of her older children, both of whom attend community college and work part-time. Ms. P. has been a resident of high-rise public housing since her children were born, but she notes substantially more concerns about the safety of her younger children and the quality of their education than she had about her older children. Ms. P. expresses concern that she must supervise her

AUTHORS' NOTE: Aspects of the work described in this chapter were initially presented at the Families and AIDS Satellite Meeting of the 11th International Conference on AIDS, July 1996. The support of the National Institute of Mental Health (5R01-MH50423, 5R01-MH55701) and the William T. Grant Foundation Faculty Scholar Award to Dr. Roberta Paikoff is gratefully acknowledged. The staff of the Chicago HIV Prevention and Adolescent Mental Health Project (CHAMP) and the CHAMP Collaborative Board are thanked for their extraordinary efforts. Finally, the families participating in our project are especially acknowledged for their time and effort. For more information about this prevention program, please contact Dr. Roberta Paikoff, Institute for Juvenile Justice, Department of Psychiatry, University of Illinois at Chicago, 1601 West Taylor, MC 912, Room 512S, Chicago, IL 60612; e-mail: roberta.l.paikoff@uic.edu.

children closely because she is afraid that her youngest son will become involved in one of the two active gangs in her neighborhood. Ms. P. is also concerned about other issues. For example, her oldest daughter became pregnant in high school, and she does not wish for her or her younger daughter to repeat this mistake. In addition, Ms. P. is aware that her community has one of the highest HIV infection rates in the city. Her brother and cousin are both infected with the HIV virus. Ms. P. indicates that she is constantly talking with her children about staying healthy and protecting themselves from pregnancy and HIV. However, she also expresses concern that "all their friends are telling them to have sex early."

Poverty, substance abuse, and community violence are disproportionately present in the lives of inner-city children (Bell & Jenkins, 1993; Garbarino, Kostenly, & Dubrow, 1991). The incidence of HIV and AIDS infection rates has risen dramatically in poor, primarily minority neighborhoods (Boyd-Franklin, Aleman, Jean-Gilles, & Lewis, 1995; Stuber, 1992). Because many of these significant stressors co-occur, it is not surprising that being reared within an inner-city environment has been associated with exposure to a wide range of health and psychological risks (Institute of Medicine, 1989). As a result, urban communities are often targeted for prevention and intervention programming. All too frequently, however, such programs encounter significant obstacles, particularly gaining community support and participation (Stevenson & White, 1994). Ultimately, when programs fail to gain community participation, children and families in need do not have access to potentially beneficial intervention and prevention programs.

In this chapter, we will describe the development and implementation of a family-based prevention program aimed at promoting health and preventing HIV risk exposure in urban, predominantly African American fourth- and fifth-grade children living in communities with high rates of HIV infection. Prior to development of the intervention, Paikoff and her team interviewed 300 urban African American families with preadolescent (10- to 12-year-old) children (Paikoff, 1993) as part of the Chicago HIV Prevention and Adolescent Mental Health Family Study. The information obtained from these families informed the development of a 12-week family-based preventive intervention, the CHAMP Family Program. The program also has been developed and implemented under the supervision of a community-university collaborative board to maximize the sensitivity of the program to the needs of urban African American families.

BARRIERS TO PREVENTION EFFORTS

Over the past 5 years, the incidence of HIV and AIDS infection rates has risen dramatically in low-income, minority neighborhoods. HIV disease has disproportionately affected large numbers of urban, minority children and adolescents. Therefore, community-based HIV/AIDS prevention programs that target youth are growing in number (Dalton, 1989; Fullilove & Fullilove, 1993; Stevenson & White, 1994). However, significant barriers to the implementation of these programs in African American communities have been identified. Specifically, Stevenson and White (1994) identified obstacles to the implementation of AIDS prevention programs that appear to be in response to real experiences of racism and discrimination. These obstacles include denial of the epidemic in minority communities and distrust of majority cultural institutions.

First, the denial of AIDS as a significant health concern has been explained by the stigma associated with AIDS for African Americans (Gustafson, McNamara, & Jensen, 1992). For example, "the Haitian experience resulted in a group of blacks being labeled punitively and disenfranchised solely because their race and nationality was associated with HIV/AIDS" (Bates, 1990, p. 343). Thus, the stigma normally associated with AIDS is complicated by reality-based fears that the disease will bring further experiences of discrimination. Second, experiences of social disrespect and a history marked by intentional deception have led many African Americans to both distrust and consider "conspiracy theories" as valid explanations for the incidence of AIDS (Dalton, 1989; Thomas & Quinn, 1991). For example, in September 1990, an article titled "Is It Genocide?" appeared in *Essence,* a Black women's magazine. The author noted,

As an increasing number of African-Americans continue to sicken and die and as no cure for AIDS has been found some of us are beginning to think the unthinkable: Could AIDS be a virus that was manufactured to erase large numbers of us? Are they trying to kill us with this disease? (Bates, 1990, p. 344)

Furthermore, in a 1990 survey conducted by the Southern Christian Leadership conference, 35% of the 1,056 Black church members who responded believed that AIDS was a form of genocide (Bates, 1990). Given the potential for reactions of both denial and suspicion from the CHAMP target community, it was imperative that a partnership with the community be developed. Without community involvement in the design, implementation, and evaluation of the intervention, it was likely that a needed and potentially beneficial HIV prevention program would not be well received.

CHAMP COLLABORATIVE BOARD

Because this community collaboration is so central to the success of this prevention program for youth, we would like to begin with a discussion of the way it was established, its composition, and the way it works. The CHAMP Collaborative Board was formed to oversee the design, implementation, and evaluation of the CHAMP Family Program. The board is chaired by the CEO of a community mental health center in a predominantly Black community near the participant community. In addition to the chair, the board comprises parent and staff representatives from each of the five schools receiving the prevention program, as well as university research staff. Since its inception, the board has met monthly. All board members are compensated for their time either through salaried positions or paid hourly consultation fees. Board members and other community parents have been trained along with mental health interns (e.g., undergraduate- and graduate-level social work and psychology students) to implement the program at schools and community sites. In addition to delivering the program, community members participate on committees that make key personnel and budget decisions, create project policies concerning personnel and data collection, design the intervention curriculum, and review proposals for research using the intervention data. In addition, community board members participated in new "professional" roles as conference presenters and as part-time and full-time project staff.

Case Study of a CHAMP Collaborative Board Member

Parents were recruited through the targeted elementary schools to serve as members of the CHAMP Collaborative Board. The goal was to involve at least two parents from each of the five schools. A current parent member came to the board with prior experience with the university researchers. This parent, a mother of seven children, had assisted in the recruitment of participants in a previously conducted research study.

M s. L. regularly attended board meetings. However, in recalling her early experiences on the board, she noted confusion about her role and some feelings of intimidation. In her words,

> When I came in there [to CHAMP] what really got me was the $10/hour. I said to Ms. F. [school principal], "I don't care what it is, just let me know what you want me to do." When I first started on the [Collaborative] Board, I thought, "How will I fit in with all these Ph.D.s and doctors and social workers? I'm just a parent." But at CHAMP everyone's an expert. No one ever made me feel like I know less than they do, or like my ideas are less important.

Ms. L. began to feel more involved and have a better understanding of the goals of CHAMP when she and her family participated in the early intervention pilot program:

> When I went through the pilot program and got my kids involved, things really started to change. When they [my kids] started, they were in it for the money, too. But as we got going, the kids started coming 'cause they got going, the kids started coming 'cause they liked the sessions; they were different every time.
>
> What really got me, the best session of the whole thing was when I thought I knew my kids but I didn't. Here I am, mother of seven children, very close with my children, monitoring them all the time. I think, know everything about where they go and who they're with, I think. Well, we did this game where the kids were in one room, parents in another room, and we each answered the same questions—one was "Name your friends" or "Name your kid's friends." Then we came back together in a room and shared our answers. When my kids named their friends I'm like, "Where did they come from?" I didn't name ANY of their friends. That really got to me, you know, and showed me I needed to get even closer with my kids and communicate more.

Over the 3 years that Ms. L. served on the board, she accepted increasing responsibilities on CHAMP. For example, she agreed to present with the staff at multiple national professional conferences regarding her experiences on the board. In addition, she began to actively follow up on the completion of her GED. Also, when a full-time position at the university became available, Ms. L. successfully applied for the job. Ms. L. continues to be an active board member while also being a full-time member of the CHAMP administrative team. Her high level of involvement in the CHAMP endeavor exemplifies the attainment of a goal of this project, strong community collaboration. In her own words, "Now look at me! I work for the university, and I feel like my CHAMP coworkers are family. I wouldn't trade this work for anything in the world."

DESCRIPTION OF CHAMP PARTICIPANTS

CHAMP serves an inner-city community that is experiencing the presence of high rates of HIV infection along with significant levels of poverty, community violence, and substance abuse (Bell & Jenkins, 1993). In addition, most CHAMP participants reside in large high-rise government-subsidized housing. The program was developed for 500 children in the fourth and fifth grades and their families. This preadolescent age was chosen on the advice of parents because only a small proportion of these children was expected to be involved in sexual behavior. One of the goals of CHAMP is to delay sexual behavior; therefore, intervening with children early is of great importance.

DESCRIPTION OF THE
CHAMP FAMILY PROGRAM

The CHAMP Family Program is intended to influence individual, familial, and social factors that affect the lives of children and their parents. More specifically, the program intends to influence (a) qualities of families, (b) parenting skills, (c) knowledge of HIV/AIDS and sexuality, and (d) social problem-solving skills. First, the program is designed to strengthen specific family relationship characteristics, such as levels of support and communication among family members. Next, the program is intended to maximize parenting skills, specifically in relation to supervision, discipline, and communication. Furthermore, parents receive information about puberty, sexuality, and HIV/AIDS. Finally, the CHAMP Family Program is meant to help children develop social problem-solving skills and assertiveness and influence positive friendship choices.

The CHAMP Family Program works with families whose children are in the fourth and fifth grades. At this age, most children are not likely to have begun activities that place them at risk for HIV exposure. These same children will also be involved in the second phase of the CHAMP Family Program when they reach the sixth and seventh grades. All families reside in high-risk contexts in which HIV infection rates are high, and when children begin to participate in risk activities early (e.g., unprotected intercourse and intravenous drug use), they are likely to engage in those activities with HIV-infected adolescents and adults. Thus, the intent of the CHAMP Family Program is to lower the incidence of behaviors and situations related to the high probability of early and unprotected intercourse and substance abuse, thereby decreasing adolescent risk for exposure to HIV.

The CHAMP Family Program is based on interviews with both parents and children from the same targeted community conducted several years prior to the development of the program (Paikoff, 1993). Parents reported a lack of comfort and communication regarding sexuality, HIV, and AIDS (relative to other risk behaviors), as well as needs for (a) support of parenting, particularly in the areas of supervision and monitoring, and (b) adult friendships to overcome a sense of isolation. Also, large numbers of children were exposed to situations of "sexual possibility" (e.g., unsupervised heterosexual private situations), and fairly large numbers of parents lacked accurate information on important aspects of HIV risk behavior. This prevention program was based on these findings and focuses both on changes at an individual level (e.g., increased basic knowledge of HIV and sexuality) and at contextual levels (e.g., improving family communication, providing support from other parents).

The CHAMP Family Program consists of 12 weekly 2-hour meetings held at school and community sites when children are in the fourth and fifth grades, with a second part of the program occurring at the sixth and seventh grades. A summary of the program is provided in Tables 4.1 and 4.2. Each meeting is cofacilitated by one or two community parents and one or two bachelor-level mental health interns, all of whom have completed a joint training program.

At the first session of the fourth- and fifth-grade program, families are introduced to the CHAMP program. Their questions are encouraged. In addition, common concerns about making a 12-week commitment are raised by facilitators (e.g., lack of time). During this first meeting, CHAMP is described as an opportunity to discuss important issues within the family and also hear from other families about how they are preparing their children for adolescence. It is always stressed that CHAMP provides an opportunity for new learning and does not "tell families how to raise their children." The CHAMP Family Program is based on a primary prevention perspective that assumes that families have strengths that can be enhanced by participation in this program and support from other parents. Respect for how families currently operate is stressed by the facilitators in the first meeting.

The next eight meetings are devoted to program content. More specifically, the third week of the program focuses on the development of talking and listening skills within families. Next, Sessions 4 and 5 provide opportunities for adult caregivers and children to talk about the importance of supervision and monitoring children to keep them safe. Families gather important information from each other regarding activities away from home, as well as safe and unsafe neighborhood and friendship contexts. The sixth and seventh weeks of the program focus on strengthening parental support networks both inside and outside the family and family rules to enhance effective monitoring of children's activities. Weeks 8, 9, and 10 are devoted to communicating accurate information about puberty, HIV/AIDS, and expectations for children as they approach adolescence.

When families are brought back together as their children enter the sixth and seventh grades, the content of the program changes. At early adolescence, goals of the curriculum are met through (a) discussion of sexual possibility situations as *likely* to occur for the majority of youth in this age range; (b) the emphasis on the important role of families in providing structure and values to assist youth in coping with these situations in their peer and friendship relationships, with the goal of staying safe and healthy; and (c) discussion of information regarding puberty, HIV/AIDS, and safer sex behavior. The early adolescent program presents a three-step approach to preventing HIV risk behavior: (a) The first goal is to encourage youth to abstain from heterosexual intercourse, (b) the second goal

(Text continued on page 77)

TABLE 4.1 Scope and Sequence of Preadolescent (fourth- and fifth-grade) CHAMP
Family Program

Session and Topic	Session Goals
Session 1	
Getting to Know the CHAMP Family Program: Working Together to Keep Our Kids Safe!	To provide clear information about the CHAMP program expectations
	To help families feel comfortable with facilitators and with each other
Session 2	
Where Are We Going? Paperwork!	To explain the purposes of research and assessment measures
	To clearly explain issues of confidentiality
	To complete pretest measures
Session 3	
Talking and Listening to Each Other	To introduce the concept of "sexual possibility situations" to parents
	To help parents identify how communication protects children from sexual possibility situations
	To help families discuss children's peer pressure experiences
Session 4	
Keeping Track of Kids—Part 1	To discuss with parents and children the importance of keeping track of children's whereabouts
	To have parents and children exchange information about each other using the CHAMP Family Game
Session 5	
Keeping Track of Kids—Part 2	To help parents identify safe and unsafe neighborhood areas
	To help parents identify their children's positive and negative peer relationships
	To help families discuss positive and negative neighborhood and peer environments
Session 6	
Who Can Help Us Raise Our Children?	To help parents identify current supports and resources for parenting
	To help parents identify ways to get the parenting support they need
	For parents to identify CHAMP group members as a support resource

TABLE 4.1 Continued

Session and Topic	Session Goals
Session 7	
Rules Keep Kids Safe	To help parents make a connection between setting clear rules and keeping children safe
	To help families discuss current rules and how to improve them
Session 8	
Growing Up: Talking About Puberty	To help parents discuss their knowledge of puberty and get information in a supportive, adult environment
	To prepare parents to talk about puberty with their children
	To prepare children to talk with their parents about puberty
Session 9	
What We Need to Know About HIV/AIDS	To give parents and children facts about HIV risk in their community
	To give parents and children accurate information about the HIV/AIDS and its transmission
	To help families talk with each other about HIV/AIDS
	To help parents answer children's questions accurately
Session 10	
Growing Up: Preparing Kids for Adolescence	To help parents anticipate their children's transitions to adolescence
	To help parents clarify their values and how those values will affect parenting decisions as children get older
	To have parents practice expressing their expectations and values to their children
	To help children think about their transitions to adolescence
	To help families discuss their expectations for adolescence
Session 11	
Where Are We Ending Up? Paperwork and More Paperwork!	To ensure that families understand the purposes of research
	To help families understand the value of their participation in research
	To complete posttest measures
Session 12	
A Celebration! Where We Have Been and Where We Go From Here	To celebrate the completion of families' time in CHAMP
	To help families plan ways to keep in touch with each other

TABLE 4.2 Scope and Sequence of Early Adolescent (sixth- and seventh-grade) CHAMP Family Program

Session and Topic	Session Goals
Session 1	
Welcome Back: Still Working Together to Keep Our Children Safe!	To explain to families why the CHAMP Family Program is working with sixth and seventh graders
	To help parents and children identify why HIV risk increases as children get older
Session 2	
Paperwork!	To explain the purposes of research and assessment measures
	To clearly explain issues of confidentiality
Session 3	
It's a Freaky-Deaky World!	To help parents and children identify sexual messages in the media and society
	To help families discuss how to prevent the negative influence of sexual messages on behavior
Session 4	
Growing Up: Dealing With Peer Pressure	To help children identify and practice handling peer pressure situations related to HIV risk
	To have parents help children anticipate peer pressure situations
Session 5	
Growing Up: Dealing With Adolescence	To help parents and children understand the changes that occur during puberty
	To help families discuss how to handle romantic feelings and relationships
Session 6	
Talking About Sex and Reproduction	To provide parents and children with accurate information about reproduction and sex
	To help children practice talking with parents about sex
	To help parents discuss reproduction and sex with their children
Session 7	
Understanding HIV	To give parents and children accurate information about HIV/AIDS and its transmission
	To discuss low-, medium-, and high-risk behaviors related to HIV/AIDS
	To demonstrate to families how to use a condom properly
	To help parents demonstrate condom use to their children

TABLE 4.2 Continued

Session and Topic	Session Goals
Session 8	
Respect Yourself and Others!	To have parents and children identify ways to demonstrate self-respect and respect for others
	To help parents communicate to children the relationship between self-respect and HIV/AIDS
Session 9	
Supervising and Monitoring Our Teenagers	To help parents identify new strategies for keeping track of teenagers
	To help parents and children anticipate changes in monitoring strategies and rules
	To help families talk about how to handle adolescent sexual possibility situations
Session 10	
The CHAMP Family Game	To review key information from each session using the CHAMP Family Game
	To help parents and children identify how each session was related to preventing HIV/AIDS
Session 11	
Paperwork!	To ensure that families understand the purposes of research
	To help families understand the value of their participation in research
Session 12	
Celebrating Safe and Healthy Families	To celebrate the completion of families' final year in CHAMP
	To help families plan ways to keep in touch with each other

is to delay sexual activity, and (c) if abstaining and delaying do not work, the goal is to encourage youth to protect themselves from HIV risk exposure through safer sex behavior.

More specifically, family-focused activities within the sixth- and seventh-grade program involve frank discussions about sexuality and HIV/AIDS. For example, parents and youth discuss lyrics to popular songs as part of the section of the program on "the Freaky-Deaky Environment," meaning that sexual messages and values are a part of everyday experience for inner-city youth. Furthermore, toward the end of the early adolescent curriculum, both parents and youth participate in condom demonstrations.

The topics are presented in a specific order for two reasons. First, the targeted aspects of family life that are thought to be the most critical to delaying adolescent sexual behavior are introduced at the beginning of the program (e.g., family communication, family monitoring, and family rules). Second, these communication and interactive skills are seen as the foundation for specific discussions around puberty, sexuality, HIV/AIDS, and planning for a child's future.

The CHAMP Family Program uses three distinct groups: (a) parent-only groups, (b) child-only groups, and (c) multiple-family groups. The rationale for having these different groups is twofold. First, there is a need for developmentally appropriate, generationally separate groups to develop shared goals, agendas, and supports outside and in addition to the relationships available within the family. In other words, parents and children need places where they can discuss their generational perspectives away from and prior to discussing them in the family. Second, some of the skills needed for the prevention of health-compromising behavior vary by generation. For example, children need practice both in family and peer dialogues. The child's role in family dialogues may stress development of conflict resolution and assertiveness skills necessary for peer interactions. Parents or adult caregivers may need more explicit practice with enforcement of rules and strategies for supervision and monitoring than is possible when children are present. Thus, individual parent and child groups precede multiple-family groups on the same topic.

Parent Support Groups

Parent meetings are meant to provide opportunities for parents to evaluate their own parenting skills and consider sensitive topics related to child development, puberty, sexuality, and HIV/AIDS in the presence of other adults. Furthermore, parent-only meetings allow adults to clarify their own behavior and values related to parenting, family life, sexuality, and risk-taking behavior without children present. In addition, these group meetings create a context for parents to obtain new knowledge about interacting with children—both from CHAMP facilitators and other parents. It is hoped that supportive relationships with other community parents are developed over the course of the 12-week program. Finally, parent-only group meetings focus on preparing for interactions with their children in multiple-family groups and at home. Each parent group meeting begins with an introduction of a new theme by the leaders. Then discussion questions guide exploration of the topic. Activities, worksheets, and information presented by group facilitators supplement discussion of selected topics. For example, in a parent meeting focused on the enhancement of parental supervision and monitoring skills, parents prepare to play a game with their children by answering questions such as the following: (a) Who is your child's best friend? (b) Where does your child go after school? (c) What is your child's biggest worry? (d) Is there a place where your child is not supervised by an adult?

Child Support Groups

Traditionally, child support groups have been conducted from a social-cognitive or social learning perspective, aimed at teaching children specific skills that are expected to promote health and reduce health risk. Although this is an aim of CHAMP, the goals of CHAMP focus on altering family interactions. Thus, an important aspect of preparing for the child support groups is considering the role of the child in altering family process. Important skills for children involved in CHAMP include talking and listening with parents and learning to negotiate their position. Again, meetings of children separately from parents allow children to consider contextual and family issues without parental input and to practice family and peer strategies in preparation for multiple-family groups. For example, in an early program meeting, children are asked to develop a list of things that worry them and potentially threaten their safety. Then they practice discussing these topics with their peers and CHAMP facilitators to increase their comfort talking to their parents about these same topics later.

Multiple-Family Groups

CHAMP meetings begin as a multiple-family group, with an introduction of the theme of the session by the program facilitators with parents and children present. A multiple-family group convenes after the parent-only and child-only group meetings. Participants are asked to share something from their separate discussions in the parent- and child-only meetings. Then, individual family activities are introduced by the leaders and related to the theme of the group meeting. Individual families then meet separately (in different corners of the room) to work on specific activities together. In most meetings, families are asked to give advice to an imaginary family, referred to as "the Johnsons." Figure 4.1 is an example of a situation in which parents and children are asked to exchange information. This figure depicts the awkwardness adolescents feel when going through puberty and the sometimes cruel way children make fun of each other. This provides a nonthreatening way to initiate discussion about adolescents, puberty, sexuality, and HIV risk.

Leaders circulate among families, providing feedback and helping families think through obstacles to productive communication between parents and children. The last 15 minutes of the multiple-family group meeting is spent as a larger group with individual families reporting on their discussions, plans, and solutions that they developed as a family. In addition, feedback from other

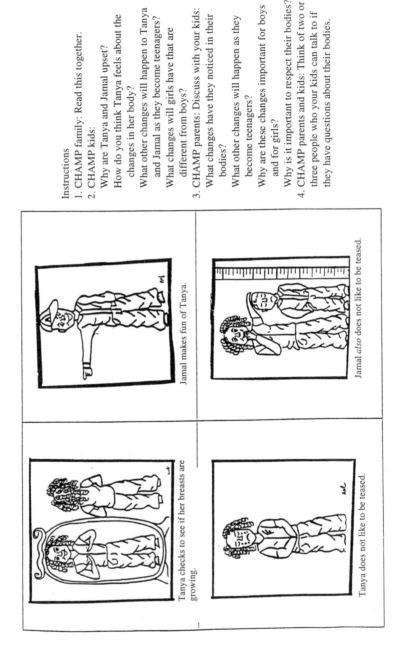

Tanya checks to see if her breasts are growing.

Tanya does not like to be teased.

Jamal makes fun of Tanya.

Jamal *also* does not like to be teased.

Instructions

1. CHAMP family: Read this together.
2. CHAMP kids:
   Why are Tanya and Jamal upset?
   How do you think Tanya feels about the changes in her body?
   What other changes will happen to Tanya and Jamal as they become teenagers?
   What changes will girls have that are different from boys?
3. CHAMP parents: Discuss with your kids:
   What changes have they noticed in their bodies?
   What other changes will happen as they become teenagers?
   Why are these changes important for boys and for girls?
   Why is it important to respect their bodies?
4. CHAMP parents and kids: Think of two or three people who your kids can talk to if they have questions about their bodies.

Figure 4.1. Examples of Johnson Family Activity

families is solicited to provide support, encouragement, and new ideas as families communicate about sensitive topics.

Benefits of This Approach

Each intervention session is meant to guide families in the process of helping them to evaluate their own strengths and needs while providing opportunities for new knowledge, support from others in the community, and practice interacting as a family within the context of the groups described above. More specifically, each CHAMP meeting focuses on raising awareness of aspects of family life that have been related to HIV risk exposure. For example, parents are encouraged to consider how frequently they discuss sensitive topics, such as puberty, sexuality, and HIV/AIDS with their children. At the fourth- and fifth-grade levels, parents are also sensitive to the term *sexual possibility situation*—those times when children are alone with children of the opposite sex. Specific skills around reducing the time children spend in these situations and parental monitoring skills are reinforced during the program. In the family described earlier, monitoring and supervision of the children's whereabouts and activities were clearly an issue to be addressed. As is the case in many single-parent families, the older children were frequently enlisted to supervise the younger children when their mother could not be present. However, at times, this was not an effective strategy.

Part of the work with Ms. P. centered on how to mobilize other adult resources to assist her with monitoring. She was able to identify her sister and a neighbor as consistent supports that could help her supervise the children after school when she needed to keep other appointments.

Within every CHAMP meeting, there is an opportunity to take an inventory of current family practices and parenting skills, such as monitoring and supervision. There is always a focus on helping families identify their own and each other's strengths and resources while also more clearly defining areas that need improvement. In addition, the CHAMP Family Program was designed to assist families in developing specific family goals and plans to accomplish these goals.

ASPECTS OF PARENTING HIGHLIGHTED BY CHAMP

Raising Awareness of How Families Can
Help Prevent Child HIV Exposure

Each week, CHAMP facilitators introduce specific information and topics related to parenting and family life that have been linked to HIV risk. For example, the goal of the fourth and fifth sessions of the program is to increase the level and effectiveness of parental monitoring. Monitoring refers to a parent or parent designee keeping track of a child's physical whereabouts, companions, and concerns. Therefore, raising awareness involves helping families to define monitoring in their own words and acknowledge its importance in reducing risk to their children. More specifically, during the fourth session of the CHAMP program, parents and children play the "Family Monitoring Game." In this exercise, parents and children complete large cards that have questions, such as, "Who is the child's best friend?" and "Where do you go right after school?" After parents and children have answered these questions separately, they come together to share and discuss their answers. In this way, parents and children practice sharing information with each other in a relaxed, supportive atmosphere.

INVENTORY OF CHILD, PARENT, AND FAMILY
CURRENT PRACTICES AND SKILLS

Following the definition of specific aspects of family life, each family is asked to assess their current practices during every meeting. A necessary foundation for highlighting and strengthening family practices is to help parents be specific and concrete. For example, in the unit related to parental monitoring skills, the goal is to help parents to identify when, where, how, and with whose help do they monitor their children. Specific activities are designed to assist families in their evaluation.

During one CHAMP meeting, Ms. P. and the other parent group members participated in an activity designed to identify potential resources for supervising children. Each parent was asked to take as many M&M candies from a jar as they had potential monitoring resources in their lives. Ms. P. then discussed with other parents how to call on those close to her—specifically, her sister and friend who lived next door—for help in watching her children more consistently.

Identification of Child, Parent, and Family
Strengths, Resources, and Needs

Every family is assumed to have strengths and competencies. These are seen as the building blocks of the intervention. Specific intervention activities are meant to help families define the "things that are working well" within their households. Furthermore, as families identify their needs, these become the specific targets of the intervention. For example, in relation to monitoring, one family might identify the need to involve more supportive people to help keep track of the children. Another parent might identify the need to supervise the activities of her children at home as her awareness of sexual possibility situations that occur rises, even when parents are at home.

Developing Family Goals and Specific
Implementation Plans

Following an inventory of strengths and needs, specific family goals and plans to accomplish these goals are developed within the intervention. An important aspect of this process is helping families to consider the obstacle to implementing their plans. Frequently, families will identify stressors or lack of time that interfere with their plans. A problem-solving approach is adopted by CHAMP leaders and other families to help a family be more successful. Again, goals will be specific to individual families. For example, for one family, a monitoring goal might be to make sure that the children are supervised after school, even if a parent cannot be available. However, for another family in the same group, a monitoring goal might involve discussing concerns and worries that a child might have on a regular, predictable basis.

INTERVENTION PROCESS WITH URBAN,
AFRICAN AMERICAN FAMILIES

The following are key process issues that we believe are necessary for engaging urban, African American families in a relationship with CHAMP and for facilitating change within families and within a larger urban community. These critical intervention elements are (a) inspiration and hope, (b) relationships and support, (c) information and knowledge exchange, (d) participation, and (e) experiences. These key processes are the focus of training for CHAMP facilitators.

Inspiration and Hope

Hope, in the face of significant adversity, is a necessity for urban families. Within African American narratives, oratories of successful African Americans, as well as stories of "how to keep hope alive," are frequent and vibrant. The CHAMP Family Program is meant to serve as another forum for hope and inspiration for families as they make active attempts to rear and protect their children.

Relationship and Support

Kinship and support networks have been identified as a historic strength of African American families (Boyd-Franklin, 1993). However, mobility, poverty, and factors associated with urban life (e.g., violence and substance abuse) can place significant strain on such relationships. CHAMP intends to help families to celebrate those networks that have remained expansive and are flourishing. Families who cannot identify helpful support networks are encouraged to develop them, possibly from within CHAMP groups.

Information and Knowledge Exchange

African American adults might approach any type of program with initial mistrust based on countless negative experiences with "helpers" (Stevenson & White, 1994). Therefore, CHAMP is committed to an honest exchange of information, knowledge, and feedback between participants and project staff. In reality, this means that goals, research questions, and hypotheses are shared with participants. Questions about the program are answered with openness and honesty. Feedback about intervention content from participants is valued and considered by the CHAMP Collaborative Board to inform future changes to the intervention.

Participation

Participation in CHAMP is meant to be an active process. Rather than having "experts" impart information to families, parents, and children are considered the "experts" of their families. CHAMP provides families with information about key aspects of the family process that we believe can help protect children from HIV risk exposure. However, families themselves are the best judge of whether this information is relevant to their family and are best to assess whether their family is successfully functioning in these specific areas.

Experience

We believe that to incorporate new knowledge that produces growth and change, parents and children have to take risks and practice new ways of relating to each other and to others in their communities. It is critical that families experience new successes and also run into obstacles to change so that obstacles can be identified and new strategies discovered.

TRAINING OF PROGRAM FACILITATORS

Training on these key intervention processes supplements training on program content and group facilitation skills. Modifying training to incorporate the unique aspects of urban life was critical, given the research that shows that even though traditional parent training groups have been associated with positive outcomes, they may not be applicable for urban parents (Guerra, in press; Patterson, 1982; Webster-Stratton, 1990). CHAMP has attempted to increase relevance of the program for urban parents by involving parents from each of the five schools as coleaders of the intervention. Both mental health staff and parent facilitators are trained jointly to develop skills in program delivery, content, and group facilitation skills. A key component of training is helping both parent and mental health facilitators learn to problem solve around obstacles within the environment that potentially could interfere with participation in the program and the efficacy of the intervention.

Ethical Issues

Issues around protection of participants' privacy arose throughout the project. For example, within CHAMP training sessions, issues of confidentiality needed to be specifically addressed because parent facilitators now had access to highly personal information regarding other CHAMP families. This was particularly important because these families were also their neighbors and their children's classmates. Strict provisions to maintain the privacy of participants were put into place within the project. Ongoing discussions reinforced restrictions of sharing information learned in CHAMP with other members of the community and with school staff.

SUMMARY AND CONCLUSIONS

The CHAMP Family Program was developed based on the input from two critical sources: basic research data from the participant community (Paikoff, 1993) and the verbal feedback from community parents and school staff. The program content was developed to bolster family organization, communication and decision making, parental supervision and monitoring, child problem-solving skills, and family knowledge about puberty, sexual behaviors, and HIV/AIDS to prevent HIV risk exposure. These targets are directly related to emerging empirical evidence for the link between family- and parent-level factors and exposure to early sexual possibility situations (Paikoff, 1993). However, the process of delivering the program activities and the training of both parent and mental health facilitators have been highly influenced by the CHAMP Collaborative Board, which is essential for a successful program (Aponte, Zarski, Bixenstene, & Cibek, 1991; Fullilove & Fullilove, 1993). The establishment of strong community partnerships is particularly important for prevention programming, which is directed toward urban, African American communities. In the words of a parent involved in the earliest stages of our collaborative board,

> I was talking to this woman in my neighborhood and she said to me, "I'm so scared," and I'm like, hey, I'm scared too, but maybe if we put all our fears together we can come up. We can come up with a little courage, you know?

REFERENCES

Aponte, H., Zarski, J., Bixenstene, C., & Cibik, P. (1991). Home/community based services: A two-tier approach. *American Journal of Orthopsychiatry, 61*(3), 403-408.

Bates, K. G. (1990). Is it genocide? *Essence, 76,* 344.

Bell, C., & Jenkins, E. J. (1993). Community violence and children on Chicago's South Side. *Psychiatry: Interpersonal and Biological Processes, 56,* 46-54.

Boyd-Franklin, N., Aleman, J., Jean-Gilles, M. M., & Lewis, S. Y. (1995). Cultural sensitivity and competence: African American, Latino, and Haitian families with HIV/AIDS. In N. Boyd-Franklin & G. L. Steiner (Eds.), *Children, families and HIV/AIDS: Psychosocial and therapeutic issues* (pp. 53-77). New York: Guilford.

Dalton, H. L. (1989). Aids in Blackface. *Daedaius, 118*(3), 205-227.

Fulilove, M. T., & Fulilove, R. E. (1993). Understanding sexual behaviors and drug use among African-Americans: A case study of issues for survey research. In D. G. Ostrow & R. C. Kessler (Eds.), *Methological issues in AIDS behavioral research* (pp. 117-132). New York: Plenum.

Garbarino, J., Kostenly, K., & Dubrow, N. (1991). What children can tell us about living in danger. *American Psychologist, 46,* 376-382.

Guerra, N. G. (in press). Intervening to prevent childhood aggression in the inner-city. In J. McCord (Ed.), *Growing up violent: Contributions of inner-city life.* Cambridge, UK: Cambridge University Press.

Gustafson, K. E., McNamara, J. R., & Jensen, J. A. (1992). Informed consent: Risk and benefit disclosure practices of child clinicians. *Psychotherapy in Private Practice, 10,* 91-102.

Institute of Medicine. (1989). *Research on children and adolescents with mental, behavioral and developmental disorders.* Washington, DC: National Academy Press.

Paikoff, R. L. (1993). *Chicago HIV and adolescent mental health project* (NIMH grant proposal). Bethesda, MD: National Institute of Mental Health.

Patterson, G. R. (1982). *Coercive family processes.* Eugene, OR: Castalia.

Stevenson, H. C., & White, J. J. (1994). AIDS prevention struggles in ethnocultural neighborhoods: Why research partnerships with community based organizations can't wait. *AIDS Education and Prevention, 5*(2), 126-139.

Stuber, M. L. (Ed.). (1992). *Children and AIDS* (Clinical Practice No. 4). Washington, DC: American Psychiatric Press.

Thomas, S. B., & Quinn, S. C. (1991). The Tuskegee syphilis study, 1932 to 1972: Implications for HIV education and AIDS risk education programs in the Black community. *American Journal of Public Health, 81*(11), 1498-1505.

Webster-Stratton, C. (1990). Predictors of treatment outcome in parents training for conduct disordered children. *Behavior Therapy, 16,* 223-243.

Chapter 5

Saving Our Children From a Silent Epidemic

The PATH Program for Parents and Preadolescents

Beatrice J. Krauss

Dorline Yee

Jennifer Tiffany

W. Rees Davis

Dennis Reardon

Jesse DeJesus

Evelyn Garcia

Celestino Rivera

Teasha Daniels

Richard Velez

Christopher Godfrey

Lloyd Goldsamt

Luis Almeyda

Edna Bula

Yolanda Jones

James Pride

Michael Pierre-Louis

Elba Troche

Joanne O'Day

National Development and Research Institutes

M r. Jones is raising his 10-year-old niece. He adopted her after her mother died from an HIV-related illness. He has been afraid to even mention HIV to his niece, not only because he is worried about her emotional reaction to her

AUTHORS' NOTE: The writing of this chapter was supported by a grant (MH R01 53834) to the first author. For more information about this prevention program, contact Dr. Beatrice Krauss, Center for Drug Use and HIV Research, National Development and Research Institutes, Inc., Two World Trade Center, 16th Floor, New York, NY 10048.

mother's death but also because he has lost so many friends and relatives himself. It is painful for him to even mention HIV. Yet he fears for his niece's future, given what he has heard about sex and drug use among the young people in the neighborhood. He also is concerned about the future of his "natural" children, who are currently living with his estranged partner, a woman injecting drugs. Mr. Jones is also anxious about the physical status of an HIV+ brother who is in jail. He is not sure if his brother is receiving the newer HIV treatments or what will happen to his brother's treatment after he leaves jail.

Mr. Jones was among the fathers recruited for our HIV-related training for parents of preadolescent children (PATH, Parent/Preadolescent Training for HIV Prevention). PATH's aim is to enable parents to be effective HIV educators for their children and in their community. Because HIV often affects more than one person in a family or social network, PATH parent trainings focus not only on prevention of HIV risk but also on understanding and coping with illnesses that may affect persons with HIV. Understanding HIV helps people safely and sensitively socialize with seropositive persons.

We hoped that PATH would give Mr. Jones a safe place to talk about HIV and would provide him with tools to assist his niece and brother to come to terms with the effects of HIV on their lives. Table 5.1 summarizes the structure of the PATH program. The PATH program recognizes that both parents and children change and mature over time in their understanding of HIV and in the ways in which they communicate. PATH asks parents to practice their communication skills, not only in parent training groups but also in guided sessions in which a parent meets alone with his or her child and a staff observer.

The PATH structure is guided by several considerations. First, parents care deeply about the welfare of their children. Because of this concern, parents already have gathered some information about HIV and sex and drug risk for HIV. Parents recognize that this information is incomplete and doubt they are giving their children the "right" information. Because sex, drugs, and HIV are sensitive topics, parents are not sure about how to talk to their children about HIV. Parent-child conversations are complicated by the fact that now most people know someone with HIV or someone who has died of AIDS. People also have attitudes, sometimes derived from street myths and misinformation, about how HIV is transmitted and who gets HIV that may have been examined but not in detail. Conversations about HIV are likely to prompt unexpected emotions and associations in both the parent and the child. To prevent the spread of HIV infection, parents and children must acknowledge and work through these emotions. Children and parents also need to be clear enough about their own values so that they do not send mixed messages and so that actions are clear and follow from those values. For parents, it is important to be able to convey the information and

(Text continued on page 94)

TABLE 5.1 Overview of PATH Group Training Sessions

Session	Timeline	Activities	Objective of Activity	Session Objective
HIV infection and transmission (3 hours)	Week 1	Kids in My Life AIDS Lifeline Feeling Circle Myths and Facts About HIV/AIDS What We Know About HIV Transmission What Kids Need to Know About HIV/AIDS One Strength I Have Is	Adults as influencers of children Personal experiences with HIV Emotions associated with HIV Clarify HIV information Apply information in new situations Understand children's risk Assess parents' HIV communication skills	Increase personal and general knowledge, identify and overcome barriers to clear communication
Parent-child communication (3 hours)	Week 2	Carousel (difficult question kids ask) I Took a Risk When. . . Safety Skills Workshop Communicating Positively Kids Share When. . . Strength Bombardment	Practice answering difficult questions Self-assessment of HIV risk Practice risk reduction Recognize teachable moments Structure teachable moments into household routines Self-esteem and child esteem building	Build skills in parent-child communication
Recognize, avoid, negotiate risk (3 hours)	Week 3	How Are Things Different for Children Now? Mapping Telephone Gender Relation Role-Plays Supporting Kids/Supporting Ourselves Empty Middle Vignettes (fill in the middle of the story)	Understand children's circumstances Recognize safe areas in the neighborhood Distinguish fact from rumor Support risk reduction norms Support safety Practice negotiating and avoiding risk	Identify risk in the child's milieu and support safety skills

TABLE 5.1 Continued

Session	Timeline	Activities	Objective of Activity	Session Objective
Safe and sensitive socializing with persons with HIV/AIDS (3 hours)	Week 4	Parent/Child/Observer Role-Plays	Practice giving clear messages	Encourage appropriate interactions with persons with HIV/AIDS
		Myths and Facts II: How HIV, TB, and Other Infections Diseases Are Transmitted	Learn universal precautions and understand the natural history of HIV	
		Caregiving/Keeping Safe Picture Cards	Practice interacting with persons with HIV	
		When Someone in My Life Has HIV...(Video)	Understand living with HIV	
		How People Who Are HIV+ Like to Be Treated	Positive versus negative social support	
		Carousel II—Concerns of Children/Parents/Caregivers	Practice answering difficult questions about illness	
		Mapping II—Community Resources	Identify local HIV resources	
		Privacy, Confidentiality, Nondiscrimination	Respect the rights of persons with HIV	
Parent-child 1 (90 minutes)	Week 5	Parent chooses activities from Sessions 1 through 4 to practice with child	Address the child's most pressing questions and needs	Parent acts as the HIV educator of their child
Parent group booster (90 minutes)	Month 3	Brainstorm about issues from everyday life	Address the parent's HIV communication needs	Parents coach one another
		HIV update	Share new HIV information	
Advanced HIV communication 1 (3 hours)	Month 15	Common Ground Bingo	Identify neutral topics for everyday communication	Advanced HIV communication: support appropriate communication with teenagers
		Update, New Information	Clarify recent HIV findings	
		Megaphone	Recognize developmentally appropriate communication styles	
		You Be the Mirror (reflecting thoughts and feelings)	Assist children in clarifying their own thoughts and feelings	
		Feelings	Expand feeling vocabulary	
		Encouragement	Support positive and safe behaviors	
		Kids and Parents in Unsafe Situations	Practice negotiating risk avoidance	

Session	Timeline	Activities	Objective of Activity	Session Objective
Parent-child 2 (90 minutes)	Month 15, Week 1	Parent chooses activities from Session 1 through 5 to practice with child	Address the child's most pressing questions, needs Practice new communication styles	Communicate more effectively about HIV
Advanced HIV communication 2 (3 hours)	Month 21	My Kid's Body Language Family Rules and Values The Magic Sentence Fill In the Blank Teaching About STIs, Drugs, and Hepatitis Kids and Parents in Safe Situations	Awareness of nonverbal communication Examine purpose of implicit and explicit household rules Practice assertive communication skills Manage unexpected reactions Examine information evaluation skills Support family safety skills	Advanced HIV communication 2: Negotiate mutual safety in the family
Parent-child 3 (90 minutes)	Month 21, Week 1	Parent chooses activities from Sessions 1 through 6 to practice with child	Address the child's most pressing questions, needs about HIV, STIs, and hepatitis Practice new communication styles	Negotiate parent and child mutual safety

skills they originally intended to convey and to know that children heard, understood, and will be vigilant in maintaining their own safety. The conversations we would like parents and children to have are a far cry from what we know is the "standard" or usual parent-child conversation about HIV. The parent makes a general admonition and warns of a negative consequence: "Don't do sex, you'll die of AIDS." The standard reply from children is a reassurance: "I won't." In this interchange, children feel cheated of the explanations they actually desire.

Children made us very aware that they are equally concerned about their parents and their parents' HIV risk. Family-based HIV prevention involves negotiating how parents and children will reassure one another about mutual safety. Mr. Jones and his niece exemplify these concerns.

Mr. Jones sat silently through PATH's first parent group training session, an overview and sharing of information about HIV infection and HIV transmission. By the second session (focused on parent-child communication), he disclosed his family history, breaking down in tears over relatives who had died. During the third session (negotiating and avoiding HIV risk), he became aware of his own as well as his niece's potential HIV risks. By the fourth group meeting (safe and sensitive socializing with persons with HIV), he was questioning the group facilitators about recent HIV treatments and steps he might take to help his brother. For the latter concern, Mr. Jones was directed to a community coordinator who made referrals and clarified some misinformation he had about HIV treatment. The community coordinator helped him arrange for his brother to be connected to a transitional prison release program for HIV+ inmates.

In the first parent-child meeting, after Mr. Jones had completed four 3-hour parent training sessions, Mr. Jones and his niece decided to role-play, asking and answering questions about family members who may have HIV. This quickly led to a discussion about Mr. Jones's sister and her illness and how his niece was handling her mother's death. She hated feeling she could never talk about her mother. "It's like she died twice." Mr. Jones says that he and his niece now talk about HIV more than they used to and about everything, including her mother, more than before. They joke around more, too, since he found out that his niece is not just "her serious side." His niece and he have become positive contributors to the PATH program. They were among those who asked for more parent-child sessions to be included when PATH expanded from four to six sessions. Because Mr. Jones discovered that his niece was worried about him—a single father who dated—he took the HIV test for the first time. Both report that she has become an unofficial peer HIV educator for her friends.

OUR PARENTS, CHILDREN, AND COMMUNITY

The parent group training that forms the basis of PATH has been delivered throughout New York State in rural areas, in suburbs, in small cities and towns, to parent groups, to church congregations, and to service agencies through Cornell University/Cornell Cooperative Extension, our collaborators (Tiffany, Tobias, Raqib, & Ziegler, 1993a, 1993b). The World AIDS Foundation recently funded PATH to adapt its program for parents in selected neighborhoods in Mexico City. In this chapter, we will concentrate on how PATH has been delivered in a community that presented particular challenges, a community highly affected by HIV. In this neighborhood, it appeared wise to offer PATH to everyone, to literally go door-to-door in person with a description of the program. The great majority (80%) of adults contacted, who were raising a preadolescent child, accepted our offer of training.

Mr. Jones and his niece live on the Lower East Side of New York City. For more than 100 years, the Lower East Side has been a haven for new immigrants from many nations and many parts of the United States. Some streets are still primarily populated by persons belonging to specific ethnic groups. The diversity of cultures, although highly related to the area's reputation as a major center for artistic creation, also means that social norms are fragmented. Because many of the residents are also abjectly poor, since the turn of the century, prostitution and drug use and trafficking have been the basis of a large illegal street economy. Always an area where sexually transmitted infections (STIs) were documented at high levels relative to other areas of New York City and the United States, the Lower East Side is now an epicenter of the HIV pandemic in the United States (New York City Department of Health, Office of AIDS Surveillance, 1996; New York City Human Services Administration, 1990). More than 1 in 10 adolescents and adults in the Lower East Side are HIV positive; children are sure they know three to four persons with HIV, one third of whom they know have died.

Mr. Jones and his niece live in one of 13,000 housing projects apartments; they may or may not be legally documented residents. Due to economic conditions, a lack of documentation, and/or a shortage of affordable housing, families "double up," sublet individual rooms, or otherwise fail to indicate their full complement of family members. Our work in the neighborhood indicates that approximately 70% of housing project residents are Latino, representing Puerto Rico and more than 30 different countries of origin; 28% African American, representing persons born in New York City, in the U.S. South, in Africa, and in the Caribbean; and 2% "other," scattered across multiple ethnic categories.

Approximately half of these families are headed by single parents, 75% of whom are women and 25% of whom are men. Partially because of preexisting child-rearing patterns and partially because of deaths of biological parents from HIV-related illnesses, a substantial portion of adults who assume the parenting role are not biological parents. We have observed a growing number of single fathers, biological fathers, or other males acting as the sole parent (e.g., uncles) due to loss of partners or siblings with children to HIV. Many parents—on the Lower East Side and throughout the United States—have dual roles regarding the children within their household (i.e., father to some, uncle to others; grandmother to some, foster mother to others). We define *parents* as adults raising children within their households on more than a temporary basis. We work equally with fathers raising daughters, fathers raising sons, mothers raising daughters, and mothers raising sons.

Youth in the Lower East Side are solicited for and sometimes engage in risk behavior at an early age. The median age for sexual initiation is 14. Local children as young as 10 or 11 are asked to join gangs involved in drug distribution. "Little Jake," for example, was adopted by a gang as a mascot when he was 9. He already wondered, at age 10, if that determined his future—he would have to sell drugs as a teenager and be a gang member as an adult. Children report drug solicitation on the way to and from school, and in school, as a daily occurrence. Children in this neighborhood also frequently experience the death and illness of friends and relatives from HIV-related conditions (Krauss, 1997). Gina's story illustrates some of the situations children in the neighborhood confront.

Gina is a beautiful 14-year-old girl with long, polished nails. She wears her hair slicked into curls. Her stepfather credits the PATH project with giving him the skills to talk his daughter into returning home after she had been lured to become a member of a "posse" headed by a flamboyant local drug dealer. Gina informed one of our interviewers,

> You wouldn't believe what goes on in this neighborhood. It is a wild place. I have a girlfriend; she is HIV positive. She's been like that since she was a baby. She's a virgin, but her friends thought, "She's 13, it's time for her to lose that." They set her up. They invited her to a party at a house; several guys were there. One of them maneuvered her into a room. Then they had sex with her. Her friends should have prepared her; they should have told her to have protection; they should have let her know what was going to happen. These were her girlfriends that set this up.

Because of early risk, our program is designed for parents of boys and girls ages 10 to 13. The children are old enough to talk openly about sex and drugs, old enough to empathize with persons with HIV, and old enough to deal with hypothetical "what-if" situations, but most are young enough to have limited exposure to HIV risks.

OUR PROJECT'S EMPHASIS ON PARENTS

In this section, we describe the reasons we decided to work with parents. We wish to emphasize that we never directly train preadolescent children. We train their parents in group sessions, give the parents several opportunities to practice teaching their children about HIV, and encourage parents to continue in their role as HIV educators, no matter how much or how little HIV education their children get from other sources.

HIV school curricula designed for New York State as a whole, for example, seem inappropriate for the immediate needs of Lower East Side youth. When our project began, New York City's public school chancellor had been forced to resign in part because of his advocacy for teaching about condom use in high schools—an age too late for effective prevention in the Lower East Side. Parents were at a loss; they felt ill equipped to provide their children with the knowledge and negotiation strategies they needed to avoid HIV risk and yet be sensitive to affected family members and friends (Krauss, Goldsamt, Bula, & Sember, 1997). In fact, our data showed that both children and parents had little comprehensive knowledge about HIV, scoring 60% and 70% correct, respectively, on a 50-item test about HIV. Their knowledge could be summarized: sex, drugs, AIDS, and condoms. This level of knowledge would be little help to the 13-year-old boy in our program who feared he had HIV because an older brother, an injected drug user, had used his toothbrush. Also, thinking only about HIV, rather than thinking also about hepatitis B and C and other contagious illnesses, would be a disservice to the health of that child.

Parents are a desirable but underused resource for HIV education. Consistently, parents are among the top two to three sources of information on sex and other sensitive topics for children; children desire to get sensitive information from their parents (Furstenberg, Herceg-Baron, Shea, & Webb, 1984; Krauss, 1997). Parents are present to influence their children over an extended period of time. Even if parents only talk about HIV 3 minutes every 5 days, as described by our community 10- to 13-year-olds, in 4 years parents would match the length of the 15-hour curriculum mandated by New York State, kindergarten through 12th grade. Parents are health educators in other areas of their children's lives. Parents can and do choose from a wide range of values and strategies to ensure health and safety in the home and in their children's lives. Parents can integrate education about HIV with other health messages. Finally, as the developmental psychologist Eleanor Maccoby (1980) argues, the lessons taught by parents are more persistent than institutional messages in part due to the emotionally charged nature of familial relationships.

THE PATH MODEL

PATH has several important components: (a) a curriculum covering six sessions of training for groups of parents; (b) a "booster" meeting of parents, after Session 4, to brainstorm about real-life issues that have arisen; and (c) interwoven with these sessions, three spaced opportunities for a parent to teach his or her child about HIV privately in the presence of an observer (see Table 5.1).

To implement PATH as it was designed, it is also important to have (a) a parent group meeting room in a safe and neutral site that can accommodate 8 to 12 parents; (b) a two-person team, one male and one female, to facilitate parent groups; (c) a community organizer to make referrals to HIV, youth, and community services; and (d) a resource, internal or external to the program, for psychological or medical referrals, if necessary.

The Curriculum

For our work with families in the community, we adapted a highly regarded HIV prevention curriculum, "Talking With Kids About AIDS," authored by a multidisciplinary Cornell University team. The curriculum is appropriate for parents with preadolescent children in their households (Tiffany et al., 1993a, 1993b). The Cornell curriculum aims to make parents effective deliverers of HIV prevention information and techniques to children, emphasizing children's need to know specific information as age and social development bring children into contact with new risks. The Cornell curriculum was also appealing because two generations—parents as "teachers" and children as "learners"—would master risk reduction skills. With the collaboration of the original authors, we expanded "Talking With Kids About AIDS" to include a unit on safe and sensitive interaction with persons with HIV and to strengthen recognition, avoidance, or negotiation of sex, drug, and other HIV risks. At the request of local parents, we added units on advanced communication skills, particularly addressed to the transition to adolescence, and on other health threats facing their children—sexually transmitted diseases, hepatitis A, hepatitis B, hepatitis C, and substance use. The last unit also assists parents in making the transition to becoming lifelong information seekers, evaluators, and teachers.

The objectives of the PATH curriculum are carefully organized at two levels: across the six parent group sessions and within each session. At each step, our program draws largely on two disciplines: life span development and social cognitive learning theory.

Life span developmental theory informs us about the roles and characteristics of parents and preadolescents. We continually visit and revisit how HIV risk and developmental tasks may interact and how discipline and communication change in a family as child and parent mature. Preadolescent and adolescent children begin, for example, to play with ideas and develop "what-if" scenarios. Asking a question, "Can you catch HIV from holding hands?" led several children in the neighborhood to think about all the ways in which you could: "If one of you has HIV and you both have cuts on your hands" and "You can share a soda with someone with HIV" are neither satisfying to children flexing their intellectual muscles nor accurate. Children in our neighborhood have responded, "But what if the person with HIV has a cold, what if I have a cold, what if they have TB or pneumonia, what if I have a disease and don't know it?" Parents need to have a broad grasp of HIV and associated illnesses and the ability to give many "for instance" examples.

In turn, as children mature, their social world becomes larger. Children have more challenges and, as they adjust to their larger world, more tools to deal with challenges. Using the insights of the developmental theorist Bronfenbrenner (1986), throughout the curriculum we examine how the larger and smaller societal and neighborhood contexts might frame tasks related to HIV risk reduction and tasks related to interacting with persons with HIV. For example, recently we found that children in the Lower East Side see HIV as only one of many very serious problems in the United States. Even though the preadolescents live in one of the nation's most highly affected neighborhoods, they saw HIV as progressively less of a problem in their neighborhood and in their family. We also found that there was very little sharing of information or talking about HIV within families. Even in this context, the two greatest HIV-related worries that children had were the following: "Someone I know has HIV and hasn't told me," and "Someone I know will get HIV." Children noted that they worried a lot about these two things. Surprisingly, so did their parents. Because of the stigmatization of HIV and attendant secrecy, children and adults were experiencing chronic grief over relatives' real or imagined illnesses and suffering. Adults and children were experiencing these feelings in isolation and in silence. The worry was in the child's and the parent's head but not shared within the family. HIV was a national and neighborhood problem but not a family problem. Parents needed to create a family environment in which conversations about HIV were expected.

Within social cognitive learning theory, we rely heavily on work in self-management and on the self-efficacy and social learning theories of Bandura (e.g., 1994). Self-management theory concentrates on mastery of skills that largely occur in private and are not publicly rewarded (Kanfer & Goldstein, 1986). Such theories emphasize physical and imaginative rehearsal of problem situations, self-reward, acceptance of some failure, and self-supports for persistence.

Elsa, a grandmother in our program, was raising her grandson, Tyrone. She had no idea how she was going to talk to him about sex, drugs, and HIV. She imagined several ways of talking to him. When she tried the first one, it didn't work so well in practice, so Elsa went on to use another strategy, and another, until she found one that worked. It turned out that her grandson was impressed most by her persistence. Tyrone saw through her repeated attempts but noted, "You really care about this."

Using role models and supporting beliefs that one can perform a behavior (i.e., self-efficacy) and that the behavior will be effective (i.e., response efficacy) consistently has been implicated in the development and maintenance of self-protective behaviors. In PATH, parents examine their own risks and risk avoidance or reduction tactics and beliefs, prior to transferring risk reduction or avoidance skills to children.

As we go through the curriculum in general and in particular, we will illustrate how these and other theories informed our choices about what to teach and how to teach it. We must emphasize, however, that the "teaching" is always collaborative with the parents. Parents are the best experts on their children and their neighborhood circumstances. Often, through thought or experience, parents have hit on solutions to common problems or tell us about problems that we were unaware existed. We can then teach solutions to others. In the Lower East Side, for example, several children in our program had been pierced by syringes that had been carelessly discarded—one syringe injured a child playing in an abandoned sandbox. We were able to develop a practical handout on what to do in this situation: Pick up the syringe from the back using a Styrofoam coffee cup, put it in a jar or can, seal the can or jar with masking or duct tape, take the child and the syringe to Bellevue or Beth Israel Hospital, have the syringe tested for HIV, and ask the doctor to decide if the child should be tested or treated after looking at the injury. In fact, some insights from the parents and children about their concerns for each other caused us to expand our thinking about HIV risk reduction.

OVERVIEW OF THE SIX SESSIONS IN PATH

In the six parent group training sessions, we lay out a developmental path that we wish parents to follow. We will lay out the sessions and then give selected examples of activities from each session, covering the first session in detail.

Within each session, the sequence of exercises is carefully planned. The sequence is based on behavior change theory (e.g., Prochaska, DiClemente, & Norcross, 1992). The first exercises are designed to raise motivation for behavior change. These are followed by exercises that anchor issues in the parent's and child's personal life. The subsequent activities involve sharing and expanding knowledge, understanding, or skills. Parents then practice applying their new understanding and skills in new settings. Parents make plans for the maintenance of behaviors in the family setting. Finally, parents enact these plans, often initially through "homework" assignments. Throughout, emphasis is placed on the primary goal: understanding HIV in our children's lives and assisting children in dealing with HIV-related issues (Krauss, Tiffany, & Goldsamt, 1997).

Session 1: HIV Infection and Transmission

In the first session, parents begin as relatively passive absorbers of HIV information, becoming aware of how many children and adults they potentially influence with their current and new HIV information. There are many activities to involve the parents.

The first activity, "Kids in My Life," is designed to foster the parents' motivation to become HIV educators of youth. Group members simply call out or write down the number of children, relatives, friends' children, and community youth who they interact with on a regular basis. A group facilitator makes a tally. Parents are often surprised to learn that a handful of adults has the potential to influence hundreds of children.

Activity 2, "AIDS Lifeline," personalizes the HIV/AIDS epidemic. Parents are guided to reflect on how "HIV/AIDS" first came into their lives. They are asked to draw a picture representing this first occasion and then to draw a chronological series of pictures representing critical episodes of how HIV has affected their lives. Parents only share these pictures with other group members if they want to, to protect confidentiality. For many parents, discussion of these drawings represents the first time they have spoken openly with others about experiences related to HIV or heard others do so. The first of these drawings often portrays an initial glimpse of HIV through a radio or TV news story about HIV in the nation or the world. Drawings from a later time in parents' lives often reflect many more personal effects—illness and death of close relatives and friends, for example. The series of drawings frequently depict stories that are quite poignant and emotional. In group discussion, parents are reminded that their children probably have similar stories to tell and feelings to discuss but that their children were born into a world in which HIV was always present.

Activity 3, "Feeling Circle," extends the personalization and identifies some barriers to communicating clearly about HIV. Parents call out all the feelings aroused by the "AIDS Lifeline" exercise and by HIV in general. They are reminded that their children are also experiencing these feelings and may need to express them and know that others have the same feelings. Emotion, a barrier to communication, becomes reframed as an opportunity for communication.

Sharing continues in Activity 4, "Myths and Facts About HIV/AIDS." Parents are given an overview of the disease, HIV infection, its transmission routes, and natural history. In trying to answer a difficult true-false test as a group, parents share information they already knew and clarify the information they just learned.

Application to new situations continues in Activity 5, "What We Know About HIV Transmission." A series of picture cards depicts sexual, social, medical, and substance use situations in line drawings. Parents are asked to sort these into piles labeled "Safe," "Somewhat Safe," "Risky," and "Need More Information." This exercise, as well as the group discussion about disagreements, clarifies HIV transmission information and brings the group to a more secure understanding of HIV risk.

Activity 6, "What Kids Need to Know About HIV/AIDS," refocuses the discussion on children. Parents brainstorm about how children at different ages are at risk for HIV and what children need to know to avoid or reduce risk at various ages.

In Activity 7, "One Strength I Have Is," parents form pairs and assess each other's strengths in passing on needed information to their own children.

Session 1 ends with a homework assignment—find an opportunity to have one conversation with your child about HIV.

Session 2: Parent-Child Communication

In this session, parents become more active. Parents add to their existing parent-child communication skills, add HIV safety skills, practice communicating with adults playing the role of children, and develop plans to have HIV-related discussions in the home. Mr. Jones, for example, found he only had to schedule a regular time to talk with his niece and model comfort in talking about HIV. He chose a simple strategy to open the door to HIV-related conversations: "I'm taking a training about talking with kids about HIV. How do you feel about that?" HIV was such a pressing issue for his niece that she was relieved to begin conversations once given permission.

An activity in this session, called "Carousel," has two objectives: (a) to give parents practice in answering children's difficult HIV-related questions and (b) to assist parents in taking a child's viewpoint in evaluating how well questions are answered. In this activity, parents become used to being bombarded with children's questions about sex and drugs through simulation and role-play. Half the parents are assigned the role of "children," and half remain parents. Parents form an inner circle (facing out), and "children" face them in an outer ring. Each "child" has a card filled with difficult questions ("Why do people become junkies?" "How do I know if I'm gay?" "When should I have sex the first time?" "What's an STD?" and many, many more). The "child" introduces himself or herself to the parent he or she is facing by stating a gender and age (e.g., "I'm an 11-year-old girl"); the child immediately begins asking the parent questions that the parent attempts to answer. A signal is given; the children shift to the right, and each parent is confronted with a new child and new problems. The process repeats several times. In another round, roles are reversed—parents become "children." At a wrap-up discussion, all the adults reflect on (a) how it felt to be a child or parent, (b) how well questions were answered, and (c) where to learn to discuss questions with children more effectively.

Session 3: Recognize, Avoid, and Negotiate Risk

The third session begins the process of understanding HIV and HIV risk from the child's viewpoint and in the child's social world. The aim of PATH is to transfer safety skills to children and to support children in maintaining safety in daily life. In this session, it becomes clear that this will only happen if the parent understands and is involved in his or her child's world. Parents brainstorm about how they can reward their children for maintaining safe behavior.

Parents explore recognizing HIV risk in the neighborhood in the second activity of this session, neighborhood "mapping." This exercise also emphasizes opportunities for HIV prevention present in the family and neighborhood ecology. A group of parents gathers around a drawing of the neighborhood. Parents have red, yellow, and green stickers available to indicate buildings, street corners, parks, and other locations that parents feel are dangerous (red), moderately safe (yellow), and safe (green) from HIV risk. Through discussion, parents come to a consensus—labeling a store "red," for example, because illegal drugs are sold there or labeling the site of a highly regarded after-school program "green." Parents are then given a guide to youth resources (tutoring, recreation, etc.) in the neighborhood, a map, and a set of stickers and are asked to repeat the exercise at home alone with their child, getting the child's perspective of the neighborhood. All parents discuss the child's-eye view maps at their next group meeting.

Session 4: Safe and Sensitive Socializing
With Persons With HIV/AIDS

This session introduces the difficult topic of how to act around persons with HIV disease. The parent's role subtly shifts to that of coach, observing performance of role-plays and reflecting on how performance could be improved. It is PATH's aim to have this reflective process eventually become internalized as well. Not every strategy and tactic will work well as parents meet unexpected circumstances. The ability to reflect and fine-tune how one handles situations is important both for the parent and the child.

To evoke discussion about safe and sensitive interactions with persons with HIV, drawings of neighborhood scenes are presented (e.g., three people—one with a cut—are playing in a park, and an HIV-affected family is coping during their daily activities; see Figures 5.1 and 5.2). The parent group is told, "One person here has HIV." Parents discuss whether the characters in the drawing are

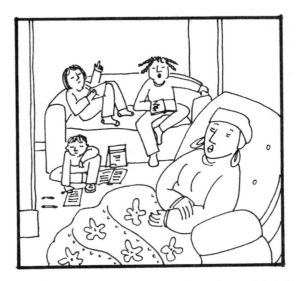

Figure 5.1. In discussing this scene, parents recognize the special challenges of living daily with HIV.

behaving safely and whether they are sensitively supporting the person with HIV. This activity represents an application of new knowledge because it follows a discussion of a list, written by HIV+ people, of how HIV+ persons do and do not like to be treated. Both activities follow a review of universal or standard precautions (medical and public health guidelines as to how to avoid transmission of all communicable diseases, including HIV).

Session 5: Parents' Role in Maintaining Safety of Children

This session acknowledges that preadolescents are maturing into young adults. Their social world is expanding. Where formerly parents could be surveillant and vigilant in discipline, safety now depends on the child's risk avoidance and negotiation skills and the child's own internalized standards. The parent's role is to assist the child to clarify and internalize standards of safety and to assist the child to behave responsibly toward one's self and others.

In a role-play, "Megaphone," parents mimic how communication is likely to change as children mature and begin to match their parents in height, timbre of voice, thoughts, and feelings. A parent pretends to be a "child" returning from school with an HIV-related worry. The "child" is greeted by a "parent" standing on a stool with a megaphone; they attempt a conversation in which the "child" tries to state his worry (a worry that is unknown to the adult playing the role of parent). The parent group discusses how the conversation is going. New skills

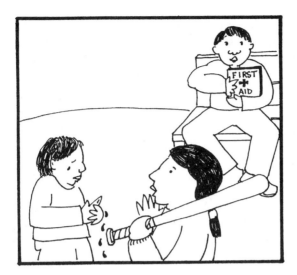

Figure 5.2. This scene evokes a discussion of universal or standard precautions.

are practiced in "You Be the Mirror." Parents learn that children need to hear their own thoughts and feelings repeated to them to understand and correct them the same way people need to see themselves in a mirror to adjust their appearance. After the practice of listening and reflection skills, the conversation is replayed with "parent" and "child" now on the same level. Adults playing the role of children find the conversation calming and often remark that they feel they are being listened to.

For Sessions 5 and 6, we were guided by the triangle model of responsibility (Schlenker, Britt, Pennington, Murphy, & Doherty, 1994) to design exercises to help parents to transfer maintenance of health-promoting behaviors to youth. The triangle model posits that a person will feel responsibility for maintaining positive behaviors if three links are in place: the individual perceives that both the means and ends of the desired behavior are consistent with his or her personal identity images and that an external or internal "audience" would judge these links favorably.

For example, HIV risk reduction is especially difficult for some of our young women because they are supposed to be "sexy" but not "sexual." They are not supposed to control when or how sex happens. Buying and carrying a condom (means) is inconsistent with their current identity image, even though being disease free (ends) is. Children and adults are both often "embarrassed to death." The short-term embarrassment of being judged as a "bitch" or "ho" by friends for demonstrating preparedness for sexual activity outweighs the long-term and somewhat remote concern for personal health. Gina, on the other hand, illustrates a less problematic identity in which means, ends, and others' supposed judgments have been brought into harmony. She states,

> When I was "out there" [on the street], I was so glad I made sure I used a condom. You'd have to be stupid not to. Now I'm back home and in school and I got choices, because I'm not pregnant and I don't have some disease. I made a mistake, but now I have a future. I'm glad my stepfather talked to me about this stuff. Those days I was out there, I still knew he cared. I came home because he reminded me I was better than that.

The triangle model shares many features with other microtheories (e.g., the theory of reasoned action; Ajzen & Fishbein, 1980) but places emphasis on personal "ownership" of, or "identity" with, a desired goal and the strategies and tactics chosen to achieve it. The theory seemed especially appropriate for adolescents who are in the process of identity formation and are especially aware of external judgments by others, including peers (Steinberg, 1991). We believe that the transition to adolescence is critical for assimilating risk reduction and avoidance into self-images, as well as planning pathways for the return to positive choices if negative choices are temporarily made (Kagan, 1992; Musick, 1991; Nurco & Lerner, 1996; Steinberg, 1991).

Preadolescents and adolescents in the community gave us a particularly salient point of leverage. Central to identity was adolescents' monitoring and concern for others (Krauss, 1997). In a neighborhood with danger, children are continually "watching each other's backs" and reassuring one another about safety. Children have these same concerns for their parents. Internalized, the concern for others becomes the script for one's own safe behavior.

Session 6: Advanced HIV Communication

In the final parent session, the parents' roles change in two ways. Parents acknowledge a new respect for their maturing children in exercises in which parents practice negotiating mutual safety, with adults playing the role of their children. The foundation of this negotiation is recognition of mutual caring, parent for child and child for parent. It is also in this session that parents become the evaluators of new information about substance use, STIs, and hepatitis A, B, and C. The session launches parents as lifelong learners and teachers.

An activity, "Fill in the Blank," elicits immediate and uncensored feelings and images about HIV and HIV prevention. Parents throw a beach ball back and forth as fast as they can. They are instructed to shout the first thought that comes into their heads when they hear phrases such as, "Girls who buy condoms are _____," "My child buying condoms is _____," "A boy who delays sex is _____," and "A person who hangs out with people with HIV is _____." The last group meeting ends with a role-play of parents catching kids in safe activities and kids likewise catching parents in safe activities. At this point, parents have learned to integrate two messages into the role-plays: (a) encouragement for safe behavior with statements of the form "I feel _____ when you _____" and (b) recognition that rules and reassurances about mutual safety need to be negotiated between parent and child because "the same way you [the child] feel relief from worry when you know your friends and loved ones are behaving safely I [the parent] am feeling about you now."

These are only a few of the more than 40 activities that parents participate in as they learn to talk to their kids about sex, drugs, and HIV in the PATH program.

Parent "Booster" Meetings

The first four sessions of parent group training occur in a relatively compressed time span—3 hours once a week for 4 weeks. These first four sessions also are filled with activities reinforcing acquisition and use of information, skills, and communication techniques. We felt that it was important for the parents to meet together in relatively unstructured time, approximately 2 months after their initial four training sessions. In this 90-minute meeting, parents could begin to act as coaches for each other about issues that had arisen in daily life. Parents could also share new information they had heard about HIV and clarify any misunderstandings. It was in just such a meeting that Gina's stepfather brainstormed with the group about how he was going to get her to return home.

This more open forum also provided PATH project personnel with an opportunity to learn about issues in the community that may not have been anticipated or may affect attitudes toward HIV risk reduction or coping with HIV. It was in these sessions that we first learned that parents were worried about a hepatitis B and hepatitis C epidemic among local injection drug users. It was this type of information that reinforced the PATH program's emphasis on universal or standard precautions against all diseases as a general risk reduction strategy. It also reinforced our notions that we should not treat HIV as a disease apart from all others but as one of a number of contagious diseases (Krauss, 1999).

Three Parent-Child Sessions

One of our more important insights was that it was helpful to schedule time for a parent to teach his or her child about HIV at our site, with a PATH staff member present who acted as a passive observer. These sessions were important for several reasons. Earlier work with the children had suggested that children wanted to approach their parents with their questions about HIV and HIV risk but were inhibited from doing so for a variety of reasons. These included fear that the parent would assume that any question about sex or drugs would imply that the child was sexually active or using drugs, fear of the parent's emotionality, concern that the conversation would drift toward the parent's own childhood rather than the child's present social circumstances, concerns about the parent's ability to keep important information confidential, and concerns as to whether the parent had the latest and most accurate information (Krauss, 1997). A further cause for apprehension was embarrassment about sexual matters, especially in conversations with a parent of the opposite sex. It was important to structure these sessions to be successful for both parent and child.

In the parent-child sessions, the parent acts as an HIV educator for his or her child. Instructions are given to the parent and child in advance. It is suggested that the parent can choose any activities from the PATH curriculum that the parent has taken to date to explore with the child. The child also can have an opportunity to ask any pressing questions about HIV. Parent and child often collude to make each other look good in these sessions; they often collaborate in the choice of exercises. The fact that the parent has already done these activities or exercises makes the parent the de facto expert.

Because the session occurs at a training site and is observed, both parent and child are likely on their best behavior. It is a safe place to discuss HIV. The presence of the observer has two further functions: First, the "silence" of the observer (observers, in fact, have rarely had to jump in and correct misinformation) validates the parent as an HIV expert and, second, the presence of an observer of the same gender as the child "desexualizes" and "professionalizes" the interaction.

Parents and children cite these sessions as among the most valuable components of PATH. Children say these sessions "break the ice" and "let us talk about HIV." Some parents have used the guided session as an opportunity to deal with very challenging issues: suspected substance use of a child, disclosure of a relative's HIV status, reassurance about an HIV+ parent's health, an opportunity to challenge a child's incorrect belief about HIV, and a chance to negotiate an agreement about risk reduction.

STRUCTURAL COMPONENTS OF
THE PREVENTION PROGRAM

Site for Prevention Program

Our intervention takes place at a rented storefront within walking distance of the residences of our parents and children. The storefront is known in the neighborhood as The Lower East Side Health Project. Our site is a converted doctor's office with a waiting area, kitchenette, meeting room, and several private offices used for interviewing. The important characteristics of the site are convenience, neutrality, and privacy. Nothing identifies the site as being associated with HIV.

Similar trainings have been carried out by Cornell University/Cornell Cooperative Extension in a variety of settings, from classrooms to church basements.

Training Staff for Prevention Program

Cornell University/Cornell Cooperative Extension and the National Development and Research Institutes offer a 3-day Training of Trainers program for PATH and its parent curriculum, "Talking With Kids About AIDS." We require this training of all staff, even auxiliary personnel.

Additional training is recommended in five areas: (a) an overview of HIV/AIDS and its treatment, (b) confidentiality, (c) grief counseling, (d) diversity, and (e) domestic violence.

Overview of HIV/AIDS and Its Treatment

Many people in the community are HIV+; any person walking through the door of our storefront site could be. Our staff's behavior with regard to protection of those who are immunosuppressed must be of the highest caliber. We have adopted the infection control recommendations of a major hospital—no one may come to work with an active cough or rash. We have the necessary materials for universal precautions—latex gloves, a sharps container, and so on. Parents or children with an active cough or rash are politely turned away and rescheduled with a brief explanation. Even the food we order for snacks during group trainings must recognize the nutrition and medication needs of participants who may be HIV+.

Confidentiality

In this high-seroprevalence neighborhood, confidentiality concerning HIV status is a major concern. Our staff is trained to avoid inadvertent disclosures and to handle all records and materials circumspectly.

Grief Counseling

Given the chronic grief in this community, we offer a brief grief workshop to the community once a year and have responded to several neighborhood incidents by offering another.

Diversity

Training on cultural diversity issues is highly desirable.

Domestic Violence

Our recruiters, community organizer, and group facilitators are in a position to overhear or learn about child abuse and neglect and domestic violence. The project director, as a licensed psychologist, is mandated in New York State to report child abuse and neglect. Victim's Services trains our staff on recognition of violence and appropriate referral; a parent advisory board made sure our referral procedures were appropriate to the community.

With the potential in the community for health or mental health problems, we have arranged to refer serious medical and mental health problems to clinicians at a large local hospital. These clinicians are available by beeper and have trained our staff in appropriate referral procedures.

Group Facilitators

The group facilitators are at the heart of the PATH project. In leading parent groups, the facilitators continually model appropriate communication styles. Because gender issues are pervasive in HIV and HIV risk reduction, it is important to have a male and female team that models respectful give-and-take, open communication, and teamwork. Because the facilitators are dealing with a diverse community and parents within that community have a multitude of values, the facilitators must be able to remain relatively value neutral. Ideally, they offer the curriculum's insights as "options" expanding the range of parent choices. They handle misinformation and conflict by suggesting other ways of interpreting information. It is important that the facilitators be trained in listening and reflection skills. Our strongest facilitators use a great deal of body language and nonverbal communication to ensure that each member of a parent training group has an opportunity to be heard. Facilitators can be members of the community where the trainings take place or highly trained professionals. Some of our most effective teams have included one community member and one professional.

It is also the group facilitators who elicit and then model the ground rules for parent groups, parent-child sessions, and the parent "booster" session. These rules usually include being punctual, not coming high, staying through the session, talking one at a time, respecting each other's opinions, not cursing or shouting, and respecting confidentiality. It is the facilitators' duty to teach parent training participants about confidentiality and to catch and correct any potential lapses.

Community Organizers

When we entered the Lower East Side with our program, HIV was our highest concern. It was not the major concern of the community (Krauss, 1997; Krauss, Goldsamt, Bula, & Sember, 1997). Early on, we made a decision to hire a community organizer not only to direct parents to HIV-related resources as needed but also to acknowledge the community's priorities by making referrals for other needs participants perceive as more pressing and immediate than HIV prevention. Our community organizer makes more than 15 referrals per week for housing, drug treatment, food, and other concrete concerns as well as referrals about HIV-related issues. Through the actions of the community organizer, our program is seen as responsive to community concerns and has developed positive relationships with a network of service providers to whom we refer.

CURRENT PROGRAM EVALUATION

To date, our data suggest that PATH positively influences parents' and children's knowledge about HIV, decreases worry about HIV, and increases intentions to avoid or reduce risk. Data suggest that PATH improves the content and context of HIV-related conversations (Krauss, Goldsamt, & Bula, 1997) and increases children's comfort in socializing with persons living with HIV/AIDS (Krauss, 1999). Parent and child clinical cases suggest even more profound effects. Children have met HIV+ relatives from whom they were formerly isolated. At least one child was treated prophylactically with AZT after receiving a puncture injury from a contaminated syringe and is not infected with HIV. A grandmother can speak to her grandson about sex and drugs and be reassured about his safety. Gina has returned home. Mr. Jones's niece talks freely about her mother.

CONCLUSIONS

The HIV epidemic cannot be disentangled easily from concurrent epidemics of sexually transmitted diseases, early pregnancy, substance abuse, poverty, and grief. Parents and children tell us that our program has gained acceptance because it addresses all of these issues, takes place in their neighborhood, enacts caring by recruiting door-to-door, builds on strengths that parents and communities already have, and sidesteps political issues about what can be told to children by empowering parents to do the telling. We also feel it hits two generations at risk and addresses primary and secondary prevention—not only is the intervention designed to prevent HIV transmission, but it is also designed to ameliorate some of the stigmatization of persons with HIV and to address the psychosocial concerns of individuals living in highly affected communities.

REFERENCES

Ajzen, I., & Fishbein, M. (1980). *Understanding attitudes and predicting social behavior.* Englewood Cliffs, NJ: Prentice Hall.

Bandura, A. (1994). Social cognitive theory and exercise of control over HIV infection. In R. DiClemente & J. L. Peterson (Eds.), *Preventing AIDS: Theories and methods of behavioral interventions* (pp. 25-59). New York: Plenum.

Bronfenbrenner, U. (1986). Ecology of the family as a context for human development research. *Developmental Psychology, 22,* 723-742.

Furstenberg, F. F., Herceg-Baron, R., Shea, J., & Webb, D. (1984). Family communication and teenagers' contraceptive use. *Family Planning Perspectives, 16,* 163-170.

Kagan, J. (1992). Etiologies of adolescents at risk. In D. E. Rogers & E. Ginzberg (Eds.), *Adolescents at risk: Medical and social perspectives* (pp. 8-18). Boulder, CO: Westview.

Kanfer, F. H., & Goldstein, A. P. (1986). *Helping people change: A textbook of methods.* New York: Pergamon.

Krauss, B. (1997). HIV education for teens and pre-teens in a high-seroprevalence inner-city neighborhood. *Families in Society, 78*(6), 579-591.

Krauss, B. (1999). Kurt Lewin Award: Kurt Lewin and action research: Destigmatizing HIV in a high seroprevalence community. *New York State Psychological Association Notebook, 11*(1), 47.

Krauss, B., Goldsamt, L., & Bula, E. (1997, April). *Parent-preadolescent communication about HIV in a high seroprevalence neighborhood.* Paper presented at the Society for Research in Child Development Biennial Meeting, Washington, DC.

Krauss, B., Goldsamt, L., Bula, E., & Sember, R. (1997). The White researcher in the multicultural community: Lessons in HIV prevention education learned in the field. *Journal of Health Education, 28*(6, Suppl.), S67-S71.

Krauss, B. J., Tiffany, J., & Goldsamt, L. (1997). Research notes: Parent and pre-adolescent training for HIV prevention in a high seroprevalence neighbourhood. *AIDS/STD Health Promotion Exchange, 1,* 10-12.

Maccoby, E. (1980). *Social development: Psychological growth and the parent-child relationship.* New York: Harcourt Brace.

Musick, J. (1991). The high-stakes challenge of programs for adolescent mothers. In P. Edelman & J. Ladner (Eds.), *Adolescence & poverty: Challenge for the 1990's* (pp. 117-137). Washington, DC: Center for National Policy Press.

New York City Department of Health, Office of AIDS Surveillance. (1996). *AIDS surveillance update: Second quarter 1996.* New York: New York City Department of Health.

New York City Human Services Administration. (1990). *AIDS, HIV infection and IV drug use estimates by neighborhood.* New York: Author.

Nurco, D. N., & Lerner, M. (1996). Vulnerability to narcotic addiction: Family structure and functioning. *Journal of Drug Issues, 26*(4), 1007-1025.

Prochaska, J. O., DiClemente, C., & Norcross, J. C. (1992). In search of how people change: Applications to addictive behavior. *American Psychologist, 47,* 1102-1114.

Schlenker, B. R., Britt, T. W., Pennington, J., Murphy, R., & Doherty, K. (1994). The triangle model of responsibility. *Psychological Review, 101*(4), 632-652.

Steinberg, L. (1991). The logic of adolescence. In P. Edelman & J. Ladner (Eds.), *Adolescence & poverty: Challenge for the 1990's* (pp. 19-36). Washington, DC: Center for National Policy Press.

Tiffany, J., Tobias, D., Raqib, A., & Ziegler, J. (1993a). *Talking with kids about AIDS: A program for parents and other adults who care (manual).* New York: Cornell University Press.

Tiffany, J., Tobias, D., Raqib, A., & Ziegler, J. (1993b). *Talking with kids about AIDS: A program for parents and other adults who care (teaching guide).* New York: Cornell University Press.

Chapter 6

Keepin' It R.E.A.L.!

A Mother-Adolescent HIV Prevention Program

Colleen DiIorio

Pamela Denzmore

Dongqing T. Wang

Jenny Lipana

Ken Resnicow

Giesla Rogers-Tillman

William N. Dudley

Deborah Fisher Van Marter

Emory University

Louise, a 35-year-old married mother of two children, attended Keepin' It R.E.A.L.! with her 12-year-old daughter, Lillian. During the second session, Louise told the other mothers in her group that she was worried about her daughter, whom she believed was sexually active. Her only evidence of her daughter's sexual activity was a discharge that she noted on her daughter's undergarments. She said that she had not yet talked with her daughter about the discharge but admitted that she was angry and feared that her daughter would become pregnant. During the discussion, Louise also revealed that she had not yet talked with Lillian about menstruation or other changes associated with puberty. She stated that she had not planned to talk with Lillian because she believed her daughter would learn what she needed to know in sex education classes offered at school.

Later in the discussion, Louise admitted that she really did not fully understand the process of menstruation and felt inadequately prepared to explain it to her daughter or to answer questions about it. Through attendance at the session and the

AUTHORS' NOTE: To protect the confidentiality of participants, names and details of the situations presented were modified. This chapter was supported by a grant from the Office on AIDS, National Institute of Mental Health (R01 MH55710). For more information about this chapter, please contact Dr. Colleen DiIorio, Department of Behavioral Sciences and Health Education, Emory University Rollins School of Public Health, 1518 Clifton Road, N.E., Atlanta, GA 30322; e-mail: cdiiori@sph.emory.edu.

discussion with other mothers, Louise learned about the menstrual cycle and that a
discharge is not uncommon shortly before a girl begins her period. The take-home
activity for this session gave Louise an opportunity to initiate a discussion with
Lillian about normal changes associated with puberty. In later sessions, Louise reported back to the group her progress in discussing sexual and reproductive topics
with Lillian. The mothers were supportive of Louise's attempts to learn and share
what she was learning with her daughter. During the final session, Louise pro-
claimed that she believed that attending the program was the most important thing
that she could have done to support her daughter.

DESCRIPTION OF PROBLEM

The increasing number of adolescents infected with HIV is a cause for concern
among public health practitioners. The increasing rate of HIV infection among
this group (Centers for Disease Control and Prevention [CDC], 1997, 1999),
coupled with its relatively high rates of sexually transmitted diseases (STDs)
(CDC, 1998) and pregnancy (Ventura, Curtin, & Matthews, 1998), suggests that
the use of condoms among adolescents is far from universal. Public health efforts to inform adolescents of HIV, STDs, and pregnancy protection have largely
focused on the adolescent, and these efforts have been largely promoted through
school systems. School-based programs about sexual health are helpful for adolescents because they introduce students to accurate information about puberty,
contraception, pregnancy, STDs, and other aspects of sexual reproduction. Yet
these same programs are often offered only once per year and generally fail to
consider the developmental needs of students. Although some students may be
ready to understand and use information following the sex education classes,
other students are not ready to adopt recommendations, and still others may not
be ready to appreciate the significance of the information they hear.

We know from educational theories that optimal learning situations are those
in which students demonstrate a readiness to learn (Maslow, 1987) and those in
which learning is reinforced over multiple times and in different ways (Driscoll,
1994; Marshall, 1992). If learning takes place under optimal conditions, the
learner is more likely to understand and use the new information (Gallagher,
1996). Creating an optimal learning environment for HIV and sex education
within school settings is difficult because it is not always possible for any
teacher or groups of teachers to be aware of the sexual health needs of individual
students. Fortunately, however, adolescents are members of other groups that
are likely to be more supportive in learning about healthy sexual development.

Perhaps the most important system within which children learn about sexual
health and reproduction is the family. Developmental specialists tell us that

learning about sexuality begins in infancy (Broering, 1991). Early in life, children learn about sex roles and intimacy through interactions with their parents, caretakers, and siblings and by observing relationships among family members (Broering, 1991). As they grow, children learn values from their parents, who also model for them behaviors that provide a context for understanding a variety of issues related to sexual health. The family system affords opportunities for parents to share information with their children and guide them in making responsible decisions about sexual health (Finan, 1997). Such dialogues between parents and children require that parents be knowledgeable about sexual and reproductive health and feel confident that they can communicate the information to their children. Moreover, parents who possess the requisite knowledge and skills can present information that is consistent with their children's developmental and learning needs.

Keepin' It R.E.A.L.! (Responsible, Empowered, Aware, Living) acknowledges the important role that parents play in promoting the sexual health of their adolescents, particularly as it relates to HIV prevention. The goal of the program is to foster parental involvement in guiding sexual development of youth and to enhance the mother's role in postponing sexual debut. We expect that adolescents whose mothers take an active role in their children's sexual development will be more likely than adolescents whose mothers take a passive role to know about risks (i.e., HIV, STDs, pregnancy) associated with sexual intercourse and be more willing to adopt HIV risk reduction practices, including the postponement of sexual intercourse.

Our program objectives are in concert with goals of Healthy People 2010 (U.S. Department of Health and Human Services, 1999). These goals, developed to guide public health programs for U.S. residents, include increasing the proportion of adolescents who discuss sexuality with their parents, reducing the proportion of adolescents who have sexual intercourse, and increasing the proportion of sexually active adolescents who use condoms.

DESCRIPTION OF POPULATION

Keepin' It R.E.A.L.! was developed for mothers and their 11- to 14-year-old adolescents living in or near the city of Atlanta, Georgia. Currently, Atlanta ranks seventh among U.S. cities in the number of cumulated AIDS cases and reported cases per 100,000 with 14,271 cumulative cases reported in the metropolitan area of Atlanta through June 1999 (CDC, 1999). Thus, adolescents who live in or near Atlanta are at a higher risk of exposure to HIV than adolescents who reside in areas with low rates of infections. To reach adolescents in the city, we joined with a community partner—the Boys & Girls Clubs of Metro Atlanta. The Boys & Girls Clubs of Metro Atlanta are an ideal partner for this HIV prevention study because most of their clubs are located in neighborhoods that are in or near the city of Atlanta where there is a high rate of HIV infection. Moreover, the Boys & Girls Clubs provide a wide range of services for youth, including health programs; they also maintain close ties with the communities they serve, and they promote parental involvement in club activities. The Boys & Girls Clubs of Metro Atlanta are part of a nationwide affiliation of local autonomous organizations whose primary mission is to help youth develop the skills they need to become productive adults, responsible citizens, and community leaders. The adolescents served by the Boys & Girls Clubs match the profile of adolescents considered at risk for early initiation of sexual intercourse and HIV infection. The youth served are primarily from disadvantaged economic, social, and family circumstances with more than 63% of young members from single-parent homes.

PROGRAM DEVELOPMENT

Theoretical Foundation

Keepin' It R.E.A.L.! is designed to promote the family's role in promoting the postponement of sexual intercourse among 11- to 14-year-old adolescents. This program that we present here is based on social cognitive theory and is designed specifically to foster discussions about sexual health between mothers and their adolescents and encourage the adoption of behaviors that enhance sexual health. Although several theoretical approaches can be used to foster the adoption of healthy behaviors, social cognitive theory has received considerable attention and has been used as the basis for a variety of adolescent HIV prevention programs. Social cognitive theory encourages the adoption of healthy behaviors through strengthening cognitive, behavioral, and efficacy skills and environmental supports. Because the focus of Keepin' It R.E.A.L.! is on families, both an individual (adolescent) and a family (mother) component were included in the program.

Social cognitive theory conceptualizes behavior as the result of interactions among personal factors, environmental factors, and the behavior itself (Bandura, 1986, 1997). Personal factors noted to be important in behavioral performance are self-efficacy (confidence that a person has the skills to perform a behavior when needed), outcome expectancies (expectations that if the behavior is engaged in, it will be successful), and behavioral goals (what a person intends to do in the future) (Bandura, 1986, 1997). For example, if an adolescent has high self-efficacy that he or she can avoid high-risk situations and that avoiding them will lead to not being pressured to engage in early sexual debut, the adolescent's goal will be to do this on every occasion that he or she attends a party.

Environmental factors also act to support avoidance of risky situations and include assistance from both family and friends and access to tangible resources. Bandura (1992) has discussed the application of social cognitive theory to HIV prevention practices. In referring specifically to safer sex practices, Bandura noted that if individuals are to prevent HIV infection, they must develop confidence in their ability to choose safe rather than risky situations and to focus on the positive outcomes associated with safer behaviors (e.g., avoiding the corner of the dance where youth are drinking and instead dancing with a friend near the band). HIV prevention programs based on social cognitive theory teach participants about avoiding risky situations and promote safer sexual practices. Effective programs must also include teaching skills such as recognizing situations that lead to unsafe behaviors, reinforcing positive behaviors, negotiating for safer sex, and using condoms (Bandura, 1992).

The approach used in Keepin' It R.E.A.L.! is to include mothers who are taught how to support their adolescents' efforts in developing HIV risk reduction behaviors. An advantage of the family approach is that the family member who learns with the adolescent can continue to provide support in decision making as the adolescent grows.

This curriculum is designed for mothers and adolescents. The primary objectives are to increase the mothers' confidence in discussing sexual health issues with their adolescents, to increase the adolescents' confidence in resisting pressures to initiate sexual intercourse before they are ready, and to enhance their confidence to use safer sex practices when they do become sexually active. We expect that adolescents and mothers who attend this program will be more likely to discuss sexual health issues with each other and will be more comfortable doing so. We also expect that adolescents who attend this program will be more likely to postpone the initiation of sexual intercourse and, when they become sexually active, to adopt safer sex practices, including the use of condoms.

Program Format

This program consists of seven group sessions held once every 2 weeks for 14 weeks. The program was designed for mothers and their adolescents. Once each group had held its first session, no new members were admitted. This format was selected so participants could form relationships with other members of their group and provide continuity to the discussions over time.

A general format was developed for the seven sessions. The group facilitator begins each session by providing an overview of the session content, and then she guides participants through a warm-up activity to build group cohesion. Except for the first session, the warm-up activity is followed by a review of take-home activities and a discussion of personal goals set by each participant at the previous session. Mothers and adolescents remain together for four sessions and meet in separate groups for three sessions. All sessions include an interactive component consisting of games, videotapes, role-plays, and skits to demonstrate and practice concepts presented during the sessions. To reinforce learning, participants are encouraged to complete take-home activities. At the end of each session, each participant sets a personal goal to improve communication between the mother and the adolescent.

Booster sessions are held to reunite the group and to foster discussion on how participants used the information and skills they learned during the seven regular sessions. This is also a time to provide updated information about HIV and AIDS.

PROGRAM DESCRIPTION

The seven sessions for Keepin' It R.E.A.L.! are summarized in Table 6.1.

Session 1: HIV/AIDS Knowledge and Attitudes

The facilitator begins the first session by providing specific information about the roles of the facilitator and the participants. The facilitator also gives a preview of the seven sessions and together with the participants establishes rules for the group to follow. These rules generally include being on time, not interrupting when others are talking, respecting the opinions of each group member, and not sharing personal information discussed within the group with people outside the group. The facilitator then engages participants in a warm-up activity for the purpose of getting to know each other's names.

Following the introductory activities, participants are guided through a skit demonstrating HIV transmission and its consequences. Adolescents assume the roles of "T cells" and "HIV virus," and mothers form a circle around them to represent the walls of the blood vessels. Through drama, the mothers and adolescents demonstrate how HIV enters the body and destroys T cells. "Bacterial cells" representing a type of pneumonia are played by adolescents who enter the "blood vessel" to demonstrate the inability of the HIV-infected T cells to fight infection. The skit generates a variety of questions about HIV and AIDS, and these questions serve as the focus for discussion about the pathogenesis of HIV, its transmission, and consequences. The skit provides an opportunity for mothers and adolescents to share with each other what they know about HIV and AIDS. When inaccurate information is presented, the facilitator can correct it and then have participants demonstrate the correct sequence of events. Because the context for discussion is drama, the focus is taken off the individual and placed on the action of the players as mothers guide them through their roles. This approach to discussing basic facts about HIV and AIDS seems to encourage mothers and adolescents to participate in the discussion with less concern about sharing what they know or do not know with each other. The spontaneous nature of this type of drama also creates an atmosphere that encourages openness in

TABLE 6.1 Keepin' It R.E.A.L.! Program Outline

Session 1	Welcome and Introduction
	HIV/AIDS Knowledge and Attitudes
Session 2	Values and Peer Pressure (adolescent groups)
	Adolescent Development (mother groups)
Session 3	Basic Listening and Communication Skills
Session 4	Talking About Sex
Session 5	Sexual Decision Making (adolescent groups)
	Parenting Challenges and Communication (mother groups)
Session 6	Putting It All Together Puppet Show
Session 7	Consequences of Early Initiation of Sexual Intercourse (adolescent groups)
	Condom Information and Skill Building (mother groups)
	Graduation and Evaluation

sharing information, thus decreasing the concern about speaking in front of a group. And the strong visual component helps the learner retain information long after the session is over.

This HIV skit is followed by a more serious discussion about people living with AIDS. To foster discussion, we begin this segment by showing a videotape of three young people who have AIDS and who discuss how they were infected and how HIV has changed their lives. Because AIDS has touched the lives of many of the mothers and adolescents attending the program, the conversation quickly shifts from the experiences presented on tape to the real-life experiences of the participants in the program. This sharing personalizes AIDS for the participants and highlights the risk of contracting HIV within the community. Both mothers and adolescents frequently comment on their sense of vulnerability. Mothers often express how "things have changed since they were young," and their concern about risk seems to focus more on their children than on themselves. This session ends with participants setting a group goal to locate information about HIV in the media.

Session 2: Values and Peer Pressures (Adolescents) and Adolescent Development (Mothers)

The second session is devoted to developmental changes of adolescents. After reviewing content presented in Session 1 and discussing the take-home activity, mothers and adolescents form separate groups and meet in different rooms. In their session, mothers discuss physiological and emotional changes associated with puberty, whereas adolescents discuss the growing importance of peer relationships. Mothers begin their session with a warm-up activity to desensitize them to words used to describe body parts and to reduce their embarrassment about discussing physiological processes. The activity begins by asking a volunteer to draw an outline of a human body on newsprint. Mothers then take turns adding "changes" to the body to depict changes boys undergo during puberty. They repeat the exercise to show changes girls undergo during puberty. The mothers generally get very involved in the activity and make a variety of comments, often humorous. This exchange serves to encourage participation and offset the embarrassment that is commonly associated with such discussions. Often mothers will use euphemisms to describe a body part. For example, a mother might use the term *thing* to refer to the penis. When euphemisms are used, the facilitator interjects the correct word for the body part. In this way, participants learn that it is all right to use appropriate terms and become comfortable using them in the discussions. As with the HIV skit in the first session, the drawing activity depends on the group rather than individuals to successfully complete the task. Thus, attention is diverted from the mother giving information to the diagram being constructed.

This exercise is followed by a videotape presentation of changes occurring in boys and girls during puberty. The presentation is very informative and explains normal developmental changes and processes, including menstruation and wet dreams. Following the presentation, the facilitator answers questions and engages mothers in a discussion of how they themselves learned about puberty and sex. A common theme emerging from these conversations is that the mothers often feel that their parents did not adequately prepare them for puberty, relationships with boys, and marriage. During this discussion, mothers often come to the realization that if they do not discuss these issues, their children will grow up to experience the same sense of deprivation. Thus, mothers leave the session with a renewed sense of motivation to overcome barriers to discussing sex and puberty with their adolescents.

It was during this discussion that Louise, mentioned at the beginning of this chapter, admitted to mothers in her group that she had never discussed sex or changes associated with puberty with her 12-year-old daughter, Lillian. Although she admitted to feeling somewhat guilty, she believed that her daughter would be adequately informed during the sex education class offered at school. Louise's primary concern was her belief that Lillian was sexually active and would become pregnant. Despite her concern, Louise had not broached the subject with her daughter and felt powerless to do anything about it. The mothers in her group were empathetic and discussed how they too felt unsure or embarrassed talking about sex with their adolescents. Some mothers described how they overcame barriers to discussing sex with their adolescents, and several noted that their concerns about their daughters' likelihood of getting pregnant prompted them to overcome any reluctance to talk with them.

Because Louise appeared to be incorrectly interpreting the reason for the discharge she noted on her daughter's undergarments, the mothers strongly encouraged her to learn more about the menstrual cycle and normal bodily processes. They believed that without other evidence, Louise might have the wrong impression of her daughter, and this distrust could destroy their relationship. Louise carefully considered the conversation, and at the end of the session, she made a goal to share with her daughter some of the information she had learned from the video that day. A take-home activity was for the mother and adolescent to name parts of the body involved in sexual functioning. This activity gave Louise an excellent opportunity to begin a conversation with her daughter.

In addition to the physiological changes associated with puberty, adolescence is a time for identity formation and growing independence from parents (Erikson, 1950). During this period, peer relationships become more important. Friendships are important for adolescents because they can provide support and instill a sense of self-confidence and stability (Marcia, 1980). Yet it is during adolescence that the number of children involved in problem behaviors, including the early initiation of sexual intercourse, rapidly increases. The influence of friends in these activities is well documented (Ary, Duncan, Duncan, & Hops, 1999). Thus, although mothers are learning about physiological changes of puberty, their adolescents discuss peer relationships. An activity that the adolescents particularly like is called "Just Say No." The purpose of this activity is to demonstrate the importance of friends in making choices. To begin the activity, the facilitator asks the entire group to stand on one side of the room and then asks for a volunteer. The volunteer is instructed to stand opposite the group. The large group petitions the volunteer to smoke a cigarette (or drink alcohol or smoke pot). The lone volunteer is told to say "no" in response. Then, one by one, the adolescents from the group join the volunteer. Each time an adolescent moves, the group petition is repeated. "Smoke a cigarette!" Each time the number of adolescents who say no gets larger. Eventually, everyone is in the "no" crowd. Following the exercise, the adolescents discuss how it felt to say no when they were in a large group saying no and how it felt to say no when they were in the small group or the only one responding. The discussion revolves around the influence of peers and why adolescents might choose to do something because their friends are doing it.

The exercises and discussion related to peer pressure are balanced with discussions and role-plays about peer power, which is defined as the opposite of peer pressure. That is, peers can serve to encourage engagement and perseverance in behaviors that promote self-esteem, academic advancement, and prosocial development. For the exercises on peer pressure, adolescents create situations, often relying on their own experiences. Using these situations, adolescents take turns role-playing peer power.

At the end of the second session, adolescents and their mothers learn more specific information about goal development and the power of goals. They each develop a goal that relates to sharing information in some way with each other. These goals include sharing information discussed in the separate groups or doing the take-home activity together.

Session 3: Basic Listening and Communication Skills

The third session is concerned with basic communication skills focusing on effective listening and assertive communication. Mothers and adolescents stay together for this session, which begins with an activity called "Pass the Word," in which the facilitator whispers a short sentence or phrase into the ear of a participant. This person then whispers it to the next person until all participants have heard the message. The last person to hear the message repeats what he or she heard out loud to the group. Inevitably, the message changes as it is exchanged from person to person, and the final one is clearly different from the original message. The purpose of this activity is to highlight the importance of listening and how easy it is to misunderstand or be misunderstood. This exercise is followed by a collection of video clips from popular television sitcoms demonstrating good and poor listening. The facilitator encourages participants to identify physical actions or facial expressions of the actors that indicate poor or good listening skills.

The video clips about listening skills are followed by a presentation on assertive, passive, and aggressive communication. Following a brief introduction on the different types of communication, the facilitator models assertive communication through the use of "I" statements. "I" statements require the speaker to take ownership of his or her emotional response to a problem behavior committed by another. The use of "I" statements contrasts with aggressive communication, in which the speaker blames another for his or her actions, or passive communication, in which a person chooses to ignore the problem behavior. Mothers and adolescents practice using "I" statements in a game called "'I' Statement Hot Potato." In this game, participants toss a beanbag to each other while music is being played. When the music stops, the person with the beanbag must respond to a given situation using an "I" statement. For example, a mother might be asked to use an "I" statement in a situation in which her son has left the bathroom in a mess. The desired response is, "When you leave the bathroom in such a mess, I get upset. I would appreciate it if, when you are finished, you would pick up the towels, put your clothes in the hamper, and put the top on the toothpaste."

An adolescent might be asked to use an "I" statement to indicate his displeasure at his mother's constant intrusion into his affairs. A desired response might be, "When you always ask me about my friends and what we do, I feel that you don't trust me." Each "I" statement is contrasted with an aggressive communication statement in which the receiver of the information is made to feel bad. Rather than telling her son how the messy bathroom makes her feel (assertive), a mother instead could tell her son that he is irresponsible, sloppy, or self-centered because he does not care that others must clean up his mess (aggressive). The son who believes that his mother is violating his privacy might tell his mother that she is too nosey and to leave him alone. Participants discuss how these aggressive statements can put the recipient of the message on the defensive and quickly escalate into an argument.

Although the mothers find assertive communication appealing, inevitably a mother vocalizes her disbelief that it can be used to change difficult behaviors of her adolescent.

Darlene, for example, is a mother of three children between 8 and 15 years of age, and she attended the program with her 13-year-old son. According to Darlene, Darryl does not like school. She must yell at him several times each morning to get him out of bed, and in the evenings, they argue about his schoolwork. She believes that if she used "I" statements, he would laugh at her, and his difficult behavior would only get worse. Other mothers agreed, insisting that aggressive communication is the only type that they can use to manage their adolescents. In the discussion that followed, the facilitator was able to show by using examples provided by Darlene that aggressive communication often leads to further arguments and resistance. She also helped Darlene and the other mothers differentiate between assertive communication, aggressive communication, and setting limits. Darlene and the participants in her group talked about setting limits in which parents decide what their adolescents can and cannot do, and then they clearly communicate the limits in firm and unambiguous language. They also agreed that adolescents should be told what the consequences of violating the limits are. Both mothers and adolescents shared their experiences. This exchange provided the facilitator an opportunity to contrast the messages associated with setting limits from those of assertive and aggressive communication.

Another concern that mothers often express is that "I" statements sound so artificial—"People don't talk like that." We agree that when taken out of the context of a conversation, "I" statements are rigid and artificial. However, to demonstrate that "I" statements can be used in normal conversation, we show clips from popular sitcoms in which "I" statements or similar forms of assertive communication are used. For a take-home activity, we encourage participants to watch sitcoms and identify the type of communication being used.

At the conclusion of this session, participants are asked to begin to write their experiences in communicating with each other in a journal. For their first entry in the journal, mothers and adolescents are asked to write letters of appreciation to each other and to discuss their letters during a "Talk Walk." Through this exercise, mothers and adolescents have an opportunity to open or enhance channels of communication.

Session 4: Talking About Sex

In Session 4, mothers and adolescents build on the communication skills they learned in Session 3. After reviewing the take-home activities from Session 3 and completing the warm-up activity, the participants join in an activity called the "Sex Barometer." In this activity, the facilitator presents to the group issues known to generate disagreement between parents and adolescents. Examples of issues are the following: "It is OK for a 16-year-old girl to have sex," and "It is OK to have sex before marriage." Mothers and their adolescents are asked to stand near the sign (with the words *strongly agree, agree, disagree,* or *strongly disagree*) that best reflects their opinion about the statement. Adolescents and mothers then discuss why they chose to stand where they did. The activity allows mothers and adolescents to hear diverse points of view about an issue and the rationale for their choices. Because mothers and adolescents sometimes take opposing views on issues and are often surprised at each other's "stance," the activity creates lively discussions. Mothers often express disbelief at their adolescents' more liberal views and wonder about the source of these views. Adolescents sometimes defend their views by noting a behavior of a family member or the reaction of the mother or father to an event.

Don was surprised to see his mother, Jewell, standing near the "strongly disagree" sign on abortion. Jewell, in turn, was somewhat dismayed to note her son's agreement with abortion. In the discussion that followed, Don noted that his mother's reaction to a friend's revelation about her recent abortion was rather mild, leading him to believe that his mother favored abortion. Jewell was surprised that her son interpreted her behavior in this way but, given what Don had said, agreed that he could misread her reaction as favorable.

The "Sex Barometer" exercise and resulting discussions allow mothers to see how their behavior can influence the development of their adolescents' sexual values. It also makes adolescents aware of the importance of discussing attitudes and feelings with their parents. The facilitator points out that values and beliefs that are openly discussed and reinforced are more likely to be adopted by adolescents than values and beliefs that remain hidden. The exercise often opens avenues for continued discussion about views between mothers and adolescents regarding sexual development of adolescents.

For the most part, the "Sex Barometer" exercise facilitates discussions between mothers and adolescents. However, in one case, the exercise created a temporary disruption of a relationship.

In this situation, the mother and daughter held opposite views about 16-year-old girls having sex. The daughter, Sarah, noted approval, whereas the mother, Nancy, strongly disagreed. In the resulting discussion, it appeared that Nancy was concerned that because her daughter agreed that it was all right for 16-year-old girls to have sex, that she too would soon initiate sexual intercourse. Nancy found it difficult to separate Sarah's view from her behavior despite her daughter's assurance that she did not plan to have sex at the age of 16. In response to this exchange, during the next two sessions, Sarah refused to participate in any discussion when her mother was present. She did, however, contribute to the discussion in the breakout sessions with the other adolescents. The conflict between the mother and daughter was the topic of conversation for the mothers in the following two sessions. During these sessions, the facilitator attempted to have Nancy recognize the need for Sarah to be able to voice her opinion without fear of reprisal. The other mothers pointed out that severe criticism of Sarah's views would cause the relationship to suffer, as Sarah would not feel comfortable talking to her mother. Indeed, Nancy admitted that this was already beginning to happen. At the final session, Nancy chose as her goal to listen to Sarah without criticizing her ideas.

Session 5: Sexual Decision Making (Adolescents) and Parenting Challenges and Communication (Mothers)

In Session 5, mothers and adolescents are challenged to discuss more difficult topics with each other. To generate discussion, the session begins with the "Hot Topics" activity. This exercise aims to increase the awareness of mothers and adolescents about topics that are more difficult for them to discuss with each other. To begin the activity, mothers and adolescents are given one index card each with a "hot topic" written on the card. Examples of hot topics include condoms, birth control, abstinence, wet dreams, and menstruation. Mothers and adolescents indicate their willingness to discuss their topic by standing near the sign that best describes how easy it would be to talk to each other about their topic. The signs are placed along the wall to demonstrate a continuum from "a breeze" to "so hard to talk, I would avoid it." After the participants have selected their places, one by one, they identify the topic on their card and share with others why they chose to stand where they did. Their comments are used to facilitate discussion that often involves an explanation of the topic. For example, Laura stood near the sign "so hard to talk, I would avoid it" for her topic on wet dreams. She stated that the reason she could not talk about it with her son Lonnie was because she did not know how she would describe wet dreams. The facilitator asked others in the group for suggestions. Both mothers and adolescents shared how they might describe wet dreams, and together the group decided on an appropriate explanation.

After the "Hot Topic" activity, mothers and adolescents separate into two groups. Mothers discuss what makes them special as parents as a way to demonstrate how parents can make a difference in educating adolescents about a very important aspect of their adolescents' lives—their sexual health. By role-playing situations, mothers practice discussing topics that they have identified as difficult or embarrassing to discuss with their adolescents. As a group, mothers help each other with real-life situations that they have identified as difficult. They explore ways in which they can encourage their adolescents to delay initiating sexual intercourse, and they discuss their feelings about encouraging their adolescents to postpone sex while providing them information on condoms and birth control.

Mothers in Louise's group used this time to check in with Louise about her reluctance to discuss puberty with her daughter, Lillian.

> Louise shared with them that she found it very difficult to initiate a conversation with Lillian about changes associated with puberty. However, because her daughter was eager to discuss these issues with her, Louise began to feel more comfortable with talks. Louise noted that the take-home activities provided topics from which to begin conversations. Louise also purchased a book on puberty for Lillian, and together they discussed some of the information that was presented in the book. Louise admitted that some topics were still difficult for her to discuss but that her anxiety about her daughter becoming pregnant had subsided.

In another group, the topic of conversation centered on Carol and her reluctance to talk with her son, Martin. In an earlier session, Carol revealed to the group that she did not think that it was her responsibility to talk to her son about sexual topics. Instead, she believed that the boy's father, who did not live with them, should assume this responsibility. Although Carol participated in the group sessions with the mothers, her participation was limited in the combined sessions with adolescents, and she did not complete the take-home activities with Martin. In the "Hot Topic " activity, it was no surprise to the group that

Carol had stood near the sign indicating that she would avoid discussing the topic of birth control with her son. Martin, on the other hand, expressed more willingness to discuss the topic "ways to prevent contraction of HIV" with his mother. In the discussion, mothers strongly encouraged Carol to talk openly with her son. They noted that because his father was not always accessible, Carol should be prepared to meet her son's needs for information and advice. As mothers themselves, they felt a deep responsibility to educate boys about assuming responsibility for their sexual health.

During their breakout group in Session 5, adolescents are given the opportunity to ask questions about HIV/AIDS that have not been answered in previous sessions. Each adolescent writes a question on an index card, which is then passed to the facilitator. The facilitator addresses each question either by providing a direct answer or by engaging adolescents in a discussion of the topic. For example, the facilitator might provide a direct answer to this question: "How old is a girl when she has her first period?" But she might ask participants to answer this question: "Can AIDS be cured?" or "Why can't mosquitoes give you AIDS?" For this latter question, the facilitator might first ask the participants how HIV is transmitted. She then might ask participants to think about which groups of people would be infected with HIV if the virus were transmitted by mosquitoes. Using information presented in Session 1, she could ask adolescents to compare these individuals with those who live in areas of high rates of HIV infection such as Atlanta. Finally, she might end with an explanation of why mosquitoes can transmit some diseases such as yellow fever and encephalitis but not HIV. This question would also give her the opportunity to point out the difference and the use of the terms *HIV* and *AIDS*.

In our experience conducting the program, we found that most of the adolescents processed about the same amount of knowledge about HIV and AIDS, STDs, and basic facts of puberty and sexual development. We quickly became aware of the fact that our participants lacked some basic information about sex despite having had sex education in school. Thus, Session 5 is often devoted to providing information about changes associated with puberty, contraception, differences between boys and girls, and HIV transmission. Some group members, however, displayed considerable knowledge about sex and reproductive health.

For example, Monica, a 13-year-old girl, was distinguished among her group for her breadth and depth of information. In Session 5, she asked questions about Pap smears and abortion, topics of which most of the other adolescents possessed little knowledge. The nature of these questions, as well as her contributions in the other sessions, made it apparent to the facilitator and the other participants that Monica was very well informed. As a result, participants often directed questions to her or listened attentively when she talked. The facilitator allowed Monica to answer the questions and monitored the answers for accuracy and clarified information as necessary.

In another group, a younger member, Josh, a 12-year-old boy, distinguished himself as a leader. He spoke with confidence on matters of sex and reproductive health, and his fellow group members listened whenever he spoke. Like Monica, he was well informed and provided accurate information. Both Josh and Monica proffered that they discussed the issues with their parents openly and felt comfortable doing so. These sessions seemed to indicate that a peer component would be good to include in the program.

Session 6: Putting It All Together

In Session 6, puppets are used to assist mothers and adolescents demonstrate the knowledge and skills they have learned in the program. The activity begins by creating realistic situations for the puppets from scripts written by adolescent participants as part of their Session 5 take-home activity. In a typical scene, a boy and his girlfriend have been to a school party and are returning to one of their homes. They find that the parents are not home and that alcohol is available. The boy is interested in drinking alcohol, whereas the girl is somewhat uncertain. Often the situation escalates, and the boy makes unwanted sexual advances. Mothers and adolescents use puppets to enact the scene, demonstrating strategies adolescents can use to cope with the situation. Because participants can play any role, a girl might assume the role of the boyfriend and use the male puppet to demonstrate how she would like a boy to act in the situation, and a mother might take the role of the girlfriend and show how a girl might act when she is under pressure to participate in risky situations. Participants also have reversed the roles of the boyfriend and girlfriend so that the girl is the aggressive suitor, and the boy is encouraging restraint. Participants are encouraged to use communication skills and resistance strategies learned during the previous sessions. As with the HIV skit presented in Session 1, the use of puppets removes the threatening aspect of the situation from the participants themselves to the action of the puppets.

Session 7: Consequences of Early Initiation of Sexual Intercourse (Adolescents) and Condom Information and Skill Building (Parents)

In the final session, after the warm-up activity, mothers and adolescents meet in separate groups for about an hour. In their group, mothers discuss condom use and practice putting condoms on penis models. The facilitator first reviews the facts about condoms and where to obtain them. She then passes a variety of condoms around the room so that mothers can feel the condoms and see the different varieties that are available. She also presents important facts about condoms such as the difference between latex and lambskin, the importance of checking expiration dates, and the use of lubricants. To increase their confidence in using condoms or showing their adolescents how to use condoms, mothers practice putting condoms on a model penis.

In their session, adolescents discuss the consequences of having sex. To begin this discussion, adolescents write one or two of their major life goals. They then explore ways in which an unexpected illness such as HIV might prevent them from reaching their goals. Adolescents then practice "positive self-talk" as a way to build their confidence. They are encouraged to use positive self-talk as a way to remind themselves of their goals when they are facing difficult situations. Following this exercise, the facilitator guides the participants through a process to developing a decision-making tree. The decision tree begins with the decision to have sex or not to have sex. Each decision then branches into other decision-making situations or consequences of those decisions. This exercise encourages adolescents to think about the long-term consequences in addition to the short-term consequences of their decisions. Adolescents are then given facts about condoms and discuss condom use as a form of HIV prevention.

Mothers and adolescents reconvene at the end of the session to discuss their experiences with Keepin' It R.E.A.L.! They reflect on what they have learned and discussed during the program. The discussion generally includes ways to help adolescents delay involvement in sexual intercourse, importance of parental monitoring and supervision, and importance of effective communication about sexual topics such as sexually transmitted diseases, including HIV, as well as pregnancy prevention. At the conclusion of this session, facilitators present participants with "diplomas" and a small gift.

TRAINING FACILITATORS

Facilitators whom we hired for the program each had a background in health education and experience in conducting HIV and pregnancy prevention programs. Two facilitators held master's degrees in public health, and two held baccalaureate degrees. We found that their previous experience in teaching about sexual health was important for this program because mothers quickly recognized that the facilitators were very knowledgeable about the subject matter and that they were comfortable presenting the information and guiding group discussions.

In addition to experience in health education, we found that the facilitators required additional training in the techniques used in the program. The program is developed to be highly interactive with general discussion, role-plays, skits, puppet shows, and other activities. Although some content is presented in a lecture format, lectures are used sparingly. As noted earlier, all four program facilitators had experience in conducting health education programs, but they had primarily used the lecture format in delivering health messages. Thus, training was required to learn how to conduct group sessions.

Our training consisted of approximately 40 hours of classroom training prior to the beginning of the program and 2-hour trainings held approximately every 2 weeks during most of the program. To facilitate training, a manual was developed for the program that contains the curriculum as well as all materials used in the programs. Throughout training, the manual served as the guide to ensure that all information is covered and that training is conducted in a systematic and consistent manner for all project staff. Throughout the project, facilitators are encouraged to refer to the manuals as necessary to address specific questions.

The training included background information about the program, the importance of fidelity to the curriculum, and elements of the program. It also included information on the nature of group discussions, how to facilitate a group, the phases of group development, and skill-building exercises. For the training on group discussion, we hired a clinical psychologist who used social cognitive theory in his practice. This instructor was ideal because he understood the theoretical aspects of our program, and he also had extensive experience in conducting group sessions. For the first several sessions, the instructor and facilitators worked on understanding the nature of groups and how to guide discussion in a group setting. After the program began, the training sessions were held every week for several months and then every 2 weeks for most of the program. In the final months of the program, the sessions were held once per month. During these training sessions, videotapes of program sessions were shown and used to critique the developing skills of the facilitators. Facilitators identified points in the discussion when they felt uncertain about what to do. These issues and other problems that arose in the groups were addressed. The training sessions were particularly helpful in learning how to deal with group conflict and understanding some of the underlying messages that participants believed important.

LESSONS LEARNED

Although we learned many things about conducting this type of program, we include here lessons most important to the implementation of the program in a community setting. One of our primary concerns about the program was the inclusion of both mothers and adolescents in the same sessions. During program development, we talked about offering separate sessions for mothers and adolescents because we thought adolescents might be uncomfortable talking about sexual issues in the presence of their mothers. However, because one of our objectives was to encourage adolescents and mothers to talk to each other about sex, we decided that it was essential to have at least some sessions in which mothers and adolescents learned together. Thus, the program consists of three combined sessions and three separate sessions, and the final session is divided equally between combined and separate sessions.

During program development, we struggled with creating the appropriate mix of joint and separate sessions. We elected to have three sessions together and three sessions separate and the final one with a mixed session. Our intention for the joint sessions was to give adolescents and mothers an opportunity to practice some of the skills in a controlled and safe environment. The reason for the separate sessions was to give adolescents and mothers the freedom to discuss issues with their peers. We found that this mix of sessions worked well. One unexpected result of having separate sessions was that they helped stimulate conversations between mothers and adolescents. After the conclusion of separate sessions, we often heard adolescents asking their mothers what they talked about in their sessions and mothers in turn asking their adolescents what they learned in their sessions.

During the separate sessions for adolescents, the facilitators noted that the adolescents were not as knowledgeable about sexual issues as we anticipated. During Session 5, the facilitators used more time than planned to discuss basic facts about puberty. Because we believed that the adolescents would have had this information in school, we elected not to include it in the program. At the time, we believed that if we included information on puberty, adolescents who might decide that the program was similar to sex education in school would elect not to attend. In retrospect, given the questions asked and the content of discussions in adolescent group sessions, it would have been helpful for the adolescents to have had the information in one of the first program sessions. Thus, as we revise the program, we will include basic information on puberty for the adolescents.

During the adolescent sessions, the facilitators also noted that an adolescent who was very knowledgeable about sexual issues was an asset to the group. The adolescent participants always seemed to be impressed with a fellow group member who seemed to know the material and who could answer the more difficult questions. The group members did not seem to be intimidated by this display of knowledge. Instead, having a well-informed group member seemed to spark the interest of other participants to learn as much as they could. Given this experience, as we revise the program, we will develop a role for a peer facilitator who can assist the primary facilitator in leading the adolescent groups.

Adolescents whose mothers consistently attended the program with them contributed more in later sessions of the program and seemed more confident in the presentation of information. We believe that mothers and adolescents who attended together were more likely to talk with each other after the sessions. Thus, these pairs of mothers and adolescents were becoming more comfortable sharing information, and the adolescents were becoming more confident in their knowledge. Although we encouraged mothers and adolescents to attend the program together, sometimes mothers were not able to, and occasionally an adolescent attended most of the sessions without his or her mother. When mothers were not present in the combined sessions, their adolescents generally contributed less to the discussions.

Summary

We found that both parents and adolescents were helped by the content of the sessions as well as by the use of separate peer sessions. However, the sessions with adolescents and mothers together were an essential way of opening lines of communication within families in a safe environment.

REFERENCES

Ary, D., Duncan, T., Duncan, S., & Hops, H. (1999). Adolescent problem behavior: The influence of parents and peers. *Behaviour Research & Therapy, 37*(3), 217-230.
Bandura, A. (1986). *Social foundations of thought and action: A social cognitive theory* (Vol. 617). Englewood Cliffs, NJ: Prentice Hall.
Bandura, A. (1992). A social cognitive approach to the exercise of control over AIDS infection. In R. J. DiClemente (Ed.), *Adolescents and AIDS* (pp. 89-116). Newbury Park, CA: Sage.
Bandura, A. (1997). *Self-efficacy: The exercise of control.* New York: Freeman.
Broering, J. M. (1991). Childhood sexual learning and sex education in schools. *NAACOG's Clinical Issues, 2*(2), 178-189.
Centers for Disease Control and Prevention (CDC). (1997). *HIV/AIDS surveillance report, 1997.* Atlanta, GA: Author.
Centers for Disease Control and Prevention (CDC). (1998). *Sexually transmitted disease surveillance, 1997.* Atlanta, GA: Author.
Centers for Disease Control and Prevention (CDC). (1999). *HIV/AIDS surveillance report.* Atlanta, GA: Author.
Driscoll, M. P. (1994). *Psychology of learning for instruction.* Needham Heights, MA: Allyn & Bacon.
Erikson, E. (1950). *Childhood and society.* New York: Norton.
Finan, S. L. (1997). Promoting healthy sexuality: Guidelines for infancy through preschool. *The Nurse Practitioner, 22*(10), 79-80, 83-84, 86-88, 97-98.
Gallagher, D. (1996). HIV education: A challenge to adult learning theory and practice. *Journal of the Association of Nurses in AIDS Care, 7*(Suppl. 1), 5-14.
Marcia, J. (1980). Ego identity development. In J. Adelson (Ed.), *The handbook of adolescent psychology* (pp. 159-187). New York: John Wiley.
Marshall, H. H. (1992). *Redefining student learning: Roots of educational change.* Norwood, NJ: Ablex.
Maslow, A. (1987). *Motivation and personality.* New York: Harper & Row.
U.S. Department of Health and Human Services. (1999). *Healthy People 2010 objectives: Draft for public comment* [Online]. Available: http://web.health.gov./healthypeople/2010Draft/pdf/intro/pdf.
Ventura, S. J., Curtin, S. C., & Matthews, T. J. (1998). *Teenage births in the United States: National and state trends, 1990-1996.* Hyattsville, MD: National Center for Health Statistics.

Chapter 7

Strengthening the Bond

The Mother-Son Health Promotion Project

Loretta Sweet Jemmott   Freida H. Outlaw
John B. Jemmott III   Emma J. Brown
Monique Howard   Brenda Howard Hopkins

University of Pennsylvania

Cora is a 46-year-old single African American mother of two sons, 24-year-old Lawrence and 15-year-old Kevin. She volunteered to participate in the Mother-Son Health Promotion Project because of her own risky sexual history and because she believes she did not adequately teach Lawrence, her oldest son, about his sexuality, including how to prevent risky sexual behaviors. She does not want to repeat this mistake with Kevin, her youngest son. She did not marry Lawrence's father because she did not want to get married "simply because she was pregnant." She did, however, move in with his father after Lawrence's birth. Shortly thereafter, she became pregnant again. Her second baby was born 2 months premature and died at birth.

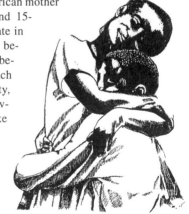

AUTHORS' NOTE: The work described in this chapter was supported by the National Institute of Mental Health (R01 MH55742). For more information about this intervention, please write to Dr. Loretta Sweet Jemmott, R.N., Ph.D., School of Nursing, University of Pennsylvania, Philadelphia, PA 19104; e-mail: jemmott@pobox.upenn.edu. This original drawing of a mother and son is reprinted with permission of the artist. It first appeared in *Fire on the Mountain* illustrated by E. B. Lewis.

Cora continues to blame Lawrence's father, a Vietnam veteran, who suffered from posttraumatic stress syndrome, for the death of the baby. According to her, he suffered from extreme anxiety, which often manifested itself in paranoid thinking or explosive anger. Consequently, she describes being constantly fearful and under stress because of his unpredictable, labile behavior. It was the persistent stress that she believes caused her to lose the baby. She separated from him shortly after the death of her second baby, and he has not been involved in their lives since the separation. Therefore, Lawrence does not know his father but, like his father, has anger control problems. Presently, Lawrence is in prison for a parole violation that occurred when he became angry with his wife at a restaurant, which triggered him to severely damage several cars parked outside by kicking in their doors and windshields.

Cora became pregnant with Kevin a few years after she moved back home with her mother. She did not marry his father either, although they have an amicable relationship. He is marginally involved with Kevin, an honor student who has professed high aspirations for his future. He has, however, recently been robbed and assaulted several times in his neighborhood. As a result, he has experienced health problems (seizures secondary to a head trauma) and depression. He was for a time afraid to go out of the house. Kevin denies being sexually active, but Cora confesses that she has been uncomfortable talking with him about sexual matters. Because her father is dead and she has only three sisters and her mother, she is concerned with the lack of a mature male presence in Kevin's life. As a result, she was eager to learn how to better communicate with her son about sexual matters, including how to encourage him to be sexually responsible by avoiding risky sexual behavior.

Cora is typical of the women who participated in the Mother-Son Health Promotion Project. She is unskilled or semiskilled, poor, and living in a housing development with one or more children, one of whom is an adolescent son. She became pregnant early in her life but never married. She has had a total of three pregnancies by two different men.

Many of the women who have participated in this project have had several pregnancies by several different men without the convention of marriage. Usually their intimate relationships are marked by episodic chaotic and dysfunctional patterns of relating, which can be directly linked to their life circumstances such as unemployment or underemployment, being on welfare, poor educational experiences, and frequent histories of alcohol and substance abuse. Many of the women have continued to be involved in destructive intimate relationships either with one or more partners or are having multiple sexual relationships over time.

The women in this project were most often personally vulnerable because of many factors, including their own risky sexual behavior, volatile intimate relationships, lack of support from their children's fathers, and lack of personal resources. However, some such as Cora are courageous and strong-willed women who would not marry "because they were pregnant." Typically, these women were primarily responsible for educating their adolescents about intimate relationships and sexual matters. Studies indicate that the family is the earliest socializing agent about sexual matters and that intentionally or unintentionally, parents are likely to have the most profound impact on their adolescents' sexual practices (Crawford, Thomas, & Zoller, 1993; Noller & Callan, 1990). Therefore, Tucker (1991) posits that direct communication is the primary means of socializing adolescents about crucial family values, beliefs, and behaviors, including sexual behavior. Furthermore, Milan and Kilmann (1987) postulated that it is not the overall quality of the adolescent-parent relationship that is related to adolescents' sexual behavior but rather the specific and frequent communication regarding sexual matters between the adolescents and their parent(s) that has a profound impact.

These findings intensify the need to strengthen the communication between mothers such as Cora and her adolescent son about risky sexual behaviors for many reasons, including the urgent need to prevent sexually transmitted HIV infection. The imperative to prevent sexually transmitted HIV infection becomes critical because the incidence of AIDS is increasing at an alarming rate among African Americans. Of particular concern to these authors is the risk of HIV infection among African American male adolescents who live with their mothers in single-parent households in low-income urban areas. Although their mothers can play a key role in reducing their sons' risk of HIV infection, effective strategies for such mothers are not well established. Moreover, as we found with mothers such as Cora, HIV sero-surveillance data indicate that the mothers themselves, because of their own sexual practices, are at heightened risk of contracting a sexually transmitted HIV infection.

DIMENSIONS OF THE PROBLEM

AIDS surveillance reports reflect the disproportionate toll that AIDS has levied on African Americans. African American women account for 55% of female AIDS cases, and White women account for only 23% of AIDS cases. In Philadelphia, where this prevention program was conducted, approximately 72% of the cumulative female AIDS cases have occurred among African American women. In addition, Philadelphia is the first urban city where the number of African Americans with AIDS in general, including the numbers of women and adolescents, increased in the past 5 years.

Evidence from several sources highlights the risk of HIV infection among adolescents, particularly low-income urban, African American adolescents. Because the risk of HIV infection among African American adolescents is strongly linked to personal behavior, it may be possible to curb their risk through the use of behavioral interventions. Therefore, this chapter will describe the Mother-Son Health Promotion Project, a theory-based, culturally sensitive behavioral prevention project designed to help unmarried African American mothers living in public housing, within urban communities, reduce their own risk of sexually transmitted HIV infection and that of their sons ages 11 to 15. This chapter covers aspects of the Mother-Son Health Promotion Project: (a) foundations of the mother-son approach, (b) the theoretical framework for the prevention program, (c) description of the Mother-Son Health Promotion Project, (d) benefits of the Mother-Son Health Promotion Project, (e) facilitator training, and (f) conclusions.

FOUNDATIONS OF THE MOTHER-SON APPROACH

Interventions with parents, particularly mothers, may be critically important to reduce HIV risk-associated sexual behavior of African American male adolescents. An emphasis on intervening with mothers becomes even more pressing when one considers the increasing numbers of divorces and out-of-wedlock births in the United States. Adolescents in single-parent households have increased risk of problems associated with sexual behavior, and it is typically the mother who provides direct care for these children. In several studies, both African American and White adolescents who lived with one parent were found to have had their first sexual experience at a younger age than did their peers who lived with both parents (Hogan & Kitagawa, 1985; Jemmott & Jemmott, 1992a, 1992b; Miller, Higginson, McCoy, & Olson, 1987). In addition, urban African American male adolescents who lived with only one parent reported less consistent condom use and were more likely to report fathering a child than were those who lived with both of their parents (Jemmott & Jemmott, 1992a, 1992b).

Mothers are potentially a great resource for communicating effectively with their adolescent sons regarding the risk of certain sexual practices. Studies examining adolescents' communication with their mothers and fathers have yielded two major findings that are particularly relevant for the Mother-Son Health Promotion Project. In general, studies have found that both sons and daughters talked more openly with their mothers than with their fathers about sexual matters because they perceived that their mothers understood and accepted their opinions and decisions more than their fathers (Crawford et al., 1993; Noller & Callan, 1990; Shoop & Davidson, 1994; Tucker, 1991; Yarber & Greer, 1986). One study found that male adolescents talked with mothers more frequently about condoms, whereas daughters talked more about menstruation and pregnancy (DiIorio, Hockenberry-Eaton, Maibach, Rivero, & Miller, 1996).

Adolescents whose mothers encouraged them to use birth control by discussing a specific method were more likely to use contraception than those adolescents who were not encouraged to use a specific birth control method by their mothers (Handelsman, Cabral, & Weisfeld, 1987). This finding suggests that parental communications about sexual practices, such as specific methods of contraception, influence the risky sexual behaviors of many adolescents. However, parents, regardless of family structure, may be reluctant to discuss sexual matters with their adolescents. This reluctance may stem from many factors, such as their discomfort talking about sexual topics, their lack of knowledge regarding the risk of different sexual behaviors, and their lack of communication skills necessary for the discussion of sexual matters with their adolescents. These factors may be intensified for single mothers who are usually responsible for discussing sexual matters with their adolescent sons.

As adolescents move toward autonomy, conflicts or rejection of parental authority might influence them to dismiss their parents as sources of creditable information. Yet surveys have indicated that parents are adolescents' most preferred source of sexual information (Sorensen, 1973), and although this research was done several decades ago, similar findings continue to emerge to support these findings. For example, recent research findings suggest that rejection of their parents by adolescents is often superficial and temporary, given that parents and adolescents usually share compatible values and beliefs (Newman, 1982; Paikoff & Brooks-Gunn, 1991. Furthermore, research also suggests that the influence of peers increases for all young people during adolescence, yet the family continues to be perceived as a stronger source of support by African American adolescents in contrast to their White peers (Clark, 1989; Handelsman et al., 1987). Other studies found that African American adolescents were more parent oriented (DiCindio, Floyd, Wilcox, & McSeveney, 1983) and perceived that they received greater social support from their families than White adolescents (Cauce, Felner, & Primavera, 1982). Hence, interventions to strengthen the communication skills and knowledge of African American parents about sexual matters may have special utility in reducing African American adolescents' risky sexual behavior.

Unfortunately, the types of parental communication skills and behaviors that may reduce adolescents' risky sexual behaviors that place them at risk for HIV infection have not been investigated. Nor have studies examined whether increasing parents' knowledge and skills at communicating with their children can reduce adolescents' HIV risk-associated sexual behavior.

A review of research and practice shows that interventions aimed at the risk of sexually transmitted HIV infection among adolescents have rarely been considered. For interventions aimed at reducing HIV risky behaviors among poor adolescent African American boys living in urban housing developments with single mothers, the prevention programs must include the teaching of sexual knowledge; both affective and cognitive components of communication, especially as it relates to sensitive topics; problem solving that includes moral and

ethical decision making; and finally, but integral to the process, directed interventions aimed at the mothers' own risky sexual behaviors.

THEORETICAL FRAMEWORK FOR THE MOTHER-SON HEALTH PROMOTION PROJECT

Efforts to develop HIV risk reduction interventions are likely to be most effective if they are based on solid theoretical foundations. Our work builds on social
cognitive theory (Bandura, 1986), the theory of reasoned action (Ajzen &
Fishbein, 1980; Fishbein & Ajzen, 1975), and its extension, the theory of
planned behavior (Ajzen, 1985, 1991). According to the theory of planned behavior, if someone has formed the intention to do something, it is more likely
that he or she will actually execute the behavior. For example, if an adolescent
has decided that he or she will use a condom at every intercourse occasion, it is
more likely that the person will carry a condom regularly and actually use it
properly. This behavioral intention is determined by both attitudes toward the
specific behavior (condom use), subjective norms regarding the behavior (my
mother expects me to do this), and perceived control over the behavior (I have
the skills to use a condom when needed). Thus, people intend to perform the behavior when they evaluate that behavior positively, when they believe significant others think they should perform it, and when they feel confident in their
ability to perform the behavior.

A valuable feature of the theory of planned behavior is that it directs attention
to why people hold certain attitudes, subjective norms, and perceived behavioral
control. Attitudes toward behavior are seen as reflecting behavioral beliefs or
beliefs about the consequences of performing the behavior. By targeting behavioral beliefs about sexual behavior, interventions may be able to change individuals' attitudes toward those behaviors. In the case of condom use, the most obvi-
ous beliefs are beliefs about condoms preventing pregnancy, sexually
transmitted diseases (STDs), and HIV infection (Jemmott, Jemmott, Spears,
Hewitt, & Cruz-Collins, 1992).

Another key consideration in the theory of planned behavior is what has been
termed *hedonistic beliefs* or beliefs about the consequences of condom use for
sexual enjoyment (Jemmott et al., 1992). Several studies have linked such beliefs to condom use or intentions to use condoms (Hingson, Strunin, Berlin, &
Heeren, 1990; Jemmott & Jemmott, 1992b; Valdiserri, Arena, Proctor, &
Bonati, 1989). A third belief that strongly influences behavior has been defined
by Jemmont and Jemmont (1992b) as partner reaction beliefs. That is, efforts to
use condoms may be influenced by whether people believe their partners would
react favorably to condom use.

Subjective norms are the collective beliefs a group has or someone thinks it
has. For example, these are the norms to which the youth looks for guidance

about whether a behavior is acceptable or unacceptable. Thus, apart from individuals' beliefs about other consequences of the behavior, they may be less likely to engage in a risky behavior if significant others (their norm group) disapprove of it. It is often argued that sexual partners are more important normative influences for women than for men and that they are especially important to ethnic minority women. Thus, the influence of sexual partners may be particularly relevant in determining condom use among single urban minority mothers. Mothers' attempts to influence their adolescent sons' behavior might be affected by their normative beliefs regarding their sons' approval.

Perceived behavioral control, like the perceived self-efficacy concept in social cognitive theory, reflects past experiences as well as anticipated impediments, resources, and opportunities (Bandura, 1986, 1989). If people believe that they have little control over performing a behavior because of a lack of requisite skills or resources, their intentions to perform the behavior may be low, even if they have favorable attitudes or supportive subjective norms regarding it (Ajzen & Madden, 1986). Obviously, condom use is not entirely under the individual's control because his or her partner's cooperation is required. Several types of control beliefs are relevant to perceived behavioral control regarding condom use because condoms are used in the context of strong emotions. Availability beliefs are concerned with the person's confidence that he or she can have condoms available when needed. Impulse control concerns individuals' confidence that they can control themselves enough to use condoms when sexually excited. Currently, individuals' confidence in their ability to persuade their sexual partners to use condoms is most often emphasized in HIV prevention programs. Technical skills are those skills that demonstrate the person's ability to use condoms with finesse without ruining the mood. By the same token, mothers' attempts to influence their sons are likely to be affected by their perceived self-efficacy, which includes their confidence in (a) their own technical skills regarding safer sex practices and (b) their ability to communicate with their adolescent sons regarding such matters. The critical factors in this theory have been used in this prevention program, which is discussed in the next section.

DESCRIPTION OF THE MOTHER-SON HEALTH PROMOTION PROJECT

The prevention program was comprised of four 4-hour sessions of sixteen 1-hour modules implemented on four Saturdays. The program also included two 3-hour booster sessions delivered 3 months and 6 months after the initial sessions. The program was implemented by African American facilitators from the public housing communities and contained culturally sensitive materials, including films, interactive activities, experiential exercises, role-play activities, and small group discussion. All of these activities were developed to build group cohesion, enhance individual learning, and enhance group discussion. The mothers lived in the same housing project just a few doors apart, yet the majority of them had never engaged in substantive conversation with one another.

The mothers in the HIV Risk Reduction Prevention Program participated in a prevention program that provided the knowledge, motivation, confidence, comfort, and skills necessary to reduce their sons' and their risk of contracting HIV and other STDs. Each of the four modules taught in the sessions imparted knowledge, assessed and changed attitudes, developed confidence and skills, and allowed participants to rehearse skills and complete and evaluate their and their colleagues' homework assignments. These activities were designed to heighten mothers' awareness of the developmental challenges and social stressors that their sons were experiencing; provide guidelines to foster positive mother-son communication; familiarize mothers with strategies to encourage their sons to make positive life choices, including positive sexual choices; and discuss ways in which they could become positive role models for their sons.

This program also was designed to help mothers examine their personal values related to sexuality, examine the extent to which the messages (both verbal and nonverbal) they conveyed to their sons were consistent with their values, and provide for them factual information about HIV/AIDS. These intervention activities were designed to enhance the mothers' skills in reducing their own personal risk of HIV infection as well as their sons'. In addition, behavioral homework assignments were used to strengthen mother-son bonds, improve their communication skills, and enhance their comfort with discussing sexual matters, which increased their willingness to talk with their sons about sexual matters, including HIV/AIDS (see Table 7.1 for an overview of the sessions for the Mother-Son Health Promotion Project).

Goals and Overview of Session 1: HIV Knowledge and Risk

The goals of Session 1 were to (a) inform the mothers about the program and build enthusiasm for the program, (b) help them become comfortable and productive in their small groups, (c) build their confidence about talking to their sons about HIV and risk reduction strategies, and (d) increase their knowledge of HIV/AIDS, HIV risk-related behaviors, and adolescent sexuality while increasing their ability to teach their sons basic HIV information.

Module 1 began with a general brainstorming discussion on issues regarding adolescent sexual behavior such as the following: Why do adolescents have sex? Why do adolescents not use condoms? What is the meaning of sex today? What kind of approval and messages have adolescents received about sex? What are their sons' attitudinal issues, gender issues, and concerns about sex?

Module 2 focused on building mothers' comfort talking to their sons about sex, including discussing barriers to talking with their sons about sex. This module included a brainstorming activity about the skills necessary for talking to

TABLE 7.1 Overview of the Four-Session Mother-Son Health Promotion Project

Session Number	Modules
Session 1: HIV Knowledge and Risk • Build enthusiasm for program • Build confidence as communicator • Increase knowledge of HIV	Module 1: Adolescent sexuality Module 2: Communications skills about sex Module 3: Increasing HIV knowledge Module 4: Teaching skills for HIV prevention

Session 2: Building Efficacy With Condoms
• Increase mothers' perceptions of sons'
  vulnerability to HIV
• Enhance positive attitude toward condoms
• Build self-efficacy about using condoms
• Build skills to teach sons about condoms
	Module 1: Review Session 1
	Module 2: Discuss risky HIV behaviors
	Module 3: Develop condom use skills
	Module 4: Role-playing teaching about
	  condoms

Session 3: Efficacy of Communication Skills
• Teaching sons that condoms are fun
• Teaching sons to abstain or use condoms
• Teaching mothers to negotiate condom use
  with their partners
	Module 1: Review Session 2
	Module 2: Increase self-efficacy and skills about
	  teaching sons
	Module 3: Focus on mothers' risk behaviors
	Module 4: Mothers' self-efficacy with negotiat-
	  ing with their partners

Session 4: Efficacy for Communicating
  With Sons
• Build self-efficacy in mothers
• Reinforce skills to talk to sons
	Module 1: Review Session 3
	Module 2: Role-playing about talking to sons
	Module 3: Tougher negotiation skills
	Module 4: Reinforce accurate information about
	  HIV/AIDS

Booster 1: Reinforce mothers' self-efficacy and skills in reducing sons' and their risk	Practicing and reinforcing communication skills about safer sex and condom use
Booster 2: Reinforce mothers' self-efficacy and skills in reducing sons' and their risk	Practicing and reinforcing communication skills about safer sex and condom use

their sons about sex, including a discussion of how to listen and a discussion about the use of teachable moments to maximize learning. A mini-lecture on human sexuality, adolescent sexuality, language used by adolescents, and basic male anatomy was also in the module. A discussion acknowledging the threat of HIV/AIDS to their lives as well as the impact of HIV/AIDS on their communities, the importance of making proud and responsible decisions, and working together to save themselves, their sons, their families, and their communities was facilitated.

At the end of this module, Tracy, a young mother with five children, including her 15-year-old son, shared that she had always thought that the boy's father would discuss sexual matters with him. In the meantime, she was concerned about his poor performance in school and his defiant behavior at home. She found that strategies that she learned in the project facilitated her being able to talk with him about sexual matters, which in turn enhanced their relationship. This newfound ability to discuss sexual matters opened the way for them to talk about other important things, such as how to improve his school performance. In addition, Tracy felt very empowered that she could talk with her son about subjects that previously she believed she was incapable of doing. Finally, Tracy has become committed to using the skills she learned to talk with her other children about sexual matters, as well as problems and concerns that they will face, such as avoiding all risky situations common to their community such as easy access to drugs, enticement to join gangs, and the expectation by teachers and peers that they will manifest poor school performance.

Module 3 focused on increasing AIDS knowledge among the women. It included information on HIV/AIDS, such as the etiology, detection, transmission, and prevention of HIV and other STDs. The risks of contracting HIV associated with injecting drugs are also discussed. Videos used in this module included *Let's Talk About AIDS,* a music video by African American rappers Salt & Pepa, and *Sex, Drugs and AIDS.* Both videos covered HIV transmission and prevention in an entertaining and educational manner. After the participants viewed the videos, a mini-lecture was provided on HIV and AIDS. The mothers participated in a brainstorming activity, "AIDS Myths & Facts," which is interactive (Jemmott, Jemmott, & McCaffree, 1995). Following this exercise, an educational brochure that reinforces learning about HIV and AIDS transmission and prevention was distributed.

Module 4 was designed to build on mothers' skills in teaching HIV prevention information to their sons. Role-playing with vignettes was the primary educational method used. At the end of the session, participants play "AIDS Basketball," reinforcing accurate information about HIV/AIDS. Mothers were assigned homework to engage their sons in a conversation about HIV/AIDS. The purpose of the homework was for mothers to find out what their sons already knew about HIV/AIDS and to teach their sons correct information using the specially designed brochure provided by the project.

Goals and Overview of Session 2: Building Efficacy With Condoms

The goals of the next session were to (a) reinforce HIV knowledge about transmission and HIV risk behaviors, (b) increase mothers' perceptions of their sons' vulnerability to HIV infection, (c) assist mothers to internalize positive attitudes and behavioral beliefs about condoms, (d) build self-efficacy and skills in the correct technique of using condoms, and (e) increase skills and comfort in teaching their sons about condoms.

Module 1 began with a review of information from the previous session. This module provided additional HIV information. It focused on mothers' salient behavioral and normative beliefs about their attempts to influence their sons' sexual behavior. Attempts are made to weaken behavioral beliefs and attitudes that prevented mothers from communicating with their sons about safer sex practices, including abstinence, and enhanced those behaviors, beliefs, and attitudes that promote communication.

Module 2 focused on discussing behaviors that place people at risk for HIV infection and the vulnerability of becoming infected by individuals who engage in unprotected sex. An entertaining video clip, *Robert Townsend STD,* depicted a couple deciding whether to have sex when they do not have a condom, highlighting the risks individuals place themselves in when they engage in unprotected intercourse. The activity, "High Risk, Low Risk, No Risk" (Brick, Charlton, Kunins, & Brown, 1989), examines and clarifies behaviors that may place women and adolescents at risk for HIV infection. The "Don't Pass It Along Activity" (Brick et al., 1989) highlights one's vulnerability to HIV/STDs infection. The video *Are You With Me?* depicts an African American mother's struggle to teach her child about the importance of using condoms while she is personally struggling with the issue of using condoms in her own sexual relationship.

Module 3 focused on building condom use skills in mothers. The mothers examined the expiration date of the condom, opened a condom package, manipulated the condom, discussed what makes condoms effective, and learned the steps and rules of correct condom use. Finally, they practiced putting a condom on a penis model. This module concluded with a discussion about where to get condoms, barriers to condom use, and barriers to their talking to their sons about condom use.

Module 4 consisted of the use of role-playing to help mothers teach their sons how to purchase and use condoms. The mothers received feedback and positive reinforcement from the facilitators during the role-play. At the end of this module, they received condom coupons for themselves and their sons, as well as their homework assignment.

Their homework assignment consisted of going to the store to redeem their coupons for condoms. While there, they gathered information that could help their sons purchase condoms. For example, they assessed where the condoms were located in the store and how much they cost. Additional homework included having mothers (a) engage their sons in conversations about condoms to find out what their sons knew, (b) assess whether their sons knew how to use condoms, (c) assess if their sons had ever used condoms, (d) teach their sons how to use condoms using a penis model, (e) have their sons apply a condom using the penis model, and (f) give their sons the condom coupons to redeem at a designated pharmacy. The mothers were asked to check if their sons redeemed their condom coupons. After the sons redeemed the coupons, the mothers were asked to discuss with their sons how it felt to purchase the condoms.

Although the project operates on the premise of normalcy with regard to mothers and sons in terms of boundaries where sexual matters are concerned, the staff were alerted to assess the feedback given by the mothers at all times for verbal or behavioral cues that might have indicated inappropriate sexual behavior by the mothers toward their sons. Ongoing monitoring by the staff about potentially nonverbal and verbal dysfunctional sexual behavior between mothers and their sons was done in a very conscious manner, using the advanced practice psychiatric nurse as a resource to the staff.

Goals and Overview of Session 3: Efficacy of Communication Skills

The goals of Session 3 were to teach the mothers knowledge and skills that increased their confidence in three areas: (a) teaching their sons how to make condoms fun and pleasurable, (b) teaching their sons how to negotiate abstinence or condom use with their sexual partners, and (c) how they (mothers) can learn how to negotiate condom use with their own sexual partners.

Module 1 began with a review of information from the previous session. The mothers also demonstrated again steps on how to use condoms correctly and how to make using them fun. This module increased the mothers' comfort and skills when talking to their sons about using condoms and assisted them in addressing their sons' concerns about negative effects of condoms on sexual enjoyment and spontaneity. An exercise on "excuses" is used in which mothers examined statements that express common negative attitudes and beliefs their sons might have about using condoms.

Module 2 was designed to increase the mothers' self-efficacy and skills in communicating with their sons regarding how to make condom use fun and pleasurable. "Talking About Safer Sex With Your Son Activity" is used to help the mothers practice talking to their sons. This is accomplished by dividing mothers into pairs for a series of role-plays, using vignettes. One vignette involves the mother role-playing herself talking to her son about the importance of using condoms, including how to make condom use fun and pleasurable. Another vignette involved the mothers role-playing a situation involving two adolescents on a date trying to make a decision regarding whether to have sex without a condom and negotiating abstinence or condom use with their sexual partner. One of the adolescents in the vignette is to be the mother's son. All information and activities are presented in a way that helps mothers to be motivated to talk to their sons and their sexual partners. The module concludes with a discussion about each vignette. Again, peer group response was useful to indicate to the mothers when they were exhibiting indicators that signaled that they were crossing sexual boundaries with their sons behaviorally, either verbally or nonverbally. Staff were alerted to have heightened awareness of such group interactions. These types of observations would then be processed at the end of the module with the master facilitator and the facilitator, and the advanced practice psychiatric nurse would also be used as a resource.

Module 3 focused on mothers' personal issues and concerns about HIV/AIDS. Mothers participated in a brainstorming activity on barriers to discussing condom use with their sexual partners and ways to overcome those barriers. A video *AIDS Is About Secrets,* which depicts African American women talking about AIDS and other STDs, their attitudes and beliefs about sex and condoms, gaining respect from their partners, and responsibility for using condoms, is showed. This video is followed by a discussion aimed at working through their attitudes and beliefs about safer sex and building self-efficacy and skills to enhance their abilities to handle risky situations.

Module 4 focused on increasing the mothers' self-efficacy and skills in negotiating with their sexual partners about using condoms. To practice how to negotiate condom use with their sexual partners, the mothers participated in a series of role-plays, using vignettes. Group members discussed each role-play. Finally, the homework assignment was to engage their sons in conversations about making condom use fun and to conduct a role-play situation in which the son negotiates condom use or abstinence with a sexual partner. Finally, the mothers had to engage their sexual partners in a conversation about HIV/AIDS and safer sex, including the use of condoms.

Goals and Overview of Session 4:
Reinforcing Skills to Talk With Sons

The goals of Session 4 were to (a) build self-efficacy in the mothers and (b) reinforce skills they needed to talk to their sons and to their sexual partners about HIV risk reduction strategies. The session begins with a review of information from the previous session. In the four modules, the mothers participated in extensive role-play regarding talking to their sons and their sexual partners. They received extensive rehearsal, reinforcement, and feedback. They were taught tougher negotiation skills, and they reviewed all information they had learned during the four sessions. At the end of Module 4, mothers played "AIDS Jeopardy," which reinforced accurate information about HIV/AIDS (Jemmott et al., 1995), and were given homework assignments. As a part of the homework assignment, they reviewed with their sons and their sexual partners all the information learned in the previous sessions. In addition, they engaged their sons in safer sex discussions using role-plays. They also continued to negotiate condom use with their sexual partners. Closure activities encouraged them to plan to participate in the 3-month booster session.

Goals and Overview of Booster Sessions:
Relating Theory to Intervention

The goals of the 3- and 6-month booster sessions were to build and reinforce mothers' self-efficacy and skills in reducing their sons' and their risk of HIV infection. The mothers were given an opportunity in the 3-month booster modules to practice and reinforce skills needed to help them and their sons engage in safer sexual behaviors. They spent a great deal of time practicing communication skills, using extensively and progressively more difficult role-play situations. They received reinforcement and feedback as well as rehearsal time related to this task. In addition, they reviewed information about HIV/AIDS. Their homework assignment included mothers reviewing with their sons and their sexual partners all of the information learned in the session. They were asked to engage their sons in safer sex discussions and role-plays. Finally, they were advised to continue to negotiate condom use with the sexual partners.

In the 6-month booster, the day began with a review of information from the previous session. The mothers had an opportunity to practice and reinforce skills needed to help their sons and themselves engage in safer sex behaviors. They spent time practicing communication skills, using extensively and progressively more difficult role-play situations focused on talking with their sons and their sexual partners. They received reinforcement and feedback, as well as rehearsal time to practice their new skills.

BENEFITS OF THE MOTHER-SON
HEALTH PROMOTION PROJECT

After the initial session, participants were beginning to exhibit group cohesion, as reflected in their beliefs that they were safe to disclose sensitive information about their lives.

Tracy, a mother of six children by four different men, was able to share with the group that she had been sexually abused as a child and that presently she was in an abusive relationship at home. Josie talked about her extensive and painful psychiatric history that included repeated episodes of major depression, posttraumatic stress disorder, and substance abuse. Over and over again, women shared that "just to get to know their sisters" was a very important secondary benefit from participating in the project. They also decided to keep in touch after the intervention ended to support each other and to reinforce with each other what they had learned in the project.

The role-play scenarios were designed to provide mothers with a wide variety of ways to use the skills for themselves as well as for teaching their sons. Each activity was brief and interactive and required that the mothers actively participate. Active participation by the mothers served to maintain their interest and attention, which may fade if the sessions are limited to lecturing and lengthy group discussions. Many of these women had never talked to their sons about sexual matters. Supportive guidance and interactive practice were needed to improve mother-son communication skills.

Compelling, educational, and culturally relevant videos depicting adolescents in various situations were viewed by mothers. The intent of the videos was to evoke feelings and thoughts in the women about risky behaviors relative to HIV/AIDS. Sessions 2 to 4 and the two booster sessions began with a review of information from the previous session. These included discussions about the previous session's homework assignment that explored (a) what happened, (b) what did not happen, (c) which part of the assignment was difficult, and (d) whether the difficulties were overcome. The sessions were structured so that there was an opportunity to address the mothers' beliefs and the ways in which their beliefs may have affected their communication with their sons. At the end of the 6-month booster session, participants were given a certificate of commitment and achievement.

Three areas contained in the curriculum have been successfully internalized by the mothers. They were (a) an emphasis on sense of community, (b) an emphasis on responsibility and accountability, and (c) an emphasis on pride in making safer choices. For example, to instill a sense of community, mothers from a specific housing development are taught together. This strategy enhances the connections they form to one another, helps them develop among themselves a sense of community, and allows them to openly share common experiences and learn to assist each other in problem solving about their intimate relationships as well as their parenting concerns. In addition, women began to develop that cultural tenet that was so prevalent in earlier African American communities where all adults claimed some responsibility for all children. Small glimpses of developing community responsibility among the mothers were evident during the Saturday sessions when the sons were present for the intervention.

One Saturday, a group of sons was observed by several mothers (none of whom were their mothers) gambling outside the building where they (all the mothers) were involved in the intervention. These mothers curtailed the activity until the particular boys' mothers could intervene in the situation. Prior to being a participant in the project, the mothers who initially intervened in the boys' gambling shared that they would not have been comfortable doing so because they would not have been able to predict how the boys' mothers would have responded to their interfering in the boys' negative activity.

The staff used such spontaneous occasions as teachable moments. That is, they praised the mothers for demonstrating supportive behaviors indicative of community spirit (intervening in the boys' negative behavior) as well as commending the boys' mothers for being receptive. In addition, the staff were able to assist mothers' discourse on larger parenting issues that focused on helping many mothers use each other to determine that gambling was not appropriate behavior for adolescent boys. At the beginning of the discussion, all mothers were not convinced that gambling was an inappropriate behavior for their adolescent sons, especially if they were winning.

The knowledge, role modeling, and support they received from the project staff and each other assisted women to internalize their responsibilities for their own sexual behavior as well as to be accountable for teaching their sons to be sexually responsible by not engaging in risky sexual behavior. The staff were committed to assisting each woman build her self-worth by providing opportunities to experience positive feedback from the group and having successful interactions with sons about important sexual matters. This ability to skillfully guide the group to embrace each other was modeled by the staff in every intervention encounter.

Joyce, who had never discussed much of substance with her 15-year-old son, ecstatically shared with the group that her son was very pleased and complimentary of her after they completed a homework assignment. She believed that she had demonstrated to her son competence about how to correctly use condoms, which enhanced her self-esteem as a mother and a teacher of pertinent, life-saving information to her son.

On an equally important level, the mothers, some of them for the first time, were overtly and covertly giving their sons messages about how to be responsible in an intimate relationship. This was an important outcome because many of the mothers admitted that they had never had a relationship in which they believed their male partner had demonstrated responsible behavior. They were therefore learning new ways of experiencing intimate relationships for themselves and to teach their sons.

Outcomes of participation in the intervention included the following: development of practical skills aimed at reducing risky sexual behavior by their adolescent sons and themselves, usage of correct language when providing sexual information to their sons, and, through their involvement with one another, learning the power and social support that can be amassed by a collective of women.

FACILITATOR TRAINING

According to the literature, single African American women living in housing developments have a plethora of stressors and unmet needs (i.e., health, financial, and employment), making it imperative to offer, among other things, job training skills that in this case were provided by one of our partners—the Urban League. Leadership training, provided by an African American female leadership consultant, and mental health assessments and referral services were provided by an African American certified advanced practice psychiatric nurse. To lessen the burden of participating in the study, a small financial incentive, child care services, and transportation tokens were given to the facilitators and mothers.

Four women residents from each housing development were identified as potential facilitators by the tenants council presidents and site managers. Two were elected after being interviewed by the project staff. The facilitators had to have a high school diploma or GED, interpersonal skills, oral communication skills, and leadership ability. They attended a two-phase facilitator training program for 11 days. Phase 1, the 4-day leadership session, included job readiness training provided by the Urban League as well as training on leadership, presentation style, communication skills, and self-esteem. The purpose of this session was to enhance their facilitation skills and increase their confidence. Phase 2 consisted of a 7-day curriculum training session. This training began with a general 2-hour meeting designed to familiarize the facilitators with the goals, purpose, and design of the study. The facilitators learned the specifics of the Mother-Son Health Promotion Project—either the HIV Risk Reduction Intervention or the General Health Promotion Intervention. The facilitators participated in all the activities that they later taught the mothers, including viewing the videotapes and completing questionnaires. They were encouraged to identify any problems with structure or content of the training and to suggest possible solutions. The facilitators and the master facilitator trainer worked together to develop common solutions to any problems that arose. Each facilitator practiced implementing the intervention within his or her group and received feedback from the group.

CONCLUSION

It is always more cost-effective to prevent a catastrophic illness than to treat it or to finance the outcomes of the devastation of the illness. In this regard, the Mother-Son Health Promotion Project is a cost-effective program that is designed to create strategies to prevent HIV infection in high-risk urban populations. It is therefore a cost containment prevention program. In the case of HIV/ AIDS, devastating outcomes of the disease include loss of wages resulting from the infected person's inability to work, as well as increased demands on health care and social services systems for persons with AIDS and their dependents as well as loss of quality of life.

Interventions such as the Mother-Son Health Promotion Project that empower families living in poor, underserved, high-risk communities benefit the community by including community members in the initial design of the prevention program, providing opportunities for community members to be trained as the experts providing the intervention to community members, and leaving resource materials such as the curriculum, videos, and posters at each housing development for future training and program endeavors. Such community partnerships are essential for the community to perceive ownership of the intervention. The creation of community partnership such as the Mother-Son Health Promotion Project is one effective paradigm that future developers of HIV interventions need to emulate.

REFERENCES

Ajzen, I. (1985). From intentions to actions: A theory of planned behavior. In J. Kuhl & J. Beckmann (Eds.), *Action-control: From cognition to behavior* (pp. 11-39). Heidelberg, Germany: Springer.

Ajzen, I. (1991). The theory of planned behavior. *Organizational Behavior and Human Decision Processes, 50,* 179-211.

Ajzen, I., & Fishbein, M. (1980). *Understanding attitudes and predicting social behavior.* Englewood Cliffs, NJ: Prentice Hall.

Ajzen, I., & Madden, T. (1986). Prediction of goal-directed behavior: Attitudes, intentions, and perceived behavioral control. *Journal of Experimental Social Psychology, 22,* 453-474.

Bandura, A. (1986). *Social foundations of thought and action: A social cognitive theory.* Englewood Cliffs, NJ: Prentice Hall.

Bandura, A. (1989). Perceived self-efficacy. In V. M. Mays, G. W. Albee, & S. F. Schneider (Eds.), *Primary prevention of AIDS: Psychological approaches* (pp. 128-141). Newbury Park, CA: Sage.

Brick, P., Charlton, C., Kunins, H., & Brown, S. (1989). *Teaching safer sex.* Hackensack, NJ: Center for Family Life Education–Planned Parenthood of Bergen County.

Cauce, A., Felner, R., & Primavera, J. (1982). Social support in high risk adolescents: Structural components and adaptive impact. *Journal of Community Psychology, 10,* 417-428.

Clark, M. L. (1989). Friendship and peer relations in Black adolescents. In R. L. Jones (Ed.), *Black adolescents* (pp. 175-204). Berkeley, CA: Cobb & Henry.

Crawford, I., Thomas, S., & Zoller, D. (1993). Communications and level of AIDS knowledge among homeless African-American mothers and their children. *Journal of Health & Social Policy, 4,* 37-53.

DiCindio, L., Floyd, H., Wilcox, J., & McSeveney, D. (1983). Race effects in a model of parent-peer orientation. *Adolescence, 18,* 369-379.

DiIorio, C., Hockenberry-Eaton, M., Maibach, E., Rivero, T., & Miller, K. (1996). The content of African American mothers' discussions with their adolescents about sex. *Journal of Family Nursing, 2*(4), 356-382.

Fishbein, M., & Ajzen, I. (1975). *Belief, attitude, intention and behavior.* Boston: Addison-Wesley.

Handelsman, C. D., Cabral, R. J., & Weisfeld, G. E. (1987). Sources of information and adolescent sexual knowledge and behavior. *Journal of Adolescent Research, 2,* 455-463.

Hingson, R. W., Strunin, L., Berlin, B., & Heeren, T. (1990). Beliefs about AIDS, use of alcohol and drugs, and unprotected sex among Massachusetts adolescents. *American Journal of Public Health, 80,* 295-299.

Hogan, D. P., & Kitagawa, E. M. (1985). The impact of social status, family structure, and neighborhood on the fertility of Black adolescents. *American Journal of Sociology, 90,* 825-855.

Jemmott, J. B., III, Jemmott, L. S., & McCaffree, K. (1995). *Be proud! Be responsible! Strategies to empower youth to reduce their risk for AIDS.* New York: Select Media.

Jemmott, J. B., III, Jemmott, L. S., Spears, H., Hewitt, N., & Cruz-Collins, M. (1992). Self-efficacy, hedonistic expectancies, and condom-use intentions among inner-city Black adolescent women: A social cognitive approach to AIDS risk behavior. *Journal of Adolescent Health, 13,* 512-519.

Jemmott, L. S., & Jemmott, J. B., III. (1992a). Family structure, parental strictness, religiosity and sexual behavior among Black male adolescents. *Journal of Adolescent Research, 7,* 192-207.

Jemmott, L. S., & Jemmott, J. B., III. (1992b). Increasing condom-use intentions among sexually active inner-city Black adolescent women: Effects of an AIDS prevention program. *Nursing Research, 41,* 273-279.

Milan, R. J., & Kilmann, P. R. (1987). Interpersonal factors in premarital contraception. *Journal of Sex Research, 23,* 289-321.

Miller, B., Higginson, R., McCoy, J. K., & Olson, T. (1987). Family configuration and adolescent sexual attitudes and behavior. *Journal of Marriage and the Family, 48,* 503-512.

Newman, P. R. (1982). The peer group. In B. Wolman (Ed.), *Handbook of developmental psychology* (pp. 526-536). Englewood Cliffs, NJ: Prentice Hall.

Noller, P., & Callan, V. J. (1990). Adolescents' perceptions of the nature of their communication with parents. *Journal of Youth and Adolescence, 19,* 349-362.

Paikoff, R. L., & Brooks-Gunn, J. (1991). Do parent-child relationships change during puberty? *Psychological Bulletin, 110,* 47-66.

Shoop, D. M., & Davidson, P. M. (1994). AIDS and adolescents: The relation of parent and partner communication to adolescent condom use. *Journal of Adolescence, 17,* 137-148.

Sorensen, R. L. (1973). *Adolescent sexuality in contemporary America.* New York: World Publishing.

Tucker, S. K. (1991). The sexual and contraceptive socialization of Black adolescent males (Black adolescent sexuality). *Public Health Nursing, 8*(2), 105-112.

Valdiserri, R. O., Arena, V. C., Proctor, D., & Bonati, F. A. (1989). The relationship between women's attitudes about condoms and their use: Implications for condom promotion programs. *American Journal of Public Health, 79,* 499-503.

Yarber, W. L., & Greer, J. M. (1986). The relationship between the sexual attitudes of parents and their college daughters' or sons' sexual attitudes or behaviors. *Journal of School Health, 56*(2), 68-72.

PART III

Adapting—Preventing Consequences of HIV Infection and AIDS

Chapter 8

Who Will Care for Me?

Planning the Future Care and Custody of Children Orphaned by HIV/AIDS

Laurie J. Bauman

Albert Einstein College of Medicine

Carol Levine

The Orphan Project

Barbara Draimin

Jan Hudis

The Family Center

Juanita is 40 years old, has lived with HIV for 10 years, and was diagnosed with AIDS a year ago. She left her husband, Carlos, who was abusive to her and her child. He resides now in Puerto Rico, and she has no contact with him. She lives with her 11-year-old son Albert and her boyfriend of 7 years, Miguel. Juanita is extremely isolated. Her family of origin consists of her mother (her father is alive but not involved) and four sisters, all of whom live nearby. Three sisters are married and have young children; the fourth is unmarried and has HIV. When Juanita disclosed her HIV status to her family, they "shunned" her and rejected all contact.

AUTHORS' NOTE: This chapter was completed with the support of the National Institute of Mental Health Grant 1 R01 MH55794 to the first author. For more information about this intervention, please contact Dr. Laurie Bauman, Albert Einstein College of Medicine, 1300 Morris Park Avenue, 7521, Bronx, NY 10461. Project Care is funded by the Ryan White CARE Act, Titles I and IV, and operates under the direction of The Family Center, a nonprofit community-based agency that specializes in permanency planning services throughout New York City. An evaluation study, using a randomized trial design, is funded by the National Institute of Mental Health Office on AIDS through a grant to the Albert Einstein College of Medicine. The study will evaluate the short-term and long-term effects of the intervention. Policy implications and ethical guidance are provided through The Orphan Project.

She has little social support and relies on Miguel for emotional as
well as economic support. She
has no custody plan for Albert
and has no idea what custody
options are available to her.
She is also unsure about
whom to choose as a care-
giver for Albert but is seriously considering Miguel,
who is extremely supportive
and knows her diagnosis.
Juanita is clinically depressed.
Her depression is severe and inter-
feres with her day-to-day activities.

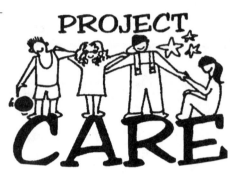

Juanita's sister had deliberately told Albert about his mother's HIV status
against her wishes. Ever since, he has been very upset. Juanita recognized his distress and took him to see a therapist, who has diagnosed him with depression. Albert has very few people with whom to share his concerns about his mother's illness. No one in his school knows Juanita's diagnosis, none of his friends know, his
godparents do not know, and he is not in contact with his aunts and grandmother.
Miguel cares for Albert very much but works long hours and is often too tired
and distracted by his own concerns about Juanita to be able to meet Albert's support needs.

◇ ◇ ◇

STATEMENT OF PROBLEM

AIDS is a family disease. Parents with AIDS face profound parenting challenges, and their children must live with a parent's chronic illness and possibly
the death of their parent. Disclosure is perhaps the most complex and painful decision parents must make—Should I try to keep the cause of my illness a secret?
Do I tell my child I may die? If I disclose my HIV to my child, will he be sad and
worried? Will he tell others about my diagnosis? How do I answer him when he
asks, "Who will care for me?"

The death of a parent in childhood increases psychological vulnerability, particularly in combination with additional risk factors. Although AIDS orphans
are an appropriate group for preventive efforts, few systematic attempts have
been made to intervene. This chapter describes Project Care, a preventive intervention designed to improve the psychological functioning of children who
survive the death of a parent from AIDS. It will accomplish this through four
specific efforts: (a) facilitating disclosure decisions and heightening communication between the ill parent and child, ill parent and future caregiver, and care-

giver and child; (b) enhancing the stability and security of the child's future through developing an appropriate and feasible custody plan prior to parent death; (c) working with the caregiver and child after parental death to ease the transition to the new family; and (d) providing access to concrete resources and social support. It is expected that appropriate disclosure to child and caregiver combined with a viable custody plan will reduce the occurrence of subsequent risk factors that have been shown to put children at risk for mental health problems. In addition, Project Care should increase the availability of protective factors, such as social support and a strong caregiver-child relationship.

Parental Death Is a Risk Factor

Several studies have examined the effects of parental death on psychological disturbance in children (see review in Osterweis, Solomon, & Green, 1984). Rutter (1966) found twice the rate of disorder among children who had experienced parental death compared to matched controls (Felner, Ginter, Boike, & Cowen, 1981; Felner, Stolberg, & Cowen, 1975). Felner et al. (1981) reported that children who had experienced parental death were more likely than children of divorced parents or a noncrisis comparison group to have symptoms of depression, anxiety, and withdrawal (Van Eerdewegh, Bieri, Parilla, & Clayton, 1982). Van Eerdewegh et al. (1982) found that 1 month after parental death, children were more likely than a comparison group to be depressed and to experience a decline in school performance; at 13 months, depressed mood was reduced, but disinterest in school, abdominal pain, and fighting were higher. Sandler, Gersten, Reynolds, Fallgren, and Ramirez (1988) report a moderate relationship between parental death and psychological symptoms, with 72% of bereaved children scoring higher than the median symptom score of a matched control group.

Most research on the effects of parental death has limited relevance to AIDS orphans for several reasons. Available data have been collected from samples of children who are living with a surviving parent. However, most mothers with HIV/AIDS are single, and little is known about how the loss of one's only custodial parent is related to psychological disturbance. Also, most research on grief in children has been conducted on Euro-American children, but almost 90% of women with HIV/AIDS are Black or Latina. Although there is a growing literature on bereavement and AIDS, it has focused almost exclusively on gay White men. Recently, attention on survivors has included children, but the literature on the impact of parental death from AIDS on children is sparse (Siegel & Gorey, 1994).

The parent's terminal illness itself is a chronic stressor that may create psychological risk (Garmezy & Rutter, 1988; Rutter, 1979, 1987). Rutter (1979, 1987) and Garmezy and Rutter (1988) found that repeated stressors (e.g., multiple hospital admissions of an ill parent) were more likely to be related to psychological disturbance in children in the context of chronic psychosocial adversity. The effects were not cumulative but exponential: Children were four times more likely to demonstrate psychiatric disorder when exposed to two stressors and 10 times more likely when exposed to more than five. Because children of parents with AIDS may have many potent risk factors for psychological disturbance *before* parental death, they may be especially vulnerable to psychological disorder after the death.

Other Risk Factors Prior to Parental Death

The literature on childhood parental loss has focused mainly on postdeath risk factors and has neglected predeath factors. The population we have targeted for intervention, children of single parents with late-stage AIDS, is disproportionately found in communities already burdened by violence, poverty, homelessness, illness, inadequate medical care, and a host of other interrelated social problems. Many of these chronic stressors have been found to affect children's mental health (Achenbach, Howell, Quay, & Conners, 1991; Florenzano, 1991; Garbarino, 1991; Jaenicke et al., 1987; Masten, Best, & Garmezy, 1990; Quinton, 1989; Rae-Grant, Thomas, Offord, & Boyle, 1989; Rutter, 1979; Wallerstein & Kelly, 1980). The multiple stressors in these children's lives are likely to have an additional but so far unstudied impact on postdeath adjustment, as Teesha's story illustrates.

Teesha's mother died from AIDS 2 years ago when Teesha was 13 years old. Teesha's mother was quite ill for some time; 2 years before her death, they moved in with Tina, Teesha's grandmother. Also in the household were Teesha's aunt and her two teenage cousins.

Her mother's last year of life was marked by physical debilitation and severe depression; during this time, Teesha attended school sporadically, and when she did attend, she was frequently in trouble. She often lied to Tina about her school attendance and began "hanging out" with a group of older teens. Teesha became sexually active shortly after her 14th birthday and started staying out until late at night, several times not coming home for days at a time. During this time, she was a part-time member of three different households. She slept and sometimes ate at a friend's house or at her grandfather's home, appearing at her grandmother's house only when she needed money or was hungry.

Despite the need to avoid upheavals after parental death, most single parents with AIDS often do not have a custody plan in place for their children at the time of parental death (LSC & Associates, 1993). Parents often assume that there are personal and cultural understandings in the family about who will care for orphaned children ("I'm sure my mother will take my children"); many simply believe that they are not sick enough and do not need to plan yet. Most have no idea how complex it is to obtain legal guardianship through the courts, and most believe that "papers" are not really needed. Finally, many mothers fear that making a plan will hasten their death—that the act of planning will bring about the death itself.

When a parent dies without a written plan, youngsters may be separated from their siblings, stigmatized by their association with HIV infection, and placed in several temporary homes before a custody arrangement is made. Because children feel helpless in the face of a parent's death, extensive changes in their environment are likely to have an adverse impact on their adjustment (Bowlby, 1980; Nagera, 1970; Rutter, 1983).

The Family Center became involved with this case after Teesha's mother died. There had been no formal custody plan put in place before the death, and it was assumed by the family that her grandmother would continue to care for Teesha, despite her problematic behavior. Family Center workers made formal plans for Teesha's two younger siblings, one of whom went to live with a cousin, the other with her father. Five months after the death, Tina obtained legal guardianship of Teesha even though she had little control over her behavior.

Risk Factors After Parental Death

Rutter (1966) suggests that for most children, psychological problems after parental death are not short-term grief reactions because many children exhibit their first serious symptoms years after the loss. Results from Elizur and Kaffman (1982) are consistent with Rutter's finding: 42 months after parental death, depression had declined, but general behavior problems had not (Kaffman & Elizur, 1983). Kaffman and Elizur (1983) found that 52% of children had severe psychological disturbance 18 months after the death of a father. Rutter argued that upheavals in the child's life after parental death created a "causal chain" from parental death to long-term disorder. These include psychological disturbance in the surviving parent, displacement from the home, and problematic family relationships. Teesha's experience is just one example of this fact.

Following her mother's death, Teesha's situation worsened. Teesha detached herself even more from her grandmother's household, and it became increasingly difficult for any one adult to monitor her whereabouts and well-being. She stopped going to school altogether and had only sporadic contact with the Family

Center social worker. Her behavior worsened, becoming increasingly confrontational with adults and peers alike. Nine months after her mother's death, she was involved in a razor slashing serious enough to require emergency room treatment and police intervention. Her grandmother, unable to control her behavior, in desperation filed a petition with juvenile court documenting her inability to supervise Teesha and requesting assistance.

Teesha continued to miss scheduled appointments with her social worker but called occasionally to report on how she was feeling and what she needed. During these conversations, she reported being sad about her mother's death and being angry that no one in the family except her grandmother seemed to care enough to ask her how she was doing. She reported that her grandmother no longer provided her with any money and that she was often hungry. She was also having trouble with sleeping arrangements. Following the razor fight, her grandfather did not want her in his house anymore. She usually slept at her friend's house, but it was uncomfortable. Her friend's father treated her like the maid, there was never enough food for her, and she rarely got a good night's sleep on the old couch in the living room.

One week short of the first-year anniversary of her mother's death, Teesha's grandfather died. Despite his increasing exasperation with her behavior, he had been an important source of support for her and had provided her with a place to sleep and with food from time to time. His death further weakened her already fragile support system, forcing her to rely more and more on friends for food and shelter. At this time, she told the social worker that her grandmother "was always in her face" and refused to meet with her when a joint session was suggested. Teesha reported that what she wanted more than anything else was to be independent and live on her own.

Following her grandfather's death, Teesha made more of an effort to stay in touch with her social worker and began to attend individual sessions more regularly. During these meetings, she continued to voice her desire to live independently but recognized this was unrealistic because she did not have any way to support herself. Her social worker encouraged her to take steps toward increasing independence, including getting her GED and investigating job opportunities. Teesha and the social worker frequently spoke about the magnitude of the losses she had experienced and the fact that those losses were forcing her to grow up and take responsibility for herself earlier than most people her age.

Over the past 6 months, Teesha has continued to make progress toward her goal of independence. She has begun to speak about her wish to have her younger brother live with her because he is not doing well with his cousin. Her desire to be a good role model for her brother and her realization that she wanted to become more self-sufficient motivated her to obtain services at a youth-focused community-based agency where she completed her GED and obtained a job in a day care center.

Teesha has made tremendous progress in the past few months but remains extremely vulnerable. She continues to work on resolving her feelings about her mother's death and has taken the first steps toward independence. In the meantime, she continues to live with her friend, sleeping in the living room with no space of her own. Although she has forged supportive relationships with professionals, her family and peer relationships are strained. She rarely sees her grandmother and has been involved off and on in an abusive relationship with a boy her age. A pregnancy 3 months ago ended in abortion.

Given the predicted rise in the number of orphaned youth, the need for preventive interventions to address risk for psychological disturbance cannot be overemphasized. Project Care has been designed to address key risk and protective factors that in turn influence psychological adjustment. It was designed to be realistic and cost-effective, and because it is implemented by a community-based agency, it is delivered in a way that is likely to be easier to replicate in other parts of the country.

THEORETICAL FRAMEWORK

The design of the intervention is based in part on the ABCX model (Hill, 1958), as modified into the "double" ABCX model by McCubbin and Patterson (1982). The model has precrisis (abcx) and postcrisis (ABCX) components (see Figure 8.1). The precrisis components are the following: (a) stressor (reality burden), which in our case is the mother's terminal illness as well as other chronic and acute stressors; (b) existing resources, including social support and relationship to the ill mother; (c) perception of the stressor (intrapsychic burden), specifically the child's perception of the mother's illness, disclosure of HIV, and perceived severity of the mother's illness; and (x) crisis, the disruptiveness, distress, and disorganization of the family around the illness. Postcrisis components are the following: (A) "pileup," which are new stressors experienced, including maternal death, placement with a new caregiver, a new home or school, and other stressful life events; (B) new resources, especially social support, relationship with the caregiver, and a stable custody arrangement; (C) perception of the situation, including the child's satisfaction with the new custody arrangement; and (X) adaptation, or fit between the demands of the crisis and existing resources, measured by child's mental and emotional health, school adjustment, and social anxiety.

The double ABCX model has several implications for intervention. First, because crises reverberate throughout the family, the family should be the unit of intervention, although the model and the long-term goals of Project Care focus on the child. Different family members may cope and adapt differently to the

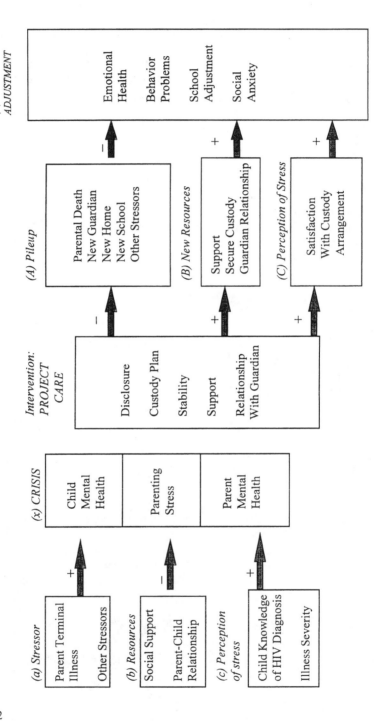

Figure 8.1. Double ABCX Model

162

same stressor, and the mental health of each family member affects the others. Therefore, both the family as a system and the unique individuals in that family need to be the targets of intervention. For example, psychological distress in the caregiver or the stress experienced by the caregiver might negatively influence the child's behavioral and emotional adjustment. Therefore, the intervention was designed to work primarily with the mother and the new caregiver but to include in the intervention topics (disclosure, custody, support, mental health) all family members. Intervention sessions explicitly raise issues for the mother about how her choices will affect the family as a unit, and the intervener seeks opportunities to build support among family members.

Second, two major areas are suggested for intervention: (a) assessing and enhancing resources that are known to help child adjustment and (b) preventing unnecessary pileup of additional stressors and risk factors. Resources are (a) support, (b) a secure family environment (a viable custody arrangement), and (c) a positive relationship between caregiver and child (Garmezy, 1987; Rutter, 1985). The intervention has been designed to enhance support from family and friends, to refer family members to support groups when needed, to provide support to the woman's supporters, and to arrange concrete support services, including homemakers and home health aids, when the mother is ill. The security of the child is key—our main aim is to help the mother to provide a satisfactory answer to her child's question: "Who will take care of me?" Many mothers believe that cultural norms and family understandings are all that is needed and that when she dies, the child will be cared for. However, in most instances, we have found that mothers are too optimistic about the willingness and ability of their chosen caregiver to provide a secure home for their children. Our intervention works with mothers to help them select the best caregivers and to obtain the caregivers' solemn agreement to become the children's caregivers in the future. We then institute the legal work necessary to ensure that the mother's plan will happen. The importance of the quality of the relationship between the mother and child as a protective factor cannot be overestimated. Children with a strong, trusting relationship with their parent are better able to handle the disclosure of the mother's serious illness and the challenges of their mother's illness. Therefore, the intervention is designed to help parents to open lines of communication with their children, to talk with them about what they think and feel, and to answer their questions.

Additional risk factors to be avoided after the death include multiple caregivers, unnecessary changes in the child's life, and separation from siblings. In the postdeath phase of Project Care, we believe that having a legal custody plan in place, plus the availability of the family specialist, will minimize the possibility that the child is shunted from family member to family member and ultimately to foster care. As part of the intervention with caregivers, we emphasize the importance of avoiding other changes in the child's life, such as moving the child to a new neighborhood or a new school, which removes the child from his or her existing support system of friends, classmates, and teachers. When siblings must be placed with different caregivers, the family specialist works with caregivers both before and after the death to obtain commitments that the children will be able to talk with each other by phone and to see each other regularly.

The double ABCX model led Project Care to target four factors: (a) Perception of the stressor should be a focus of the intervention; specifically, disclosure of parental illness (but not necessarily HIV) to child and caregiver is necessary to prepare the child for parental death and to develop a custody plan. It is a necessary component to encourage open communication so that the child can talk about his or her feelings and fears. (b) To avoid unnecessary pileup after maternal death, we should develop a viable custody plan with the mother; in particular, this will help avoid unnecessary multiple placements after death. In addition, new caregivers will need counseling on the importance of maintaining a stable, regular routine for the child, including assuring contact with friends and siblings. (c) New resources need to be arranged after maternal death by identifying financial and housing services for new caregivers; in addition, the social support systems of both the caregiver and child need to be assessed and enhanced because emotional and practical support has been shown to be related to a child's adjustment to stressors. (d) Adaptation will be enhanced by facilitating a positive relationship of caregiver and child because Garmezy (1987) and others have found that childhood resilience is in part determined by the presence of a caring adult. Note that the intervention is delivered to the mother alone—it is she who is the client of the agency. Although Family Center staff may speak with the child from time to time and short-term counseling may be provided, the intervention works through the mother and then the new caregiver to accomplish its mental health effects. Thus, the theory of the intervention is about the child, but the intervention is with the mother, which highlights the fact that family, particularly the mother, is the most important influence on child adjustment and development. Consequently, a very effective way to improve outcomes for children is to improve their family context and the transition to a new family.

PROCESSES THROUGH WHICH PARENTAL LOSS MAY RESULT IN PSYCHOLOGICAL DISTURBANCE

Some research suggests how the "causal chain" from parental death to disorder might emerge. Some of the processes are (a) disclosure and lack of open communication, (b) stability and custody, (c) relationship with caregiver or new guardian, and (d) resource and protective factors in children facing parental death.

Disclosure and Lack of Open Communication

Adults hold myths and misconceptions about children's understanding of death. These myths tend to deny children opportunities to talk about their grief or to mourn with the help of a supportive adult. These misconceptions, in turn, are integrally tied to adults' poor understanding about what children of different ages understand about death. A child's understanding of the meaning and causes of death is closely associated with developmental stage. Several researchers (e.g., Koocher, 1981; Lonetto, 1980; Orbach, Talmon, Kedem, & Har-even, 1987) have documented the developmental trends in children concerning death. Young children may be unable to grasp the abstract concept of death, but they do understand and grieve a loss (Sekaer, 1987). However, by age 7 or 8, children generally understand that death is final, and by age 10 or 11, they can understand the causes of death (Osterweis et al., 1984). Although children can understand death and do grieve, children do not mourn like adults. They may acknowledge loss of the parent in the real world but try to maintain a relationship with the dead parent in their inner world (Siegel & Freund, 1995).

Adults need to handle a child's grief reactions and concerns in a developmentally appropriate way. However, recent studies on bereavement in children indicate that our society is replete with myths about children's lack of ability to comprehend and absorb the reality of death (Wortman & Silver, 1989). Consequently, adults may be afraid to deal directly with a child in explaining the death of a loved one, not realizing that children are capable of understanding and expressing a wide range of reactions to someone's dying (Kranzler, Shaffer, Wasserman, & Davies, 1990). Lack of communication may deprive children of the needed opportunity to express feelings of loss and anger, ask questions, and adequately process their grief reactions. The subsequent suppression of feeling can deepen depression and so delay the resolution of the bereavement process.

Environments that foster disclosure and open communication of feelings such as guilt, loss, anger, and sadness have been shown to enhance the adjustment of children to parental death (Black & Urbanowicz, 1987; Bowlby, 1980; Brice, 1982; Cain & Fast, 1965; Furman, 1964, 1974, 1983; Hilgard, Newman, & Fisk, 1960; Kliman, 1973; Miller, 1971; Nagera, 1970). However, fostering open communication is difficult in families experiencing what Doka (1989, 1994) defines as "disenfranchised grief," that is, grief that cannot be openly acknowledged and socially supported. The grief experience with AIDS is analogous (Doka, 1989, 1994), and the stigma and secrecy that surround AIDS in families can be expected to have a negative impact on children's ability to mourn openly and to make an appropriate adjustment to a new living situation (Dane & Miller, 1992). Well children may worry that they have acquired AIDS from their parent and need to be reassured (Siegel & Gorey, 1994). Support to the new family at this critical juncture can be extremely valuable. Here is a case example of how lack of communication between the new caregiver and bereaved children affects child adjustment and how intervention can be helpful.

Harold, Trevor, and Gerard are 8, 5, and 3 years old, respectively. Their mother, Toni, died of AIDS 2 years ago at the age of 23. The three boys live with their

52-year-old grandmother, Ingrid, who is their legal guardian. Ingrid first learned that Toni had HIV when she moved to New York City from Jamaica to care for her daughter during the last few months of her life.

Following Toni's death, Ingrid focused on the details of the transition the family was making with her as head of household. She made sure that the children's benefits remained in place, moved to a larger apartment, purchased furniture, and enrolled the youngest child in day care. She was overwhelmed by her own feelings of loss for her daughter and wanted to ensure that the children did not feel sad. She never cried in front of them and could not bring herself to speak about Toni in their presence, fearing that she would be too overwhelmed. She believed that she could not expose her feelings and at the same time be the "pillar of strength" that her family so desperately needed.

Not long after Toni's death, the boys were having difficulty dealing with the loss of their mother. Ingrid sought counseling for the children but was reluctant to address her own feelings around the death and the burdens of her unexpected role as caregiver for three very active, young boys. The family specialist worked with Ingrid to help her feel more comfortable in explaining and talking about death in age-appropriate ways with all of the children and to dispel the personal and cultural myths that expressing feelings of grief is a weakness. In this process, Ingrid began to work through her own feelings about the loss. Beginning to relieve this burden allowed her to trust her ability to share these feelings without feeling overwhelmed and to facilitate the children's expression of their own grief. She also realized that she was the children's primary link to their mother and that it was appropriate in this role that she actively engage them in remembrances. In a particularly poignant home visit by the family specialist, Ingrid brought out a box of photos of Toni before she became ill, and she and the boys spent time fondly remembering their happy years together.

Over the course of the work, Ingrid reported that the boys had fewer episodes of unprovoked crying, were better at managing their anger, and were doing better in school and day care. She also reported that 5-year-old Trevor, who had been unable to sleep by himself, was sleeping through the night in his own bed. Harold, the 8-year-old, was less withdrawn but continued to show signs of continuing distress. As the oldest child, he had had the longest relationship with his mother, and her death affected him most strongly. He was referred to long-term treatment in the community for continued bereavement counseling, with particular attention to how his unresolved grief was negatively affecting his social development.

Stability and Custody

The literature on bereavement supports the need for consistency and stability after parental death (Furman, 1974, 1983; Nagera, 1970; Osterweis et al., 1984; Rutter, 1966). Children deserve a well-considered, carefully evaluated, and realistic answer to the poignant question, "Who will take care of me?" "Meeting children's basic physical and emotional needs is a necessary precondition to mourning. If these needs are unmet, mourning may be inhibited because anxiety leads them to deny the loss" (Siegel & Gorey, 1994, p. 568). Furthermore, as noted earlier, avoiding disruption in the postdeath phase is key to better adjustment in children (Rutter, 1966).

Yet few parents with AIDS have a realistic custody plan in place for their children. Helping parents with AIDS to plan for the future custody of their children is complex. Ensuring that caregiver arrangements are feasible and legalistic is immensely complicated and intricate. Establishing a stable new family may be hampered by the lack of systems that bridge AIDS-specific services and entitlements with services and entitlements for which new caregivers and surviving youngsters may be eligible. In New York City, more than 3,000 families receive comprehensive, coordinated case management services through the Division of AIDS Services Income Support, a program of New York City's Human Resources Administration. However, once the parent with AIDS dies, most cases are closed within 1 to 2 months of the client's death, and no system exists for following children afterward.

Planning and executing long-term guardianship for children are complicated further by the complexity of the service systems that must be coordinated for the development of a feasible plan. Families and their social service providers must be able to negotiate both the legal and entitlement systems, at the same time meeting the changing psychosocial needs of the ill parent, children, and other family members.

Relationship With Caregiver or New Guardian

The caregiver-child relationship is key to children's future adjustment. Research documents that the family and the "parent"-child relationship are protective factors. Among inner-city children, the quality of parent involvement was positively related to children's social competence (Reynolds, Weissberg, & Kasprow, 1992). Other family factors that may buffer against the harmful effects of parent death include protective parenting styles (Alvy, 1987) and family resourcefulness and adaptability (McAdoo, 1982).

The caregivers' level of chronic stress and psychological health will influence child adjustment through a variety of mechanisms (Billings & Moos, 1983; Gordon et al., 1989; Hammen et al., 1987; Hammen, Ellicott, Giltin, & Jamison, 1989; Hetherington & Martin, 1979; Holahan & Moos, 1987; Maccoby, 1980; Maccoby & Marin, 1983; Main, Kaplan, & Cassidy, 1985; Rutter & Quinton, 1984). Caregivers often take on the newly bereaved child with good intentions but rapidly learn that the transition to a new family structure is difficult. Building of the new relationship is influenced by the quality and length of the previous relationship between the caregiver and child (if any), who else lives in the household, child characteristics and temperament, child psychological and emotional distress, and housing and financial problems.

Frances is a 44-year-old mother of six and grandmother of four. She joined Project Care to work on guardianship for two of her grandchildren, Terry and Shawnee, who came to live with her after their mother, Elizabeth, died of AIDS. At the time of her death, Elizabeth had been in Project Care for 4 months working on a permanency plan for her children. Elizabeth was willing to have her mother involved but was adamant that she not know her HIV status or the fact that 9-year-old Terry also was HIV+. She believed that her mother would care for the children regardless of Terry's HIV status and did not want to worry her about HIV. Elizabeth did inform her mother that she and Terry were sick, choosing to tell her that they had sickle cell anemia rather than AIDS. Elizabeth began discussing the various planning options available in New York State when she died suddenly, without any written documentation of her wishes for her children's future care.

As Elizabeth assumed, Frances did take her grandchildren into her home. With no other good option for the children, she decided to care for them as long as she could, despite her own ill health. At the time of her daughter's death, Frances was informed by the hospital about her grandson's HIV status and given information necessary for his continued medical care. She was shocked by the suddenness of Elizabeth's death and surprised to learn of her and Terry's HIV status. She was soon overwhelmed by all of the decisions she had to make following her daughter's death and by the obstacles she encountered in accessing the children's entitlements and in enrolling them in school.

The Family Center lawyer and family specialist assisted Frances with letters to the Board of Education and Department of Social Services, and the children began receiving benefits and were enrolled in school in time for the new academic year. Frances met with the lawyer to review the guardianship process and decided to pursue this avenue for legalizing her caregiving role with Shawnee and Terry. The guardianship process takes about 4 months to complete when everything goes smoothly. In this case, the process met with a number of obstacles, including Shawnee's father, who saw his daughter regularly and whose consent to the plan was needed. Shawnee's father did eventually consent to the plan, and 18 months after Elizabeth's death, the paperwork was ready for submission to the court. In the meantime, Frances was increasingly ambivalent about pursuing the guardianship because she feared that the court-ordered home study (the usual procedure in these proceedings) would find her apartment too crowded. In addition to Frances, Shawnee, and Terry, the household includes four of Frances's daughters and four of their young children in a cramped three-bedroom apartment. Frances and two of her daughters had been on waiting lists for alternative public housing for several years, but there was no way of knowing when any of them might move. Frances has refused assistance from The Family Center in the form of bunk beds, new bureaus, and other furniture that could allow the family to maximize the space. She is difficult to reach and does not answer phone messages or respond to letters.

Although Frances did not directly convey her ambivalence about pursuing the guardianship further, she has made it clear that it is not her first priority. With the children in school and in receipt of benefits, there is no immediate need for the legal paperwork. Frances clearly has reservations about subjecting herself and her family to the scrutiny of the court. She is still overwhelmed by her added responsibilities, and she is angry that Elizabeth did not do more to secure a custody plan before she died. If Elizabeth had planned in a way that realistically informed Frances that she would be taking care of Shawnee and Terry, it is possible that better housing arrangements could have been obtained. It is also possible that had Elizabeth included her mother in the planning process, Frances would now be more motivated to complete the guardianship and might be more open to receiving assistance from The Family Center.

Resource and Protective Factors in Children Facing Parental Death

All children with multiple risk factors do not go on to develop psychiatric disorders: Many demonstrate that they are "stress resistant" (Rutter, 1979). Factors that characterize resilient children and their families include biological (e.g., intellectual ability, developmental age), dispositional (e.g., use of proactive coping strategies, self-efficacy, and self-esteem), family-related (e.g., having a good stable relationship with at least one caregiver), and community-related variables (e.g., school and educational climate; social support from outside the family, particularly at least one adult mentor or confidant) (Hurrelman & Losel, 1990; Masten et al., 1990; Rae-Grant et al., 1989; Rutter, 1979; Werner & Smith, 1982). These resource or protective factors appear to hold in samples of minority inner-city children in poverty as well. The strongest correlates of resiliency and competence were (a) positive self-esteem; (b) intelligence; (c) family support, warmth, and cohesion; and (d) an adult authority figure. Although some of these factors cannot be manipulated in an intervention, others can be enhanced using known technologies.

DESCRIPTION OF INTERVENTION

Project Care is a home-based program delivered in two parts: (a) after parental diagnosis with AIDS (or late-stage HIV disease) and (b) after parental death. The Project Care intervention team is composed of social workers, attorneys, and "family specialists" who are college graduates with intensive training. Family specialists meet with the family approximately every 2 weeks and access lawyers and social workers as needed.

In Part I, interveners provide in-home sessions to (a) assist ill parents with disclosure issues, (b) develop a custody plan, (c) obtain the nominated caregiver's consent to care for the child, (d) meet with the future caregiver to assess needs and access services, (e) finalize a legal custody plan, and (f) evaluate and enhance informal supports. Part I is implemented over a 6-month period prior to the mother's death. The time period can be compressed if the mother's health worsens precipitously or extended if the intervention goals have not been met. Most families have completed the core intervention within 6 months, but typically court proceedings take longer. It is important to continue the intervention for as long as necessary to develop a viable custody plan. After Part I has been completed, we maintain bimonthly telephone contact with the family to assess whether the custody plan remains viable and to monitor the mother's health status.

Following parental death, Part II of Project Care works with the new caregiver and child to (a) assist in the transition to a new family; (b) provide access to concrete services when available, such as new housing and financial assistance; (c) evaluate and enhance social support; and (d) assess children's mental health and provide counseling or referral as needed. The postdeath intervention is provided in four to six sessions over a period of 4 months, spaced as the family requires and prefers.

Project Care staff have written a series of modules ("guided conversations"), which correspond to the program of services and provide a flexible framework and resource for the interveners throughout Parts I and II. Some of these psychoeducational materials address emotionally neutral topics such as healthy eating and stress management and relaxation. They are included because some mothers and caregivers find it too difficult to begin emotionally laden topics immediately, and these enable the family specialist to cultivate rapport before embarking on more difficult subjects. In addition, the materials break down the chosen topics into manageable steps and present numerous opportunities for the client to role-play with the family specialist and to acquire problem-solving skills.

Description of Population

Project Care serves families in which the mother with AIDS is receiving case management services from the Division of AIDS Services Income Support (DASIS), a program of New York City's Human Resources Administration. To be eligible for these services, a client must have a Centers for Disease Control and Prevention (CDC)-defined AIDS diagnosis or symptomatic HIV that requires home care services, be Medicaid eligible, and reside in of one of the five boroughs of New York City. Almost 90% of parents with AIDS in New York City receive services from the Division of AIDS Services Income Support; therefore, this project has access to a majority of the entire population of eligible New York City families. Most DASIS clients are African American and Latino, and many have a history of drug use; their needs for social services are extremely complex.

The AIDS Serviceline, well known by medical and social service providers throughout New York City, is the single point of entry for DASIS services. More than 70% of clients call the Serviceline after a hospitalization: The rest are referred by private physicians, correctional facilities, shelters, AIDS service organizations, and others. Project Care services are appropriate for children of any age, but for evaluation purposes, we are recruiting mothers with children ages 8 to 12.

Overcoming Reluctance to Join Project Care

Women who are invited to receive Project Care services refuse for four main reasons: (a) They do not think they need a custody plan because informal understandings exist in the family, (b) they think they already have a legal plan, (c) they say they are not sick enough, or (d) planning is too threatening and painful. Timing is key to approaching mothers about the need to plan custody for their children. For some mothers, planning commences only in the terminal phase of their illness, when they must acknowledge the need to plan. For other mothers, however, custody planning is less threatening when they are not ill, and they are feeling optimistic. One approach that works is to universalize the need for a plan—that is, all parents should have a custody plan. Even though they are doing well and feel healthy, having a plan in place is something important they can do to protect their children's future.

To encourage mothers to join Project Care, we developed a 7-minute videotape that features mothers talking about Project Care and its services. It shows family specialists delivering services in the mothers' homes, and mothers who have been through Project Care explain why it is important. The video is designed for in-home use and does not refer to HIV in any way. The purpose of the video is to reduce mothers' fears about the program and encourage them to take the first step.

SUMMARY OF PROJECT CARE

Content of the Program

Project Care has two parts. Part I, which occurs prior to maternal death, focuses on disclosure and communication, custody planning, and working with the new caregiver. Although the focus of Part I is with the ill mother, the family specialist meets with the children and proposed caregiver as well. During this phase of the service, the family specialist makes biweekly home visits, lasting 60 to 90 minutes. These visits focus on assistance with entitlements and discussions about disclosure and custody planning, and when the client is ready, they include an attorney to discuss legal options and provide the legal services necessary to execute the mother's chosen plan. The family specialist provides support to the mother and other family members through this difficult work and offers the services of the clinical staff when appropriate. Project Care aims to meet client-defined needs related to child well-being as well as covering custody matters. There, at the first session, the mother completes a needs assessment form that lists topics covered under each component of Project Care. Mothers are encouraged to choose which aspects of the program to start with. The interveners thus start the program "where the client is" addressing her most pressing concerns. This builds trust and meets client-defined needs first, which makes the mother more receptive to deal with other pressing but difficult issues such as disclosure and custody planning.

When the mother is ready to discuss disclosure, the family specialist works with her to develop a strategy to prepare her family for the possibility that she will die and to lay the groundwork for the development of a custody plan. With mothers who choose not to disclose their HIV status, family specialists discuss the alternatives of disclosing serious or terminal illness. In doing this work, the family specialist and mother discuss the pros and cons of disclosure, assess the current extent of disclosure within the family, identify barriers to further disclosure, discuss the hazards of not disclosing, and role-play possible disclosure scenarios. In these discussions, the family specialist helps the mother assess her existing supports and develop strategies for maintaining and enhancing those supports throughout the disclosure process and afterward.

The custody component of Project Care assists mothers with the actual preparation of plans for their children's future. During this phase of the work, the family specialist assists the mother in identifying a possible caregiver for each child. In doing this, the family specialist assists the mother in identifying each child's special attributes and needs and helps her to articulate her wishes and dreams for each of her children. This phase of the work also takes into consideration other circumstances that might influence the viability of the plan. For instance, if the proposed caregiver is elderly and the child is young, the family specialist would work with the mother to anticipate what might happen if the caregiver was no longer able to care for the child and might suggest that a backup plan be made. At this point in the work, the family specialist also assesses the child's feeling about the proposed caregiver and works with the family on emotional and behavioral issues that might threaten the plan. With the mother's permission, the family specialist may involve a clinical staff person to assess these issues and to provide short-term individual or family counseling if appropriate.

When the mother is ready, the family specialist brings in an attorney to explain the various custody options. Mothers are well prepared to choose the option that is best for their family after meeting with the lawyer. After the choice has been made, the lawyer executes all of the paperwork associated with putting the plan in place and makes sure that all needed signatures are obtained. If the mother chooses to have the plan legalized in court, the lawyer will accompany her to all court dates.

The family specialist encourages the mother to include the proposed caregiver in the planning process as early as possible and works with her to arrange a meeting of the three of them to discuss the plan. The purpose of this meeting with the new caregiver is to ensure that she fully understands that she is agreeing to take custody of the children after the mother's death and to speak with her about what she perceives to be the strengths and weaknesses of the plan. This meeting also gives the family specialist an opportunity to work with both the mother and caregiver to anticipate concerns and problems that may arise after placement and to assess the caregiver's eligibility for services that may be needed. This meeting also serves as a time for the family specialist to talk with the caregiver about her support system and to strategize with her about how she might enhance those supports if needed.

At the time of maternal death, Part II commences. This part focuses on new family adjustment. Its aim is to assist the new family during the transition period, when the custody plan is most at risk, and to provide children and their caregivers access to the family specialist on a regular and "as-needed" basis. Part of the effort is supportive, to assist the child and the caregiver with the grief process. More than half the time, the caregiver will be a relative of the mother and therefore will be grieving herself. The family specialist often works with the clinical staff at this point in the intervention to help the family recognize the issue of bereavement as a source of distress and to assist the caregiver with recognizing the wide variety of bereavement reactions that may emerge. At the same time, the family specialist assists the caregiver with accessing services to stabilize the family's income, housing, and other concrete needs and follows up to determine whether the family has accessed the referrals. If the caregiver has no previous parenting experience, the family specialist will help the caregiver develop dependable routines, work on consistent discipline styles, and otherwise foster a sense of security for the children. The family specialist and clinical staff work with all caregivers to help them mobilize supports for themselves and the children. When necessary, the attorneys will go to court with the new caregiver to fully implement the custody plan.

Intervention Team

Project Care is delivered primarily by "family specialists." Most are bachelor-level counselors with 2 years' experience with AIDS projects at The Family Center. They are supervised by a social worker who has worked extensively with families with AIDS. In addition, three kinds of specialists review each case with the family specialists and become directly involved in service provision in specified circumstances: (a) A social worker visits families as necessary to assess children's mental health, provide short-term counseling, and make referrals for therapy if necessary. The social worker may also make a home visit to assess barriers to custody planning or to facilitate a family discussion. (b) One of three attorneys provides legal assistance to clients in the home to explain legal options, draw up wills, handle standby guardianships, draw up custody petitions, and/or begin adoption proceedings. They also represent family members in court in guardianship proceedings. (c) A benefits and housing specialist is available for family specialists to consult on financial, housing, health, or other concrete services.

Referral Network

Linkages to community resources are an important part of Project Care. The Family Center has a close working relationship with the New York City Administration for Children's Services. In fact, The Family Center assisted the Administration for Children Services in designing its Early Permanency Planning Project, which helps mothers prepare a foster home for their children. In our project, foster care was selected as a custodial arrangement for a few families. The Family Center has an excellent network of relationships with mental health providers citywide and can refer adults and children for services throughout the five boroughs.

Training

Training and support for all intervention staff are intensive. All family specialists, attorneys, and social workers are trained intensively in Project Care philosophy and how to use each of the 18 modules for Phase 1 and the 5 modules in Phase 2. The content of each module is thoroughly reviewed and discussed, role-play is used to illustrate standard and problem situations, and sample "scripts" are provided to give family specialists examples of responses to their clients' needs. A big part of training is developing the working team relationships. The Project Care team consists of family specialists, attorneys, social workers, and benefits specialists. Although each must know how Project Care is delivered, they must learn their roles and responsibilities and how their jobs differ. In particular, there are delicate issues to negotiate between attorneys and other staff concerning "who is the client," what information is privileged, and what legal information a layperson can provide and what an attorney should provide. Team members also need to agree on when to call on other team members to enter a case. Role boundaries are difficult to negotiate at first, and there are informal and formal discussions during training about these issues as well as case presentations to illustrate team roles. For example, although family specialists can help mothers think through the custody planning options available, it is the attorney's job to explain the legal implications of each option and assess whether the mother's choice is appropriate given the specific circumstances. All staff are trained in skills and techniques that can be used to assist clients in addressing difficult and painful issues, bereavement counseling, breaking through resistance, custody planning options in New York State, eligibility requirements for social service entitlements and services, referral resources, and the recognition of depression in mothers and children. All new staff go on family visits to observe experienced staff. In addition to content, all staff are taught how to do an intake, how to do a genogram, New York State HIV confidentiality laws, how to recognize and report abuse or neglect, emergency interventions (violence, suicide), and how to conduct a home visit. Field safety is reviewed, and organizational issues are covered such as communication among staff within the program, communication with service providers outside the program, how to complete client contact forms, how to maintain a chart for each family, how and when to make referrals, and how to maintain contact with clients. All staff meet with their supervisors weekly for personal case conferences and ongoing clinical supervision. Group supervision is conducted weekly, including case presentation.

CASE STUDY OF JUANITA'S PROJECT CARE EXPERIENCE

Recruitment

Juanita was invited into Project Care services by telephone by our recruiter, who explained the program and services available. She agreed to accept the service, and at the first appointment, Mashariki Kudumu, her family specialist, completed an intake form to obtain pertinent family history, current service use, and medical status. She explained the service and the major areas of the Project Care intervention (custody planning, disclosure, support system) and began to build client-intervener rapport.

Visit 1. Mashariki used this visit to take a history of Juanita's illness and her relationships with her immediate family and to assess her readiness to begin custody planning. Juanita first tested positive for HIV in 1990 and was diagnosed with AIDS more than 1 year ago. She left her husband, Carlos, who was abusive to her and her child. He resides now in Puerto Rico, and she has no contact with him but fears he may return and try to take her 11-year-old son Albert away. She lives with Albert and her boyfriend of 7 years, Miguel. She has no custody plan at this time and has no idea what custody options are available to her. She is unsure about whom to choose as a caregiver for Albert but is seriously considering Miguel or

Albert's godparents. Miguel is extremely supportive of her and knows her diagnosis; the godparents do not know that she has AIDS, but she wants to change that.

Juanita is extremely isolated. Her mother and four sisters all live in the New York area, but when Juanita disclosed her HIV status to her family, they rejected all contact with her. Juanita seems quite depressed, and Mashariki learned that Juanita had been diagnosed with depression, is on medication, and is seeing a therapist. Mashariki encouraged Juanita to consider joining a support group for women with HIV and promised to find a possible group for her to attend. Mashariki briefly reviewed Project Care services, and Juanita chose to begin with custody planning.

Visit 2. Mashariki began the first custody planning module, "Choosing a Future Caregiver," which is designed to help the client consider several aspects of choosing a caregiver. The work began with a discussion of the reasons for naming a caregiver and addressed what might happen if a caregiver is not chosen and Juanita became too ill to care for Albert. Because Juanita had taken that difficult first step and decided to choose a caregiver, Mashariki assisted her by helping her describe what she wants the caregiver to be like and what she wants the caregiver to be able to do for Albert. Then, Mashariki did a genogram to identify all of Juanita's family members and friends and Albert's godparents. Together, they used the genogram to systematically review possible caregivers for Albert. Because her family rejected her after she disclosed her HIV status, and because there is a lot of bickering and abuse among her family members, Juanita would not consider any of her immediate family as possible caregivers for Albert. She reiterated her interest in either Miguel or Albert's godparents as possible caregivers. At this point in the module, the family specialist assesses whether the client has talked with the chosen caregiver. Juanita had talked extensively with Miguel, who wants to adopt Albert. However, she had not spoken to the child's godparents because she had not told them she was ill. At this visit, Mashariki referred Juanita to the support group, but Juanita would not go because she was afraid that she would not fit in and would "be judged." She was so traumatized by her family's reaction to her being HIV+ that Mashariki was unable to reassure her.

Visit 3. Mashariki continued the same module to help Juanita choose a caregiver. At this time, Juanita finally admitted that she was reluctant to allow Miguel to adopt Albert because "all the records would change and he would have to change his name." Mashariki explained that there were other ways for Miguel to have custody aside from adoption, and Juanita was very relieved. She agreed that Mashariki should meet together with her and Miguel next time to discuss caregiver options. Mashariki also explained that because Albert's father was alive, he should be contacted about the guardianship proceedings.

Visit 4. Mashariki asked Juanita about how things had gone since the last visit. Juanita reported that she had had a conversation with Albert's godparents about HIV to start to feel out whether they would be supportive of her or reject her if she disclosed her HIV status to them. She did this by telling them that her sister was HIV+ and that she was worried about her. The godparents were shocked, and their reaction scared Juanita. Mashariki initiated the module "Talking to Others About Your Illness." This module helps clients decide whether to disclose information about their illness and provides specific guidance about how to disclose. Issues that are covered include the pros and cons of disclosure, the burden of secrecy, the risk of inadvertent disclosure, the impact of disclosure on social support, the "process" of disclosure and the fact that it continues over a long period, deciding how much to tell, and the pros and cons of "partial" truths. Although Juanita had wanted to disclose to Albert's godparents, she chose not to pursue this at this time. Had Juanita decided to disclose, Mashariki would have used role-play to rehearse what she would say and would review with her possible short-term and long-term reactions, including denial or changing the subject, anger, distress, blaming, and inquisitiveness.

Because Miguel was unable to attend, Mashariki completed a different module, "Talking to Your Child About Your Illness." This module is designed to assess what the mother has told her child about her illness. During the course of this module, the family specialist provides guidance as the parent decides whether to disclose and how much to say. This includes helping the parent create a safe environment in which to talk about his or her illness, helping the parent to choose the words to describe the illness that are appropriate for the child, and preparing the parent for the range of emotional responses that may result. The emphasis throughout all of this work is to maintain effective communication both during the disclosure itself and after the disclosure takes place. When working with a parent on disclosure to a child, the family specialist first assesses what the mother has told the child herself, what others may have told the child, and what she believes the child knows and understands about her illness. Once this foundation has been laid, the discussion then turns to what the mother wants to tell the child, the pros and cons of disclosing, and the choice of words appropriate to the child's level of understanding. Role-playing is an important part of this work and helps the mother fine-tune the language she wants to use and to anticipate the child's reaction both immediately and longer term.

Juanita told Mashariki that her sister had deliberately told Albert about his mother's HIV status against her will. Ever since Albert had been told of his mother's HIV status, he had been very upset. Mashariki then implemented the module titled "How Are Your Children Doing?" The goal of this module is to assess the child's behavior so that the family specialist and client can decide whether the child needs formal evaluation and referral. The module has separate sections for different developmental stages from toddlers through adolescence. With older children, the family specialist may speak directly with the child. Mashariki engaged Juanita in a conversation about Albert, asking first for Juanita's description of Albert's behavior or affect and following up with specific questions about school performance and problems, somatic symptoms, moods, friendships, and relationships with siblings and other family members. Finally, Mashariki assessed whether Albert had ever received counseling or therapy. Juanita was extremely worried about Albert. She was so concerned that she had obtained a referral to a therapist, who diagnosed Albert with depression. Albert will not talk to anyone about his mother's illness except his mother and his therapist. Furthermore, the therapist referred Albert to a special education class, and as a result, Albert is doing a bit better in school. No one at Albert's school is aware of Juanita's health problem.

Visit 5. Miguel and Juanita met with Mashariki to discuss caregiver options, the custody planning module called "Permanency Planning Options." This module is designed to provide the client with a basic understanding of the range of planning options available, to help her decide which one is most appropriate for her family, and to assist in formalizing the plan if necessary. In addition, the family specialist assists the mother to locate important documents such as birth certificates, which will be necessary for the formal custody planning options. Ultimately, the client is prepared to meet with an attorney to discuss the specifics of the plan and prepare legal documents.

Mashariki reviewed the four main custody planning options: a last will and testament, standby guardianship, the early permanency planning project within the foster care system, and adoption. They chose standby guardianship as the best fit for their needs. Mashariki then told Juanita and Miguel that biological parents are assumed by the courts to be the natural guardians of their children. Because Albert's biological father is alive, according to New York state law, he must be informed of any legal proceedings concerning custody of his child. Juanita was extremely worried about contacting Albert's father, Carlos. He had physically abused both Juanita and Albert and was an active drug user. He had made no effort to contact them in many years and had not sent child support to Albert. Mashariki explained that it was important to contact the legal biological father but also reassured them that under the circumstances, even if the father wanted custody of Albert, the court would be unlikely to grant it. Juanita was very worried that by contacting him, she and Albert would be vulnerable to abuse again or that he would demand custody. Mashariki found it difficult to reassure her, and the meeting ended with Juanita still quite anxious. Immediately after this visit, Mashariki met with Sarah Orr, a Project Care attorney, to discuss Juanita's legal needs and her request for a standby guardianship petition.

Visit 6. Mashariki and Sarah met with Juanita and Miguel to plan the standby guardianship petition. Again, Juanita voiced her fear of her abusive husband and her concern about contacting him. She admitted that the lack of involvement of Albert's father with Albert reminds her of her own abandonment by her father, and she became very emotional. Mashariki provided support and again explained why the father had to be contacted and that the history of abuse could be documented. Sarah completed her own assessment of Juanita's custody plan and reviewed court procedures for standby guardianship. Sarah told Juanita that she would begin working on the petition and suggested that she also work with Mashariki to complete other important legal work soon, including completing an advanced directive and arranging power of attorney.

Visit 7. Mashariki initiated the module called "Advance Directives," which helps the mother choose someone to act as a health care proxy and identifies exactly what interventions she wants at the end of her life. Mashariki explained what a health care proxy is and talked with her about the people she might trust with this responsibility. She explained how a health care proxy works and when it is implemented, the importance of discussing it with her physician, why it is important to think about it before it is needed, issues of disclosure of HIV by physician to the proxy, and how a proxy is prepared. Juanita selected Miguel as the primary proxy and a sister as the alternate. Mashariki told them she would have Sarah prepare the paperwork for Juanita to sign at the next visit.

Visit 8. Juanita began the visit with Mashariki by saying that she was unhappy that Miguel would not always practice safe sex. Recently, she had told Miguel that she would not have sex with him unless he used a condom, and he became very angry. She is worried about making him upset because she is isolated—he is her only support person, and she is dependent on him financially. Mashariki validated her concerns and praised her strength in trying to practice safe sex. Mashariki asked if Juanita would want to change the custody plan if Miguel was HIV+. Juanita resolved that Miguel should be tested and would raise the issue with him.

Juanita changed the subject and described how sad she was because a pet had died and her own losses—and her own mortality—were weighing on her. She became tearful and said that she did not want to die and that she wanted to continue to raise her son. Mashariki provided support, validated her concerns, and praised her for doing the custody plan as a way of continuing to care for Albert after she was no longer able to. Juanita also showed Mashariki a paper she had received about her housing that had upset her. Miguel is not listed as a legal tenant in the apartment, and Juanita was concerned that Miguel could not stay in the apartment otherwise. However, listing him might jeopardize her eligibility for the apartment. Mashariki referred the problem to the benefits specialist, who looked into the issue. He subsequently determined that Miguel could be added to the lease now without jeopardizing their eligibility, and this was arranged.

Visit 9. Mashariki showed Juanita and Miguel the completed health care proxy and witnessed its signing. She reviewed the purpose with Miguel. She also arranged to have it translated into Spanish for Miguel.

Visit 10. Mashariki met with Juanita and her sister to review the purpose of the health care proxy and explain it. Mashariki also initiated the module on "Should I Have a Will?" Mashariki described how a will is made and the advantages of having a will, including that it would state her wishes for the future care of Albert, how she wants her personal belongings distributed, and her preferences for funeral arrangements. Juanita decided that she wanted her custody preferences stated in a will, along with funeral arrangements and property distribution. She selected Miguel as executor and promised to make a list of her possessions for next time.

Visit 11. Mashariki and Sarah worked with Juanita to complete the provisions for the will. Sarah also reviewed with Juanita the specific provisions of the standby guardianship petition. Sarah reassured Juanita that she would accompany her to court to file the petition and promised to have the papers ready in 2 weeks. Mashariki followed up on whether Miguel was tested for HIV and learned that Miguel had been tested for HIV and that his test was negative. Miguel stated that the testing counselor had been quite effective, and Miguel was now more receptive to using condoms consistently.

A few days later, Juanita called Mashariki and was very upset. Albert had been badly burned on Thanksgiving Day while helping to cook the turkey with Miguel. He was in the hospital, and a children's services worker had questioned her about a possible abuse situation. Mashariki reassured her that this was standard practice, and Mashariki encouraged her to contact the worker to see if there was a chance that charges might be pressed. Two days later, Juanita called to say that the child was much better and would be released and that children's services was not going to press charges.

Visit 12. Sarah, Mashariki, Juanita, and Miguel met to review and sign the legal papers (will, guardianship). At that meeting, Miguel stated that he might be leaving to take a seasonal job in Minnesota. He was not sure that he would go or, if he went, for how long he would be away. Mashariki and Sarah decided to go ahead and complete the legal work but not to file the papers in court until Miguel returned. Mashariki and Sarah implemented "Going to Court" with Juanita and Miguel. Because the standby guardianship petition would need to be court approved, it is important that both Juanita and Miguel understand what would happen. Family court is frustrating and unpredictable, and preparing clients for the process can be very helpful. Sarah explained how the court works (e.g., what is an "intake," what is a "part," who must be present, filing the case, waiting to be called, who are court officers, how long they would have to wait to see the judge). She described what the courtroom would look like and who the people were, as well as the fact that at least two appearances would be needed. She also explained that although some parts of the process were standard, many were variable, and, depending on the case and the judge, different things might happen. In most cases, the standby guardianship petition process includes "checks" that are made on the suitability of the guardian (home visit, checking abuse/neglect state registry, interviewing the child, etc.). In some cases, a law guardian (an attorney) is appointed to represent the child's interests, speak to the child, and provide a report about the suitability of the custody arrangement from the child's point of view. Sarah explained that the judge is not permitted to inquire about Juanita's HIV status but that, on occasion, HIV confidentiality has been compromised, and she should be prepared for that small risk. Sarah then explained again that Albert's father must be notified about the matter, and Juanita decided to file an affidavit of abandonment.

Visit 13. Sarah, Mashariki, Miguel, and Juanita met. Miguel would be going to Minnesota for several weeks. Juanita was very upset that he was leaving. They finalized the affidavit of abandonment and agreed to file it with the custody papers when Miguel returned. Sarah reviewed with them where important papers were, including the importance of obtaining a copy of the child's birth certificate. At this late stage in custody planning, Sarah and Mashariki learned for the first time that Miguel is technically married, although he has been separated for many years. He had been reluctant to reveal this when Sarah had first taken a legal history but now trusted her enough to disclose this. He asked Sarah to handle the divorce, and she agreed to handle a simple divorce and prepare the forms. When Miguel returned from Minnesota, the papers were signed and filed by Sarah in court.

Visit 14. Juanita signed her will in the presence of witnesses. Mashariki completed the "Joint Visit With Caregiver and Parent" module with Miguel and Juanita to assess Miguel's readiness to parent Albert. This meeting focuses on the positive and potentially problematic aspects of the custody arrangements. This module is not intended to persuade or convince anyone to become a guardian; in fact, it is sometimes used by potential caregivers to say no if they feel reluctant. Mashariki was assured by Miguel that he wanted to be Albert's guardian, and Mashariki talked with them about Miguel's relationship with Albert now and how it might change in the future. The module guides a conversation among the family specialist, the client, and the caregiver about parenting issues and how the mother wants to see her child raised. Mashariki then reviewed practical issues that might arise, such as how Miguel would care for Albert alone, whether there were others who could help care for Albert after school when Miguel was working, and whether he would have enough money and space to care for him alone. Miguel will be staying in the same apartment with Albert, which will provide stability for Albert and keep him in the same school with his same peer network. Mashariki also introduced the issue of parenting and determined that Miguel had already been acting as a parent to Albert and that he felt comfortable in that role. Mashariki also implemented another related module, "Services and Entitlements," to identify services that Miguel might need and be eligible for when he became Albert's guardian. This module uses a semistructured interview format to assess Miguel's needs and assesses eligibility for services.

Postscript. Two months later, the court approved Miguel as guardian. Several months afterward, Miguel's divorce was granted. Juanita is doing well and has had no HIV-related illnesses.

This case study uses one family's experience to describe how Project Care services are delivered step by step. The case is typical of most families in that Juanita is not extremely ill, and she has only one child. She was unusual in that she was more receptive than most to custody planning services. When families have multiple children with different fathers, more than one custody plan may be prepared. Also, some mothers are currently using alcohol and drugs, have pressing unmet concrete needs for housing and food, or find custody planning too threatening and hard to complete.

Note also that we have described the case in linear fashion as though the process unfolded sequentially. In reality, there are many "horizontal" themes, and the process is more like weaving warp and woof—and sometimes the patterns shift and colors are added and discarded with little control by the weaver! Finally, this case is typical in that there is a major surprise fairly late in the planning. Although the exact nature of the surprise varies idiosyncratically from family to family, in almost all instances there has been an important fact or problem that comes to light after many months of working with the family. It took 6 months to complete the 14 Project Care visits and 2 additional months to obtain court approval for the plan.

ETHICAL ISSUES

Because of the complex and unusual ethical issues involved in delivering Project Care, an ethics board was formed, chaired by Carol Levine and composed of Mindy Fullilove, M.D.; Nancy Dubler, L.L.B.; and Kathy Powderly, R.N. This board at first focused attention on the issue of what constitutes a viable custody plan and what minimal criteria should be used for a plan. Soon after, in the discussions between the ethics board and the Project Care staff, it became apparent that three additional issues were most troubling: discrepancies between what clients and staff perceived as a viable custody plan, conflicts between social workers and attorneys serving the same family, and custody plans that depended on vulnerable new caregivers.

Staff were committed to promoting the mother's autonomy by ensuring that her views about future custody were implemented. However, at times, promoting her autonomy came into conflict with the value of beneficence, enhancing the well-being and interests of the mother and especially her children. Early discussion of cases in which clients failed to disclose to the potential new caregiver the serious nature of her illness or failed to ask the potential new caregiver whether she would agree to take on this responsibility led to the development of 10 questions to ask about the viability of custody plans (see Table 8.1).

Another ethical problem concerned the differing perceptions between social workers (and other mental health workers) and attorneys working with the same family. Social workers and attorneys, by virtue of their different training, differ in their professional codes of ethics, the legal requirements of reporting child abuse, boundaries of confidentiality, ability to work on a multidisciplinary team, the definition of who is the client (and obligations to that client), and general outlook toward their responsibilities, especially concerning the children's interests. Thus, attorneys and social workers may view the same family and the same custody plan very differently. Confused and conflicting loyalties and ambiguous responsibilities may not only make it more difficult to work on a team but also may be detrimental to the basic goal of helping a family make a viable custody plan. Discussions begun in the ethics board and with the staff were brought to a larger group, the Permanency Planning Network, which is a coalition of 50 direct service providers in the New York metropolitan area. The topic met with such a positive response that a second, more formal program was planned with a case study and a panel moderated by Alan Fleischman, M.D., of the New York Academy of Medicine. This, in turn, led to a half-day conference, attended by

TABLE 8.1 Ten Questions to Ask About the Viability of Custody Plans

---

1. Is the plan intended to be permanent?

2. Will children be placed in a household where neither the caregiver nor anyone else will subject them to abuse or neglect?

3. Has the parent discussed his or her serious illness with the proposed caregiver in realistic and not hypothetical terms, and has the caregiver agreed to the plan?

4. Is the caregiver in good enough health to care for the children?

5. Can the caregiver support the children financially, with assistance if needed and available?

6. To the extent possible, have the children participated in and agreed to the custody plan?

7. Will the children be placed with siblings or at least kept in contact with them?

8. Does the plan keep the children in familiar neighborhood and school surroundings, or, if this is not feasible, is there a plan for an orderly transition?

9. Does the proposed housing meet basic standards of safety and privacy?

10. Are there any barriers to legalizing the plan (e.g., caregivers' previous felony conviction or previous record on child abuse/neglect)?

---

more than 100 people from several states, at the New York Academy of Medicine and a publication (Retkin, Stein, & Draimin, 1997).

Finally, concerns were raised about custody plans that rely on a vulnerable new caregiver, especially an adolescent or young adult. Plans that rely on an elderly person or one with health problems can, with strong advocacy, be made more secure by obtaining community services for the elderly or disabled to assist with child care. Elderly people often have community resources, such as church groups, to assist them. This is a subject that will be increasingly important as older caregivers become overwhelmed and unable to care for more children. A related problem is placement of children with someone who also has HIV/AIDS. When a caregiver's health is fragile or the long-term ability to care for the child is questionable, we have developed two-step custody plans. That is, we arrange a second custody plan that will be implemented if the new caregiver is no longer able to care for the child.

The problems of adolescent caregivers are more complex. There are practically no community services for youth who care for their siblings. Their age peers are usually engaged in other activities and are unavailable in assisting the young caregiver. Some young new caregivers have babies of their own to care for. Although mothers recognize the burden they are imposing, many HIV+

mothers desperately want their oldest child, especially a daughter, to take care of her siblings so that they will not be separated or so they will not be placed with their father or their father's relatives. These wishes potentially place the mother's autonomy in conflict with the best interests of the new caregiver and perhaps of other children as well.

The ethics board is not only an important sounding board for resolving individual ethical dilemmas. It also has served as a broader discussion forum for Project Care, has served as a resource for other providers, and has contributed to the larger world of law and ethics.

IMPLICATIONS

Health Policy

Children of mothers with HIV/AIDS are the province of no existing social service system. They typically fall through the cracks of AIDS services because once the mother dies, all HIV-related income and assistance terminate. Because few of the children are HIV infected, they no longer qualify for the services they have come to rely on.

Caregivers are the single most underserved population we have worked with. There are few support groups, no income supports, and no services for parenting and bereavement assistance, and foster care services are unavailable unless the caregivers become foster parents, which requires that they turn custody over to the state.

These very vulnerable families rarely come into contact with an agency until they are in deep trouble. The health care system is the only service system that the mother is likely to interact with on a regular basis, but there is little effort on the part of adult practitioners to address the problems of the children. Systematic structures need to be built into adult HIV medical services that assess and assist HIV-affected children.

Cost-Effectiveness

Custody planning is labor intensive and prolonged, requiring the special expertise of attorneys to complete well. It is not an inexpensive program. Yet the consequences of not intervening are much more expensive, considering the potential future costs of foster care placement, school failure, health risk-taking behaviors (smoking, use of alcohol and drugs, early sexual debut, unprotected sexual activity), prison and institutional placement, and mental disorder. There are many opportunities for these children to begin down a wrong path, paths that lead to preventable morbidity and mortality, societal dependency, or illegal activity. The research evidence is clear that a secure placement with loving care-givers who will monitor and guide children is protective against a variety of poor child outcomes and will therefore be cost saving in the long term. Moreover, it is the decent, right thing to do—to provide a clear and reassuring answer to each child's poignant question, "Who will care for me?"

SUMMARY OF PROJECT CARE

It has been estimated that 85,000 to 125,000 children will be orphaned by HIV/AIDS by the year 2000. Many children do not have a legal custody plan in place at the time of parental death and may bounce from caregiver to caregiver without the security of a long-term placement. Project Care is a home-based intervention that assists mothers with late-stage HIV/AIDS in their decision about whether to disclose their illness to their children, provides custody planning services (including an attorney), and assesses and refers children for mental health services. After maternal death, the project assists new caregivers to make the custody plan legal, provides bereavement services, and assists children to make the difficult transition to a new family. Our goal is to reduce the risk of poor mental health outcomes in children.

REFERENCES

Achenbach, T., Howell, C., Quay, H., & Conners, C. (1991). *National survey of competencies and problems among 4-16 year olds: Parent's reports for normative and clinical samples.* Chicago: University of Chicago Press.

Alvy, K. T. (1987). *Black parenting: Strategies for training.* New York: Irvington.

Billings, A., & Moos, R. (1983). Comparisons of depressed and non-depressed parents: A social environmental perspective. *Journal of Abnormal Child Psychology, 11,* 463-485.

Black, D., & Urbanowicz, M. (1987). Family intervention with bereaved children. *Journal of Child Psychology and Psychiatry, 28,* 467-476.

Bowlby, J. (1980). *Loss.* New York: Basic Books.

Brice, C. (1982). Mourning throughout the life cycle. *American Journal of Psychoanalysis, 42,* 315-326.

Cain, A., & Fast, I. (1965). Children's disturbed reactions to parent suicide. *American Journal of Orthopsychiatry, 36,* 873-880.

Dane, B., & Miller, S. (1992). *Intervening with hidden grievers.* Westport, CT: Autumn House.

Doka, K. (1989). *Disenfranchised grief: Recognizing hidden sorrow.* Lexington, MA: Lexington Books.

Doka, K. (1994). Suffer the little children: The child and spirituality in the AIDS crisis. In B. O. Dane & C. Levine (Eds.), *AIDS and the new orphans: Coping with death* (pp. 33-41). Westport, CT: Greenwood.

Elizur, E., & Kaffman, M. (1982). Children's bereavement reactions following death of the father: II. *Journal of the American Academy of Child Psychiatry, 21*(5), 474-480.

Felner, P., Ginter, M., Boike, M., & Cowen, E. (1981). Parental death or divorce and school adjustment of young children. *American Journal of Community Psychology, 9,* 181-191.

Felner, P., Stolberg, A., & Cowen, E. (1975). Crisis events and school mental health referral patterns of young children. *Journal of Consulting and Clinical Psychology, 43,* 305-310.

Florenzano, R. (1991). Chronic mental illness in adolescence: A global overview. *Pediatrician, 18*(2), 142-149.

Furman, E. (1974). *A child's parent dies: Studies in childhood bereavement.* New Haven, CT: Yale University Press.

Furman, E. (1983). Studies in childhood bereavement. *Canadian Journal of Psychiatry, 28,* 241-247.

Furman, R. (1964). Death and the young child: Some preliminary considerations. *Psychoanalytic Study of the Child, 19,* 321-333.

Garbarino, J. (1991). What children can tell us about living in danger. *American Psychologist, 46*(4), 376-383.

Garmezy, N. (1987). Stress, competence and development. *American Journal of Orthopsychiatry, 57,* 159-185.

Garmezy, N., & Rutter, M. (1988). *Stress, coping, and development in children.* Baltimore, MD: John Hopkins University Press.

Gordon, D., Eurge, D., Hammen, C., Adrian, C., Jaenicke, C., & Hiroto, D. (1989). Observations of interactions of depressed women with their children. *American Journal of Psychiatry, 146,* 50-55.

Hammen, C., Adrian, C., Gorden, D., Burge, D., Jaenicke, C., & Hirohito, D. (1987). Children of depressed mothers: Maternal strain and symptom predictors of dysfunction. *Journal of Abnormal Psychology, 96,* 190-198.

Hammen, C., Ellicott, A., Giltin, M., & Jamison, K. (1989). Sociotropy/autonomy and vulnerability to specific life events in patients with unipolar depression and bipolar disorders. *Journal of Abnormal Psychology, 98*(2), 154-160.

Hetherington, E., & Martin, B. (1979). Family interaction. In H. C. Quay & J. C. Werry (Eds.), *Psychopathological disorders of childhood* (2nd ed., pp. 30-82). New York: John Wiley.

Hilgard, G., Newman, M., & Fisk, F. (1960). Strength of adult ego following bereavement. *American Journal of Orthopsychiatry, 30,* 788-798.

Hill, R. (1958). Generic features of families under stress. *Social Casework, 49,* 139-150.

Holahan, C., & Moos, R. (1987). Risk, resistance, and psychological distress: A longitudinal analysis with adults and children. *Journal of Abnormal Child Psychology, 96,* 3-13.

Hurrelman, K., & Losel, F. (1990). *Health hazards in adolescence.* Berlin: Walter de Gruyter.

Jaenicke, C., Hammen, C., Zupan, B., Hiroto, D., Gordon, D., Adrian, C., & Burge, D. (1987). Cognitive vulnerability in children at risk for depression. *Journal of Abnormal Child Psychology, 15*(4), 559-572.

Kaffman, M., & Elizur, E. (1983). Bereavement responses of kibbutz and nonkibbutz children following the death of a father. *Journal of Child Psychology and Psychiatry, 24,* 435-442.

Kliman, G. (1973). Facilitation of mourning during childhood. In S. C. Klagsbrun & W. Kliman (Eds.), *Preventive psychiatry: Early intervention and situational crisis management* (pp. 59-82). Philadelphia, PA: Charles Press.

Koocher, G. P. (1981). Social support and psychological distress: A longitudinal analysis. *Journal of Abnormal Psychology, 90,* 365-370.

Kranzler, E. M., Shaffer, D., Wasserman, G., & Davies, M. (1990). Early childhood bereavement. *Journal of American Academy of Child and Adolescent Psychiatry, 29*(4), 513-520.

Lonetto, R. (1980). *Children's conceptions of death.* New York: Springer.

LSC & Associates. (1993). *Report on the lives of Chicago women and children living with HIV infection.* New York: Author.

Maccoby, E. (1980). *Social development*. New York: Harcourt Brace.

Maccoby, E., & Martin, B. (1983). Socialization in the context of the family: Parent-child interaction. In E. M. Hetherington (Ed.), *Handbook of child psychology* (Vol. 4, pp. 1-102). New York: John Wiley.

Main, M., Kaplan, N., & Cassidy, J. (1985). *Security in infancy, childhood and adulthood: A move to the level of representation*. Chicago: University of Chicago Press.

Masten, A., Best, F., & Garmezy, N. (1990). Resilience and development: Contributions from children who overcome adversity. *Development and Psychopathology, 2,* 425-444.

McAdoo, H. (1982). Stress absorbing systems in Black families. *Family Relations, 31,* 479-488.

McCubbin, H., & Patterson, M. (1982). Family adaptation to crisis. In I. Hamilton & H. McCubbin (Eds.), *Family stress, coping, and social support* (pp. 26-47). Springfield, IL: Charles C Thomas.

Miller, J. (1971). Children's reactions to the death of a parent: A review of psychanalytic literature. *Journal of the American Psychoanalytic Association, 19,* 697-719.

Nagera, H. (1970). *Children's reaction to the death of important objects: A developmental approach*. New York: International University Press.

Orbach, I., Talmon, O., Kedem, P., & Har-even, D. (1987). Sequential patterns of five subconcepts of human and animal death in children. *Journal of the American Academy of Child and Adolescent Psychiatry, 26,* 579-582.

Osterweis, M., Solomon, F., & Green, M. (1984). *Bereavement: Reactions, consequences and care*. Washington, DC: National Academy Press.

Quinton, D. (1989). Adult consequences of early parental loss. *British Medical Journal, 299,* 694-695.

Rae-Grant, N., Thomas, H., Offord, D., & Boyle, M. (1989). Risk, protective factors and the prevalence of behavioral and emotional disorders in children and adolescents. *Journal of the American Academy of Child and Adolescent Psychiatry, 28*(2), 262-268.

Retkin, R., Stein, G. L., & Draimin, B. H. (1997). Attorneys and social workers collaborating in HIV care: Breaking new ground. *Fordham Urban Law Review, 24*(3), 533-565.

Reynolds, A., Weissberg, R., & Kasprow, W. (1992). Prediction of early social and academic adjustment of children from the inner city. *American Journal of Community Psychology, 20*(5), 599-624.

Rutter, M. (1966). *Children of sick parents: An environmental and psychiatric study*. London: Oxford University Press.

Rutter, M. (1979). Protective factors in children's responses to stress and disadvantage. In M. W. Kent & J. E. Rolf (Eds.), *Primary prevention in psychopathology: Social competency in children* (Vol. 3, pp. 49-74). Hanover, NH: University Press of New England.

Rutter, M. (1983). Coping and development: Some issues and some questions. In N. Garmezy & M. Rutter (Eds.), *Stress, coping and development in children* (pp. 1-42). New York: McGraw-Hill.

Rutter, M. (1985). *Child and adolescent psychiatry: Modern approaches*. Oxford, UK: Blackwell Scientific.

Rutter, M. (1987). Continuities and discontinuities from infancy. In J. D. Osofsky (Ed.), *Handbook of infant development* (2nd ed., pp. 1256-1296). New York: John Wiley.

Rutter, M., & Quinton, D. (1984). Parental psychiatric disorder: Effects on children. *Psychological Medicine, 14,* 853-880.

Sandler, I., Gersten, J., Reynolds, F., Fallgren, C., & Ramirez, P. (1988). Using theory and data to plan support interventions. In B. H. Gottlieb (Ed.), *Marshalling social support* (pp. 53-83). Newbury Park, CA: Sage.

Sekaer, C. (1987). Towards a definition of childhood mourning. *American Journal of Psychotherapy, 41,* 201-219.

Siegel, K., & Freund, B. (1995). Parental loss in latency-aged children. In B. Dane & C. Levine (Eds.), *AIDS and the new orphans: Coping with death*. Wesport, CT: Greenwood.

Siegel, K., & Gorey, E. (1994). Childhood bereavement due to parental death from AIDS. *Developmental and Behavioral Pediatrics, 15*(3), S66-S70.

Van Eerdewegh, M., Bieri, M., Parilla, R., & Clayton, P. (1982). The bereaved child. *British Journal of Psychiatry, 140*, 23-29.

Wallerstein, J., & Kelly, J. (1980). *Surviving the breakup*. New York: Basic Books.

Werner, E., & Smith, R. (1982). *Vulnerable but not invincible: A study of resilient children*. New York: McGraw-Hill.

Wortman, C., & Silver, R. C. (1989). The myths of coping with loss. *Journal of Consulting and Clinical Psychology, 57*(3), 349-357.

Chapter 9

Helping Adolescents and Parents With AIDS to Cope Effectively With Daily Life

Mary Jane Rotheram-Borus   Marguerita Lightfoot

University of California, Los Angeles

Teresa is from a Dominican family and is the oldest of five children. She was 17 when her mother disclosed to her that she had AIDS. At the time, she had no idea her mother was sick and therefore was very shocked. Teresa says she was glad her mother told her she had AIDS; however, she wished she had not been the only one of the siblings who was informed. She did not know anyone else who had a family member living with AIDS, and although she tried to keep it a secret, it was very difficult for her. Teresa found it hard to concentrate at school and felt socially isolated, feeling that no one understood her, her struggles, or her pain. She felt she needed to talk to someone about her mother's condition, so she told a cousin. She later regretted this decision because the cousin told her own mother (Teresa's aunt), and Teresa's aunt told others. Teresa's mother was very angry at her for not "keeping the secret." Again, Teresa felt alone while continuing to feel very uncer-

AUTHORS' NOTE: This chapter was completed with the support of National Institute of Mental Health Grant 1 ROI MH49958-04 to the first author. We thank the parents, caregivers, and adolescents who participated in this study, as well as those who assisted in it, including the staff of The Family Center/MHRA and Housing Works, our interviewers and group leaders, and Coleen Cantwell, Tri Cisek, Betty Crenshaw, Jen Elliott, Hsin-Hsin Foo, Laura Franzke, Nionne James, Kris Langabeer, Noelle R. Leonard, Patrice Lewis, David Litke, Tanko Mohammed, Laura Rosen, and Nim Tottenham. For more information about the intervention, please contact Dr. Mary Jane Rotheram-Borus, Professor, Director, Clinical Research Center, UCLA Neuropsychiatric Institute, 10920 Wilshire Boulevard, Suite 350, Los Angeles, CA 90024-6521; e-mail: mjrotheram@npimain.medsch.ucla.edu.

tain about her future. During this time, Teresa also had the added burden of being told by her mother that if anything "happened to her," she wanted Teresa to take care of her younger siblings. At the age of 17, Teresa knew that she needed to take care of not only her mother but also her younger siblings as well.

Now, at age 22, Teresa lives with her husband and 1-year-old daughter. Since her mother Laura died of AIDS a year ago, her two younger sisters, ages 9 and 6, have also lived with her, and for a brief period, her 17-year-old brother, Anthony, lived with her. The family lives in a two-bedroom apartment in New York City.

The number of families affected by HIV/AIDS is increasing. Approximately 650,000 to 900,000 Americans are living with HIV/AIDS (Centers for Disease Control and Prevention [CDC], 1999), and a growing proportion of new HIV infections occurs among women. These women and men (typically injecting drug users) are likely to have children whose lives are affected daily by their parents' HIV infection. With the introduction of antiretroviral therapies, persons living with HIV are likely to live longer (Kaplan, Masur, Jaffe, & Holmes, 1995; Sharp, 1996). Therefore, parents with AIDS will have to cope for many years with many physical health symptoms, caring for their children and family, being identified in their community as having a stigmatizing illness (Herek & Capitanio, 1993), and knowing that they have a life-threatening illness. Parents with AIDS typically do not live in two-parent, middle-class families but are more likely to be struggling financially (often on public assistance because of their health), are single parents, and involved in substance use subcultures (either from their own behavior or that of their partners). Children are more likely than their peers to experience higher levels of depression, anxiety, and social withdrawal (see Sandler et al., 1992, for a review). The goal of this chapter is to describe an intervention designed to help parents and their adolescent children cope with AIDS and the stressors associated with HIV, both while the parent is alive and after the parent dies.

As Teresa's story illustrates, having a parent living with AIDS has a pervasive impact on a child's life. A parent's illness and death during adolescence result in a serious life crisis, one that occurs at the same time that the youth faces the challenge of forming a personal identity, physical changes brought on by adolescence, fundamental shifts in his or her ability to cognitively process information, shifting peer groups, and societal expectations regarding the youth's social roles (Balk, 1991; Osterweis, Solomon, & Green, 1987; Rotheram-Borus, Miller, Murphy, & Draimin, 1997). Grieving for a parent can impede the youth's successful completion of these developmental tasks and interfere with a successful transition to adulthood (Balk, 1991). Teresa was required to "grow up too fast" and did not have the opportunity to focus on her own adolescent developmental tasks but instead had to focus on family tasks. Teresa's accelerated maturity led her to feel socially isolated, stressed, and as if her life course was no longer under her own control.

Clinicians' work with bereaved youth lead us to expect that when a parent dies, the adolescent's life is likely to be significantly disrupted for at least 1 year and typically for 3 years, with grief reactions continuing throughout their lifetime, particularly at anniversaries and special events (Osterweis et al., 1987). However, after interviewing adolescents in about 150 families in which the parent has died from AIDS, Murphy, Lightfoot, and Rotheram-Borus (1999) found that the youth report depression and distress in the period right after the parent dies but appear to do well within about 6 months. Despite the difficulties inherent in bereavement, there may be positive aspects to coping with death at an early age. Some youth report that the loss of a family member gives them a deeper appreciation of life, helps them show greater caring for their loved ones and experience stronger bonds with their parents, and results in greater personal emotional strength (Oltjenbruns, 1991). It may be that tasks such as selecting a career, establishing an intimate romantic relationship, and parenting one's own children are the areas that are most likely to be affected by having a parent die.

Parents with AIDS must make many decisions about how to deal with illness-related challenges, particularly disclosure, custody, and coping with stigma. Most parents find out that they are HIV seropositive about 1 year before being diagnosed with AIDS (Wortley et al., 1995). The parent then must decide how and when to disclose his or her HIV/AIDS diagnosis and whether and how to discuss the implications of the illness over time with their children. In 1994, parents living with AIDS could anticipate that they might die within about 2 years after learning of their diagnosis. Now life spans are likely to be much longer, and an HIV diagnosis may mean living with a chronic illness, further complicating the decisions about whether to disclose their serostatus to their children.

Furthermore, a viable custody plan may serve to prevent negative outcomes in their children. Children of parents who die unexpectedly without having made custody plans are at higher risk for negative outcomes compared to prepared children (West, Sandler, Pillow, Baca, & Gersten, 1991), and the legal complications are greater (Levine & Stein, 1994). However, a parent living with AIDS may not want or know how to deal with these issues. Making custody plans indicates that the parent living with AIDS recognizes that he or she may die. Especially since the introduction of antiretroviral medications, parents living with AIDS can anticipate a longer life, and therefore the making of custody plans may seem less important. Parents living with AIDS who have a history of substance abuse (84% of a sample of parents that participated in our program) have historically feared interacting with the legal system; lawyers and social service agencies may have attempted to take children away from them in the past. To seek help from the legal system is often not an easy task. These issues are reflected in the case of Rolanda.

Rolanda is a 35-year-old African American woman who was diagnosed with AIDS after the birth of her third child, Jameel. Jameel was tested for HIV at birth as part of routine procedures and was found to be seropositive. At the time of her child's birth, Rolanda's blood tests showed that her immune system was already significantly compromised (e.g., she had a T cell count below 200), even though she had not experienced AIDS-related opportunistic infections or symptoms. Rolanda held a full-time job in an office but later had to stop working due to the emergence of AIDS-related symptoms. Consequently, she not only had to struggle with her shattered image of herself as a healthy person but also with her decreasing ability to provide for her family. Rolanda went on permanent disability and experienced a significant reduction in socioeconomic status. Although many infants either seroconvert or do not show health problems for many years, Rolanda's baby Jameel was quite sick throughout his infancy and died at the age of 2. Rolanda was devastated by Jameel's death and suffered a debilitating depression for a long time afterward. Rolanda not only had to grieve the death of her youngest child from AIDS but also had to continue to struggle with the challenge of raising her two other seronegative children.

One of Rolanda's primary concerns when she was first diagnosed with AIDS was that her family would be devastated if they were to find out. She partly feared that her children would reject her, perhaps blaming her for contracting HIV. She also wanted to protect her children's innocence; she wanted them to "have a normal childhood" but feared that the news of her illness would burden them. Her two older boys, ages 10 and 13, were well adjusted, active in sports, and doing well in school. Following her own positive test, she knew the older boys should be tested for HIV at their next medical checkup. However, Rolanda dreaded the disclosure of her and Jameel's status to the family doctor, who happened to be a family friend.

Rolanda felt that her AIDS diagnosis was very stigmatizing. She perceived that not disclosing her HIV status to her children would shield them from experiencing negative reactions from others. In the face of family upheaval and multiple stressors, Rolanda decided not to disclose her HIV status to her children. She strongly believed, or wanted to believe, that her children were unaware about her current health problems, particularly about her having AIDS.

AIDS is a relatively unique infection whose disease course is unpredictable, and, therefore parents living with AIDS do not receive much guidance from persons with other diseases or illnesses concerning complex decisions regarding custody and disclosure. Ultimately, only Rolanda could make these decisions. As clinicians, we have observed many families in which disclosing had disastrous consequences for the family (e.g., families evicted from apartments, children isolated at school, parents fired from jobs), observations that are similar to other researchers (Armistead, Klein, Forehand, & Wierson, 1997). Especially after her baby died, Rolanda's disclosure of her serostatus may not have been beneficial. Even trained mental health professions may be unsure how to advise families such as Rolanda's because little is known about the impact of disclosure on the child's present and future adjustment or on subsequent adjustment. A study conducted by our research team found that adolescents who knew about their parents' HIV infection were more likely to engage in sexual risk acts and report conduct problems at school and with peers (Rotheram-Borus, Draimin, Reid, & Murphy, 1997). In general, the field lacks clear guidelines regarding disclosure issues.

Families need a forum in which they can discuss disclosure, custody, and other HIV-related issues and decide on the best course of action for their family. This chapter describes an intervention that was designed for parents living with HIV, their adolescent children, and subsequent caregivers of the youth once the parent has died. The intervention is based on cognitive-behavioral principles. The primary goal of the intervention is to reduce long-term negative social, behavioral, and mental health consequences associated with parental death for adolescents by increasing the parent's and adolescent's coping skills.

GOALS FOR PROJECT TALC (TEENS AND ADULTS LEARNING TO COMMUNICATE)

The intervention was designed to help parents make decisions regarding disclosure and custody, as well as to increase a family's ability to maintain positive daily routines while the parent is ill. Coping skills—the ways an individual and a family deal with stress—are important for families adjusting to HIV. The coping skills of parents living with AIDS, their adolescent children, and other family members are intertwined, influencing and reinforcing each other.

Goals for Parents

Therefore, to facilitate their adolescent's long-term adjustment, Project TALC enables the parents to

1. recognize and label their feelings and establish and maintain emotional self-control with children when distressed by their own illness and imminent death;
2. manage the daily family routines in an effective fashion by establishing rules regarding positive interactions;
3. problem solve stressful situations, particularly any arising from stigmatization of HIV;

4. recognize useful styles of coping and identify when a coping style is not working well;

5. maintain their roles as caretakers, rather than becoming dependent on their adolescent children to become the family's caretakers;

6. help provide skills to their children to avoid substance use and HIV and to do well in school;

7. decide when, how, and to whom to disclose their illness; and

8. make custody arrangements for their children.

Goals for Adolescents

Adolescents who attend the intervention know of their parents' HIV serostatus. Parents living with AIDS can attend without allowing their children to attend or without disclosing to their children but not vice versa. To help the adolescents adjust well over the long term and to help their family as their parents become increasingly ill, the intervention helps the adolescents to

1. recognize and label their feelings and establish and maintain emotional self-control in stressful situations;
2. begin to explore the youth's personal identity and the social roles that the youth assumes in the family and with peers;
3. identify a set of family rules that help youth and the person with AIDS (PWA) accomplish daily tasks (such as cleaning the house) without high tension and frequent negative interactions;
4. maintain a healthy lifestyle that does not include substance use, unprotected sex, high rates of truancy, or contact with the criminal justice system; and
5. cope with symptoms of emotional distress concerning their PWA and their own future.

The intervention is based on the assumption that a series of critical behavioral skills underlies the parent with AIDS' successful management of his or her infection, coping with daily stressors, completing parenting tasks such as disclosure of illness and custody planning, and providing support for each other. A skill is the ability to perform an action at a reasonable level of competency. The skills are reflected in the actions that participants take, not only when confronted with problems but also when they take charge of their lives and are working on their own goals. Skills are categorized as intellectual (solving a problem), emotional (managing anger), social (solving a family conflict), and physical (putting on a condom correctly). For example, coping with negative emotional states such as anxiety and depression is a skill that assists in resolving problems (e.g., who will take care of the children after the parent's death?). Facing problems by taking action, seeking social support, and having hope or spirituality are positive styles of coping, whereas problem avoidance, self-destructive, or depressive styles may not only be ineffective but also compound the problems (Monat & Lazarus, 1991).

Choosing whether to disclose one's serostatus and custody planning are two primary goals related to coping with HIV. For example, gathering information regarding the existing legal and personal options for potential custody arrangements is necessary for effective custody planning (Draimin, 1993). Although the prevention program focuses predominantly on family issues, implementing condom use as a means of preventing further transmission of HIV is also an issue for seropositive parents and is addressed.

PHASES AND SESSIONS FOR PROJECT TALC

In the coping-skills intervention, Project TALC has three separate phases related to the stages of the PWA's illness and involves sessions in which the parent and adolescent meet together and separately (Rotheram-Borus, Miller, et al., 1997). Each phase is composed of 8 to 16 sessions, with each session lasting 2 hours. Each phase of the intervention addresses different issues with different domains of knowledge, attitudes, and skills relevant to the parent's illness. The intervention is designed to be delivered in two sessions per day (e.g., 9 a.m. to 4 p.m. on Saturdays, with one 2-hour session in the morning and another 2-hour session in the afternoon [following lunch]). Table 9.1 summarizes the sessions in each phase of the intervention.

Phase I: Taking Care of Myself

In Phase I, parents meet in small groups without their adolescent children. During this phase, parents use their skills in coping with their illness, make decisions about and build skills around disclosure of serostatus, and begin thinking about their children's future needs.

Before parents can help their adolescents adjust to their illness, they must themselves adjust to living with AIDS. Thus, the eight sessions in Phase I have the following objectives: (a) to enhance the PWA's ability to cope in a positive manner, despite the negative emotions generated by having AIDS; (b) to assist the PWAs in finding meaning, maintaining control, and repairing self-esteem in response to their illness; (c) to assist the PWAs in making and implementing decisions about disclosing that they have AIDS to their children, family, and others; and (d) to help them establish a future orientation in coping with their children.

TABLE 9.1 Sessions in Each of Three Phases of the Intervention

Parent With AIDS	
Phase I: Taking Care of Myself	
Session 1	Coping with illness
Session 2	Coping with fear
Session 3	Coping with anger
Session 4	Coping with sadness
Session 5	Coping with the meaning of my illness
Session 6	Deciding to disclose
Session 7	Disclosing
Session 8	Planning for the future

	Parent With AIDS	*Adolescent*
Phase II: Illness Phase		
Session 1	Awareness of my children's needs	Making sense of my PWA's illness
Session 2	Caring for my children	Disclosure of PWA having AIDS
Session 3	Making custody arrangements	Dealing with stigma
Session 4	Starting my custody plan	Dealing with fear
Session 5	Listening to my children	Coping with sad feelings
Session 6	Sharing with my children	Coping with anger
Session 7	Reducing problem behavior	Acting constructively
Session 8	Creating a positive home	Creating a positive home
Session 9	Resolving home conflicts (Part 1)	Resolving home conflicts (Part 1)
Session 10	Resolving home conflicts (Part 2)	Resolving home conflicts (Part 2)
Session 11	Selecting a custodian	Selecting a custodian
Session 12	Dealing with drugs and alcohol	Dealing with drugs and alcohol
Session 13	Preventing pregnancy/fatherhood	Preventing pregnancy/fatherhood
Session 14	Making a custody plan	Encouraging safer sex
Session 15	Encouraging safer sex	Encouraging safer sex
Session 16	Setting legacy and the youth's goals	Setting my future goals

TABLE 9.1 Continued

Caregiver and Adolescent (Except Where Noted)	*Adolescent*
Phase III: Adjustment Phase	
Session 1 Youth and caregiver needs	
Session 2 Caregiver's role and expectations	
Session 3 Dealing with loss and grief (Part 1)	
Session 4 Raising an adolescent (caregiver only)	Planning for my future (Part 1)
Session 5 Dealing with loss and grief (Part 2)	
Session 6 Improving communication (Part 1)	
Session 7 Helping someone cope with loss	
Session 8 Improving communication (Part 2)	
Session 9 Caregiver support (caregiver only)	Planning for my future (Part 2)
Session 10 Dealing with anger	
Session 11 Coping with sadness	
Session 12 Dealing with problem behavior (caregiver only)	Dealing with fear
Session 13 Safer sex and reducing drug use	
Session 14 Resolving conflicts	
Session 15 Creating a positive atmosphere	
Session 16 Looking to the future together	
Young-Adult Version (Bereaved Youth Only)	
Phase III: Adjustment Phase	
Session 1 How have things been going?	
Session 2 Planning for the future	
Session 3 Dealing with loss and grief	
Session 4 Getting help and support	
Session 5 Dealing with loss and grief	
Session 6 Coping with loss and helping others cope	
Session 7 Planning for my future	

TABLE 9.1 Continued

Young-Adult Version (Bereaved Youth Only)	
Phase III: Adjustment Phase	
Session 8	Communicating effectively
Session 9	Dealing with anger
Session 10	Relationships and sex (Part 1)
Session 11	Relationships and sex (Part 2)
Session 12	Coping with sadness
Session 13	Making decisions about pregnancy and parenthood
Session 14	Dealing with fear
Session 15	Reducing substance use
Session 16	Looking to the future

There are three major themes addressed in the eight sessions of the first phase. First, a search for meaning and a new social identity are initiated to help parents answer the question, "Why did this happen to me, and how significant is this situation for me?" The impact of the parent's identity as living as a parent with AIDS is explored, and the new social roles and responsibilities associated with this identity are explored. Second, parents must develop a sense of personal control by confronting these questions: "How can I manage what has happened to me? Can I prevent it from getting worse or happening to someone else I love? Can I manage daily life tasks? Can I parent my child?" Therefore, managing distressing emotions is crucial, and the intervention employs cognitive-behavioral techniques to enhance parents' skills for handling strong negative emotions. Third, the intervention helps parents repair the damage to their self-esteem that is inevitable when confronting a life-threatening situation, especially HIV infection. Therefore, the intervention reinforces parents' strengths, including helping parents perceive their interpersonal strengths.

Juanita participated in most of the sessions in Phase I of Project TALC and engaged well with other group members. Juanita expressed concern about the present well-being of her children and for "protecting" them from her AIDS diagnosis. Juanita lived in fear of the stigma and potential prejudice that her AIDS diagnosis posed; she herself held many misconceptions and misinformation about HIV and AIDS. Juanita also feared that her children would blame her and "hate" her for contracting HIV. During the course of the intervention, it was clear that Juanita herself harbored intense guilt about contracting HIV and "killing Ortiz," one of her children who became HIV infected. Juanita also expressed feelings of helplessness and uselessness because she was no longer working. Her personal identity was built on the foundation that she was a strong and independent woman. However, her current lifestyle was in sharp contrast to her perception of herself.

The emphasis in the eight sessions of Phase I is on PWAs taking care of themselves and coping with the feelings, demands, and tasks that living with AIDS imposes. The first session helps the PWA recognize that other families are experiencing similar challenges. This session was particularly important for Juanita. By hearing the experiences of other group members, she was able to feel that others understood her conflicts and that she was not alone. For Juanita, like many PWAs, this was the first time she was able to express her feelings about her struggles of living with AIDS.

The next three sessions of Phase I enhance recognition of feelings and control of emotional expression. Parents are encouraged to express their feelings and learn techniques for coping with fear, anger, and sadness. For example, in Session 2, parents tell each other what their worst fears are, thereby normalizing their feelings and creating a supportive environment. The parents share ways to deal with their fears and are taught relaxation techniques. When the group confronted anger, Juanita was able to express for the first time her anger toward her deceased husband, who had infected her. Using the empty chair technique, Juanita cried, yelled, and cursed at the empty chair about the pain that contracting HIV had caused her and her children. This was very cathartic for Juanita; she later characterized the experience as having "a weight being lifted from me." Not only was the expression of "never-acknowledged" emotions therapeutic for the parents, but receiving support and recognizing the association between these feelings and behaviors also allowed the parents to gain self-awareness of their behavioral styles and gain motivation to deal constructively with difficult feelings for themselves and their children. Once the parents express their feelings and learn techniques to cope with the feelings, Session 5 focuses on the parents clarifying their life values, developing positive meaning about their illness, identifying areas in which they could exercise self-control, and creating visions of their future. These activities help parents develop a new social identity as a parent living with AIDS and identify social roles to cope more effectively with family and friends to meet their long-term goals.

The PWAs must make a series of decisions about how much responsibility to place on their adolescent children. Many of the youth in families with a PWA are forced to assume adult roles, a process called *parentification* (e.g., maintaining household chores, giving advice to parents, parenting others). Adolescents are not typically emotionally or developmentally ready to manage these roles successfully. In our sample of PWAs, more household chores were done by daughters with PWAs and both daughters and sons of substance-abusing parents (Stein, Riedel, & Rotheram-Borus, 1999). Parents with more severe physical symptoms and illness had children who were more likely to give advice and reverse roles with their parents. Giving advice was also more common among children with younger parents and male adolescents.

The impact of parentification on adjustment also was examined over 6 months. Performing more household chores predicted greater internalizing symptoms of emotional distress among adolescents; giving advice predicted more sexual behavior and higher self-esteem. Adolescent role reversals predicted more alcohol and marijuana use among adolescents. These results suggested that parentification is not beneficial; therefore, our intervention focused on helping parents maintain their roles and generate family rules that left responsibility and control of daily routines with the parent (Stein et al., 1999).

Sessions 6 through 8 focus on skills and decisions regarding disclosure of illness. Problem-solving skills are introduced as a general tool for PWAs in making decisions about whether to disclose their HIV status and to whom, when, and how to tell their HIV status. Role-playing, modeling, and examining anticipated consequences around the issues of disclosure of HIV status assist parents in making decisions about disclosure. In addition, the parents' plans and goals for their relationships with their children, family members, friends, and partners are explored. Scripts for positive self-instructional thoughts help prepare the parents for disappointments and for coping with strong emotional reactions to anticipated loss by their children.

In our study of parents with AIDS and their adolescent children, both mothers (87%) and fathers were significantly more likely to disclose their serostatus to adolescents (73%), compared to younger children (23%). However, only 44% of PWAs disclosed their serostatus to all their children; 11% disclosed to none. Adolescents informed of their PWAs' serostatus engaged in more sexual risk acts, smoked more cigarettes, reported more severe substance use, and reported greater emotional distress than uninformed adolescents. One year later, about 75% of PWAs had disclosed their serostatus to all children in the family. At 2 years, about 85% had disclosed to all of their adolescents. Therefore, although we focused on disclosure within our intervention, it appears that eventually almost all families disclosed parental serostatus.

In planning for custody for their children, parents confront their mortality and loss of family. Turning to prayer and spiritual beliefs was one strategy parents used in our study to help provide meaning to the implementation of the custody and future plans for their children. This was particularly difficult for Juanita because it required her to explore what it means to "protect" her children from AIDS, given that she knew they were going to eventually grieve her "unexpected" death. Juanita had been struggling with disclosure to her children; she had not told her children about her HIV status and was very fearful regarding the children's reaction. However, she was also forced to confront how she and her children were going to deal with the reality of her deteriorating health. Rolanda was able to express in the Project TALC intervention group her thoughts and feelings about disclosing to her children while receiving feedback and support in a safe environment. Phase I ends with identifying strategies for creating a positive future for the PWAs and their adolescents.

Phase II: Illness Phase

In Phase II, youth who know their parents' HIV serostatus begin attending the intervention, first in small groups with other youth and then by joining parents in a small group. In the youth groups, the youth first work together to enhance their ability to cope with their parents' illness, deal with stigma about AIDS, and make decisions about when and to whom to disclose their parents' HIV status. Youth and PWAs also learn relaxation skills and how to set and meet goals for the future. In the parents' group, parents focus on the future, including walking through the steps of making a viable custody plan and building skills to address the psychological barriers to custody planning. In the adolescents' group, there is greater emphasis on the avoidance of problem behaviors (sexual risk, substance use, truancy, criminal justice contact, illegal activities). PWAs also learn how to help their children avoid problem behaviors. Finally, at the end of Phase II, PWAs and youth work together to establish positive daily routines and to finalize the custody plan.

Both parents and youth attend the 16 sessions in Phase II; parents and adolescents attend 7 sessions separately and 9 sessions together. Because the intervention deals specifically with HIV/AIDS issues, only youth who have been told by their parents that the parent is HIV+ can participate in this part of Project TALC. Youth who are not informed about their parents' illness should be provided with referrals to other types of programs for families. Although they would not receive assistance specific to their parents' HIV status, the youth could benefit from therapeutic support. Parents may attend the group workshops regardless of whether they have disclosed to their children.

At the time PWAs participated in our study of Project TALC, the PWAs were already seriously ill and experiencing further declines in physical health. When PWAs are ill, their adolescent children face many challenges: their own emotional reactions to their PWAs' illness, anticipatory loss of their parents, fear for their own futures, decisions about disclosure to their friends and family, coping with stigma, responding to increased care demands for younger family members as well as the PWAs, and planning for their own futures. Thus, the second phase of Project TALC focuses on the social identities, rules, roles, and skills (behavioral, affective, knowledge) required to facilitate adolescent behavioral, social, and mental health adjustment.

Teresa participated in Project TALC for 4 years, first with her mother and brother (Phase II) and then as a bereaved youth and new caregiver (Phase III). Teresa's mother, Laura, disclosed her HIV status to Teresa when she was 17 years old. Her brother Miguel, who is a year younger than Teresa, was told more than a year later, and her brother Anthony was told only a few months before Laura died, when he was 15. Teresa's two sisters do not know what caused their mother's death. Teresa now has custody of her two sisters, and, similar to her mother, Teresa does not think her sisters need to know the nature of their mother's illness.

First Laura and then Teresa and Miguel participated in the Project TALC groups. Anthony did not attend because Laura had decided not to tell him that she had HIV, and thus he was ineligible. Teresa reports that the groups made it easier to talk about "what was going on with me" and allowed the youth and their mother to plan for the future. Laura had spoken to Teresa and Miguel previously about caring for the younger siblings if she became too sick, but while attending the Project TALC group, Laura realized that she needed to make legal arrangements for their care. She planned to go to court and start the paperwork, but because she was still feeling strong and healthy, she put it off, feeling there was no need to rush. She also felt somewhat superstitious about making the plans legal, as though doing so would hasten her death. She hoped that her spoken request would be sufficient if anything happened. These issues were addressed in the program because other mothers had similar experiences, and at the end of the group cycle, she made an appointment with a lawyer to discuss her options.

Teresa was glad she was told that her mother was terminally ill because knowing that one day she would probably have to take care of her siblings made her more responsible. For example, she made sure she went to school and tried hard to be a good role model for her siblings. She was glad that her mother trusted her enough to tell her that she had AIDS, although Teresa thinks she would have guessed it even if her mother had only told her she was sick. Knowing that her mother was ill helped Teresa prepare herself mentally for her mother's death.

Adolescents such as Teresa deal with the issues of coping with their parents' illness, making home life better, avoiding risk behaviors in daily settings at school and in the neighborhood, and planning for their future living situation and personal goals. To cope with the impact of their parents' illness in Project TALC, youth explore the meaning of the illness in their own lives. For Teresa, this meant examining both concrete and abstract issues. Concretely, Teresa had to become more responsible and try to be a role model and mother figure to her other siblings. She also had to come to terms with abstract issues such as her feelings regarding her mother's past behavior and her mother's responsibility for their present life situation.

From this exploration, youth begin to confront the issues of disclosure and stigma. In Sessions 2 and 3, concrete problems are addressed, such as making decisions about disclosure of the parents' AIDS diagnosis and coping with stigma. Youth are taught problem-solving techniques to assist them in making their decisions regarding disclosure of their parents' illness. Youth practice confronting situations in which the stigma of being a member of an AIDS household is an issue. The youth also learn to cope by rehearsing internal dialogues and using techniques, such as relaxation and deep breathing, to reduce their emotional distress. Teresa expressed fear about the anticipated reactions of others on telling them of her mother's illness. She was afraid that her family would desert her and she would be ridiculed. Not only did Teresa have her own fears to cope with, but she also carried the fears of her mother, who insisted that Teresa keep "the secret." Teresa's fears were apparent in her reluctance to disclose and her impulsive disclosure to her cousin. During the intervention, Teresa was able to think through the benefits and consequences of disclosing and, in this process, was able to choose whom to disclose to. Thinking through the disclosure also allowed Teresa to obtain the support she needed.

Developing emotional self-control around and increasing comfort in expressing fear, sadness, and anger are the focus of Sessions 4 through 7. These sessions also emphasize self-esteem, self-efficacy, and believing that one can survive difficult times. Youth explore their feelings through cognitive-behavioral exercises. For example, youth are asked to write their fears on index cards, share them with others in the group, and problem solve dealing with those fears. One of Teresa's biggest fears was that she was not going to be able to properly care for her brother and sisters. As Teresa and the group processed this fear, Teresa was able to identify how the fear played out in her everyday life. For example, Teresa would be hypervigilant concerning her siblings' appearances. This resulted in daily conflicts between Teresa and her siblings, who would subsequently avoid Teresa. Teresa would then feel angry and hurt by her siblings' actions. The group was supportive in helping Teresa realize her limitations, identify her unrealistic expectations, and problem solve ways to keep her behavior from being fueled by her fear.

While the youth meet, the parents meet separately and focus on their children's needs and plan for the future. Sessions 1 through 4 of this module focus on custody planning, an essential area for effective future outcomes for children. In our study of PWAs and their adolescents, most PWAs (80%) discussed custody plans; however, only 30% initiated legal plans, typically for younger children. Legal custody arrangements were not associated with adolescent adjustment at recruitment or follow-up (Rotheram-Borus, Draimin, et al., 1997). About one third of PWAs (31%) in both conditions had made custody plans for at least one adolescent at the time of recruitment (the baseline interview), and 28% had made custody plans for all adolescents in the family. At 1 year, 54% had made custody plans for at least one adolescent child (50.5% for all adolescent children). Two years following recruitment, 67% of the PWAs had made plans for at least one adolescent, and 63% made plans for all of their adolescent children.

The intervention sessions are constructed to assist parents in building the skills to overcome psychological and legal barriers to custody planning. For example, in Session 2, mothers increase their feelings of comfort with the idea of making a plan, outline the pros and cons of making a plan, and identify characteristics of a desirable new caregiver. In subsequent sessions, parents obtain information about the types of legal options available to them (e.g., guardianship or kinship foster care). In a later session, a lawyer, who is an expert in custody planning issues, is invited to the group to answer questions. Parents also work toward solving problems that arise in planning, such as not having anyone to approach to take custody of their children or making decisions about splitting up their children.

Phase II also focuses on improving the daily interactions between the parents and youth. Parents and youth meet together to improve their relationship and home life and to make a plan together for the future. In Sessions 8 through 16, creating a positive atmosphere at home is accomplished through identifying strengths in the family's heritage and personal history. Parents and youth also identify ways in which to create a positive home atmosphere, resolve conflicts at home, and reduce youth's potential drug and alcohol use, HIV risk acts, and pregnancy or fatherhood.

A major focus of these sessions is on improving communication by teaching active listening, expression of positive feelings, and management of behavior problems. In addition, the sessions address the PWAs' legacy for their youth (e.g., values and mementos of their life together), youth's acceptance of the legacies, youth's sharing of their goals for their future, and the PWAs' endorsements of confidence in their children's competence and shared love. This part of the intervention is extremely important to the families. Teresa and her mother, Laura, found this part of Project TALC invaluable. Although Teresa and Laura communicated with each other fairly well, they avoided certain issues. Although they had a custody plan, they never talked about Laura's death. During these sessions, Laura was able to express her desires for her funeral. Teresa shared her hopes, dreams, and fears for the future and received reassurance from her mother. Simultaneously, Teresa was able to reassure her mother about her ability to survive. Laura could then create a comforting picture of how and what her child would grow to be. The intervention cycle ends with a graduation ceremony in which participants are given a certificate of appreciation and speak individually about their experiences in the program.

Phase III: Adjustment Phase

In Phase III, youth whose parents have died attend the intervention. There are two versions of Phase III: one for bereaved adolescents living independently (young-adult group) and another for youth living with new caregivers (Gwadz et al., 1999; Rotheram-Borus, Miller, et al., 1997). The goals and content of these two versions are similar, although the young-adult group emphases a young person's adjustment and long-term goals rather than caregiver-youth relationships.

The adolescent has four primary tasks to complete in the adjustment phase: (a) to grieve; (b) to participate in building a new, positive family unit; (c) to prevent lingering depressive feelings and negative emotions from becoming ongoing problem behaviors; and (d) to plan for the future. Caregivers have an independent set of goals: (a) to grieve, if they were close to the deceased; (b) to support their adolescents in coping with the loss and in making new adjustments; and (c) to obtain social support from other caregivers while confronting unfamiliar parenting demands.

In May 1997 and prior to an appointment with a lawyer, Laura (Teresa's mother) suddenly was admitted to the hospital with pneumonia, where she remained until her death in July. Unfortunately for Teresa, there was no time to grieve. At the funeral she learned that her stepfather intended to obtain custody of her two younger sisters. Teresa had no knowledge of the legal system, including where she should go to ensure that her mother's wishes were respected, but she knew she needed to act, even though she was in shock from the loss.

The day after the funeral, Teresa was in family court, where she applied for custody of her sisters and brother. This custody battle caused problems with other family members as well, as people started to take sides. However, she successfully obtained custody of her three siblings, and they moved into her one-bedroom apartment where her husband and newborn daughter also lived. Her brother, Miguel, who had agreed to help with their care, lived separately and did not go to court with her on that day, although he said he would be as supportive as possible.

Teresa truly appreciated the opportunities she had to spend with her mother during Project TALC, especially the time spent planning for life after Laura's death. Teresa said, "If the plans are all made ahead of time, the children feel more stable, more secure. Mommy's not here, but she fixed everything." However, Teresa says she wishes they had made additional preparations. For example, according to Teresa, although it was helpful that she made a custody plan and communicated it to family members, it would have been better if she had completed the legal documents and saved some money to help pay for the care of her siblings.

Laura thought the children would continue getting the same level of benefits after she passed away, but this was not the case. They get a little each month, mostly Social Security survivor benefits because Laura worked in the past. Teresa, her husband, her daughter, her brother, and her two sisters live primarily on her husband's salary, and finances are tight.

Although she wanted to care for her siblings and thought she was the best person to do so, some problems occurred. Not surprisingly, 17-year-old Anthony saw her as a peer rather than an authority figure, and so her attempts to discipline him were generally unsuccessful. He started skipping school and staying out late. Eventually, everyone agreed that having three children, one teenager, and two adults in a one-bedroom apartment was intolerable. Teresa particularly missed having "alone time" with her husband. They barely had time to adjust to their new roles as parents.

In Phase III, youth and caregivers engage in activities to grieve and to establish a supportive new family environment. In the first session, caregivers and youth meet separately to discuss the changes that have occurred in their lives and how their relationships with their new families are developing. In Session 2, caregivers and youth meet together to discuss the changing nature of their roles vis-à-vis each other—for example, from being the indulgent grandparent to the strict disciplinarian or the spoiled and perfect niece to acting-out youth. Caregivers and youth also learn how to clearly communicate their expectations in behavioral terms. In Session 4, participants begin to work on grief, starting with identifying normal grieving processes, talking about the deceased parent, expressing feelings about the deceased parent, and identifying concerns about the grieving process. Youth and their new guardians share mementos from the parent and special events. In Session 5, caregivers and youth focus again on grief, continuing to talk about the deceased parent and identify what can be helpful to the grieving youth. Caregivers build skills to help youth deal with grief while identifying ways they can build their own support systems. Youth work on identifying what would be helpful to them in dealing with grief. Other sessions focus on enhancing coping (e.g., with anger and sadness) and on building and improving the new family relationship, as well as looking to the future. Emotional expressiveness and self-control are revisited. Coping with fear, sadness, and anger is taught using the reality of the recent death as the stimulus event.

Consistent with the model presented to PWAs and youth, the caregivers and youth are presented with a model of a positive relationship of appreciating, listening to each other, expressing feelings, directing requests to each other, and solving problems. Youth develop goals and share them with guardians who have identified what they want for their adolescents. Without denying the pain of losing a parent, positive future plans are identified.

Four Techniques Used in Each Session

Four techniques are used in each session to facilitate group interaction and skill development. First, participants are reinforced for their interactions within the group by giving each other tokens of "thanks" (colored poker chips) when they like what another participant said or did or when they have positive feelings toward others during the session. Second, participants are taught to be aware of the intensity of their affective reactions through the use of the "Feeling Thermometer," a self-report (paper-and-pencil) tool to self-monitor one's emotional state. Affective reactions provide motivation to participants, signal the need for action, and facilitate perceptions of social connections. Third, participants consistently reintroduce themselves to the group in a positive way, acknowledging their own strengths, characteristics, convictions, and needs. These introductions build a new sense of personal identity as a positive contributor to an important activity. Fourth, relaxation skills are practiced throughout as a primary means of coping with illness, daily hassles, losses, and anticipated death.

Addressing Problems at Multiple Levels

Problems are addressed at multiple levels in the participants' lives. First, the key aspects of the parents' social identities were reviewed. Parents with AIDS' identities included themselves as parents, children to their own parents, friends, siblings, workers, religious congregants, women or men, members of their ethnic groups, and, now, persons with AIDS. Any new behaviors that were to be addressed needed to have meaning to one of these social identities of the parent living with AIDS. For example, being a "parent with AIDS" indicates a role of planning and caretaking for children and is likely to be associated with family rules regarding disclosure of parental serostatus to nonfamily members (or not). In addition, the parents must help their families to adjust to their health status. We focus on change at multiple levels because we want behaviors to be maintained over long periods of time. Specific behaviors (e.g., making breakfast every morning and family members eating together) cannot be maintained unless these behaviors are set within a broader set of meaningful roles and identities. Therefore, as specific behavioral successes occur, the meaning of enacting the behavior within the scope of family relationships and one's long-term social identities are discussed and considered.

Furthermore, examination of social identities allows parents and adolescents to form scenarios for their life trajectories, scenarios that invoked images of "ideal" selves and "possible" selves (Marcus & Nurius, 1986). The parents and adolescents are then challenged to answer these questions: Is acting in certain ways consistent with the person's self-perceptions? Does the adolescent believe his or her parent is well and healthy when, in fact, the parent is ill? Can the person identify future goals to act differently today? These are central belief systems or attitudes that emerge from the social identities and role perceptions among intervention participants.

PARTICIPANTS IN PROJECT TALC

The average age of the parents who participated in this prevention program was about 38 years old—some were as old as 70, and the youngest parent of an adolescent was 25 years old. Most belonged to ethnic minorities: 45% were Latino and 34% were African American. Most parents living with AIDS (81%) were mothers. When fathers were identified as the parent with AIDS, there was typically a mother or a new romantic partner who was actually caring for the child. There was substantial effort to recruit the fathers, and the group format had to be modified for fathers. Given the feedback from fathers, we anticipated that individual family sessions may be more acceptable to fathers. The family received substantially more benefits from the city of New York if there was a parent with AIDS; therefore, some families had the fathers temporarily take official custody of the children to qualify for enhanced benefits, even though the mother remained the primary caretaker of the children.

A second group that was very difficult to reach were Spanish-speaking mothers. All intervention and assessment materials were adapted for Spanish-speaking mothers, yet few wanted to participate. Mothers with AIDS who completed the intervention program were hired as peer recruiters to encourage other Spanish-speaking mothers to attend, but even these same-ethnic peers were not successful at recruiting Spanish-speaking mothers. Only 2 of 15 mothers who only spoke Spanish attended the intervention (about 40% overall were Latino and could speak both English and Spanish). In the future, alternative intervention modalities must be designed for fathers and Spanish-speaking mothers.

About half (54%) of the parents living with AIDS had graduated from high school. Only a few parents living with AIDS had children who were temporarily in foster care placements, group homes, or incarcerated. Only about 1 in 4 parents with AIDS had an adult romantic partner. Another 20% lived with their own parents or other relatives.

About one third of the parents living with AIDS (37%) had injected drugs over their lifetimes, but only 5.6% injected drugs in the previous 3 months. Fathers were significantly more likely to be injecting drugs compared to mothers. Over their lifetimes, PWAs had a mean of 35 partners, although 50% of the mothers had fewer than 8 partners. Only 3.8% always used condoms, yet many had no sexual partners now that the parents were aware of their HIV status. Over their lifetimes, many parents had engaged in high-risk behaviors, including having sex with partners who bartered sex (23%), injecting drugs (65%), and having partners who were HIV seropositive (60%) or were bisexual (23%). Recently,

58% of parents abstained from sexual activity; among the sexually active, most had one sexual partner (91%), and more than half reported 100% condom use. Parents were very ill, and most had an average of 15 physical symptoms over the previous 3 months, symptoms that resulted in moderate distress.

Similar to their parents, 49% of the adolescents were Latino and 38% were African American; 53% were female. The mean age of the adolescents was 15 years old; 89% were currently in school.

HOW WELL DID THE INTERVENTION WORK?

An evaluation of Project TALC was conducted to determine how the intervention helped the adolescents of parents living with AIDS over 2 years.

As a result of participating in Project TALC, problem behaviors and conduct problems decreased among the adolescents, and these changes were sustained for 2 years. This is particularly important because multiple problem behaviors and conduct problems are likely to substantially increase the societal costs of AIDS-related conditions (e.g., by increasing the percentage of youth in jail).

The intervention also helped the adolescents cope with their life situations. The emotional distress of youth participating in Project TALC rapidly decreased after 1 year and remained at about the same level after 2 years. Similar to the findings for emotional distress, family-related life stressors decreased significantly among the adolescents who participated in Project TALC. In addition, the self-esteem of the youth increased. These changes were substantial; we continue to monitor whether these reductions will persist and lead to lower rates of psychiatric disorders over time.

There were similar benefits from participating in Project TALC for the parents living with AIDS. Emotional distress rapidly decreased after 1 year and remained at about the same level after 2 years. In addition, the participating parents' self-reports of anxiety symptoms also decreased. Similar to their adolescent children, the parents' problem behaviors decreased over 2 years.

The current evaluation suggests the importance of providing assistance to families with a parent living with AIDS before the parent's death. Participating in Project TALC resulted in improved rates of adolescent behaviors associated with negative outcomes in early adulthood as well as factors that promote resiliency (e.g., self-esteem, family stressors).

CONCLUSION

AIDS has presented society the challenge of caring for the large number of children whose parents are living with significant health problems and dying prematurely. There has been little research on children of parents with long-term chronic diseases—particularly adolescent children—prior to the death of their parents. Currently, 13 million children are orphaned by AIDS internationally, with about 80,000 in the United States (Shaw, 1999). Unlike children affected by other diseases, these children come from disenfranchised African American or Latino families in inner-city neighborhoods permeated by substance use. The challenges facing the parents, their children, and the children's new guardians are substantial. There has been little research that can guide the implementation of programs to assist these families. The stigmatization and prejudice that surround AIDS increase the families' stress. Only with shifts in national norms regarding our perceptions of collective responsibility toward children and destigmatization of illnesses such as AIDS can we begin to adequately address the problems associated with parental AIDS. This intervention is aimed at helping families until the day that these major structural interventions can be implemented.

REFERENCES

Armistead, L., Klein, K., Forehand, R., & Wierson, M. (1997). Disclosure of parental HIV infection to children in the families of men with hemophilia: Description, outcomes, and the role of family processes. *Journal of Family Psychology, 11,* 49-61.

Balk, D. (1991). Effects of sibling death on teenagers. *Journal of School Health, 53,* 14-18.

Centers for Disease Control and Prevention (CDC). (1999). HIV/AIDS Surveillance Report. U.S. HIV and AIDS cases reported through June 1999. Atlanta, GA: CDC.

Draimin, B. (1993). Adolescents in families with AIDS: Growing up with loss. In C. Levine (Ed.), *A death in the family: Orphans of the HIV epidemic* (pp. 13-23). New York: United Hospital Fund.

Gwadz, M., Rotheram-Borus, M. J., Franzke, L. H., Lightfoot, M., Tottenham, N., & Leonard, N. R. (1999). *Picking up the pieces: Caregivers of adolescents bereaved by parental AIDS.* Manuscript submitted for publication.

Herek, G. M., & Capitanio, J. P. (1993). Public reactions to AIDS in the United States: A second decade of stigma. *American Journal of Public Health, 83,* 574-577.

Kaplan, J. E., Masur, H., Jaffe, H. W., & Holmes, K. K. (1995). Reducing the impact of opportunistic infections in patients with HIV infection: New guidelines. *Journal of the American Medical Association, 274*(4), 347-348.

Levine, C., & Stein, G. (1994). *Orphans of the HIV epidemic: Unmet needs in six U.S. cities.* New York: The Orphan Project.

Marcus, H., & Nurius, P. (1986). Possible selves. *American Psychologist, 41,* 954-969.

Monat, A., & Lazarus, R. S. (Eds.). (1991). *Stress and coping: An anthology* (3rd ed.). New York: Columbia University Press.

Murphy, D. A., Lightfoot, M., & Rotheram-Borus, M. J. (1999). *Adolescent outcome following parental death from AIDS.* Manuscript submitted for publication.

Oltjenbruns, K. A. (1991). Positive outcomes of adolescents' experience with grief. *Journal of Adolescent Research, 6,* 43-53.

Osterweis, M., Solomon, F., & Green, M. (1987). *Bereavement: Reactions, consequences, and care.* Washington, DC: National Academy Press.

Rotheram-Borus, M. J., Draimin, B. H., Reid, H. M., & Murphy, D. A. (1997). *The impact of illness disclosure and custody plans on adolescents whose parents live with AIDS.* Manuscript submitted for publication.

Rotheram-Borus, M. J., Miller, S., Murphy, D. A., & Draimin, B. H. (1997). An intervention for adolescents whose parents are living with AIDS. *Clinical Child Psychology and Psychiatry, 2,* 201-219.

Sandler, I. N., West, S. G., Baca, L., Pillow, D. R., Gersten, J. C., Rogosch, F., Virdin, L., Beals, J., Reynolds, K. D., Kallgren, C., et al. (1992). Linking empirically based theory and evaluation: The family bereavement program. *American Journal of Community Psychology, 20,* 491-521.

Sharp, D. (1996). Vancouver AIDS meeting highlights combination attack on HIV. *Lancet, 8*(9020), 115.

Shaw, A. (1999, September 16). AIDS eclipses war, orphaning millions of children, U.N. says. *Washington Times,* p. A14.

Stein, J. A., Riedel, M., & Rotheram-Borus, M. J. (1999). Parentification and its impact among adolescent children of parents with AIDS. *Family Process, 38,* 193-208.

West, S. G., Sandler, I., Pillow, D. R., Baca, L., & Gersten, J. C. (1991). The use of structural equation modeling in generative research: Toward the design of a preventive intervention for bereaved children. *American Journal of Community Psychology, 19,* 459-480.

Wortley, P., Chu, S. Y., Diaz, T., Ward, J. W., Doyle, B., Davidson, A. J., Checko, P. J., Herr, M., Conti, L., Fann, S. A., Sorvillo, F., Mokotoff, E., Levy, A., Hermann, P., & Norris-Wakzak, E. (1995). HIV testing patterns: Where, why and when were persons with AIDS tested for HIV? *AIDS, 9,* 487-492.

Chapter 10

The Family Health Project

Strengthening Problem Solving in Families Affected by AIDS to Mobilize Systems of Support and Care

Bruce D. Rapkin   Jo Anne Bennett
Paulette Murphy   Michele Muñoz

Memorial Sloan-Kettering Cancer Center

The Victor family: "Helping Ourselves as Well as Others." The members of the Victor family participating in our program included a 29-year-old person with AIDS (PWA), his 45-year-old mother, and 48-year-old stepfather. In discussing the problems this family faced, it soon became clear that the mother and stepfather were the major source of support and stability for an extensive family network. In addition to the PWA, this couple had two other sons (ages 24 and 21) who were having difficulty holding jobs and becoming independent from the family, as well as a daughter (age 26) who was relying on her parents for support during her first pregnancy. Both mother and stepfather also actively cared for their own parents and siblings with various serious health problems, including AIDS, epilepsy, and substance use. During our first session, the son stated that he signed up for this program in hopes of getting some help for his parents. Things had come to a head several months earlier, when the stepfather had several minor strokes and was under

AUTHORS' NOTE: The development of this chapter was supported by an NIMH grant (R01 MH55770) to the first author. For more information on this prevention program, please contact Dr. Bruce Rapkin, Sloan-Kettering Institute for Cancer Research, 1275 York Avenue, New York, NY 10021; e-mail: rapkinb@mskmail.mskcc.org.

medical advice to limit his activity. Furthermore, although the son was now doing well on a combination therapy, he was concerned that his own condition would deteriorate and that he would need to rely more on his parents. He stated, and the parents agreed, that coming to a program "for" the PWA was the only way he could ever get them to come for help, to find ways to relieve some of the demands on them, and to learn to help themselves as well as others.

Paul's and Jake's family: "Three Men and a Baby." This family centered on a gay African American male couple (Paul and Jake), both in their 40s and both PWAs. After living together as a couple for a number of years, Paul's and Jake's lives became quite disrupted when Paul's brother and his girlfriend had a baby and moved in with them. The brother's job took him out of town for days at a time. The girlfriend was actively using crack and was also out of the house quite a bit. This left Paul and Jake saddled with the child care responsibility and all of the household chores. During our first session, Jake stated that he and Paul had been fighting with one another a great deal because the house was dirty all the time, and no one was taking responsibility for what needed to be done. Paul and Jake realized that they were taking all of these burdens on themselves because they were not sure how to approach Paul's brother or his girlfriend about sharing tasks without making matters worse. They were particularly concerned that the girlfriend would leave and take the baby (at that time, almost 11 months old) if they asked too much of her. Finding a way to work with Paul's brother to ensure a safe and stable home for the baby while regaining some control over their home became the initial focus of Paul's and Jake's work in our program. The urgency of this situation was heightened by Paul's and Jake's own health concerns. In particular, Paul complained of chronic fatigue as well as pain associated with untreated dental problems. Both men were worried about how added household demands made it more difficult for them to take care of themselves and one another.

AIDS places an enormous strain on family systems. Families—such as the Victor family and Paul's and Jake's family—are challenged by an unpredictable illness while managing other sources of chronic and acute stress, with little or no training, guidance, and support. Given the scope and uncertainty of the challenges they face, families affected by AIDS need flexible coping skills that can be applied to a variety of circumstances. This chapter describes a new family problem-solving (FPS) program being tested to determine whether social problem-solving training can help HIV-affected families cope with problems and obtain vital supports and resources. The FPS program adapts a well-established social problem-solving model to the special needs of low-income, multiproblem families. The premise for this approach is straightforward: By working together as a problem-solving unit, family members should be better able to anticipate and respond to adaptive challenges. The FPS approach emphasizes family competencies and encourages members to support one another's coping efforts. Ultimately, this program is intended to prevent or reduce difficulties that families often experience in obtaining care, responding to changes in illness, and renegotiating household roles and responsibilities.

The two families introduced at the beginning of this chapter were chosen to highlight how this program can work with diverse families facing multiple problems. We will refer to these examples throughout this chapter to illustrate how families learn the problem-solving model and how they can make use of it to cope with multiple challenges and problems. For confidentiality purposes, details of each case have been obscured or omitted.

RATIONALE FOR A PROBLEM-SOLVING APPROACH FOR FAMILIES AFFECTED BY HIV/AIDS

As the two cases demonstrate, families affected by HIV/AIDS face multiple health care and psychosocial problems. Problems may include complex medical management and caregiving issues, disruption of family roles and routines, and concerns about the family's future as illness progresses. Illness trajectory and treatment efficacy are unpredictable, making it impossible to anticipate what problems families will confront and when. The problems of coping with illness are compounded by the stigma of AIDS. PWAs and their families may experience rejection from friends, loss of jobs, and harassment (Bor, Miller, & Goldman, 1993). Concerns about disclosure may cause families affected by AIDS considerable difficulty in seeking support (Hays, Chauncey, & Tobey, 1990; Smith & Rapkin, 1995). Even years after disclosure, family members may still be angry or ashamed about a PWA's history of homosexuality, substance use, or infidelity.

Problems related to AIDS co-occur with other issues facing the family. Given high levels of poverty, substance use, unemployment, and poor health care, AIDS-related problems may not even be the most pressing faced by these families. Indeed, both the Victor family and Paul and Jake presented with problems that were related to the needs of their extended families. As these examples demonstrate, PWAs may be called on to help other family members resolve serious problems, at times to the detriment of their own health and well-being.

To solve these problems effectively, families must often overcome significant obstacles. These obstacles include geographical distance (Weissman & Epstein, 1989), lack of knowledge about how to be helpful (Good, Good, Schaffer, & Lind, 1990; Starrett, Bresler, Decker, Waters, & Rogers, 1990), and often a history of negative interactions (Fiore, Becker, & Coppel, 1983; Fobair et al., 1986; Shinn, Lehmann, & Wong, 1984). As we found in our work with the Victor family, even the most capable problem solvers may have difficulty balancing competing demands for family members' time, energy, and resources

(Stoller & Pugliesi, 1989). The emotional and psychological status of the family also impedes problem-solving efforts. As illness advances, family members may withdraw due to physical or emotional exhaustion or overidentification with the patient (Carl, 1986; Dunkel-Schetter & Wortman, 1982; Flaskerud, 1987; Namir, Alumbaugh, Fawzy, & Wolcott, 1989; Peters-Golden, 1982). Family members also may be reticent to discuss problems with PWAs, for fear of making them sicker by worrying them. By the same token, PWAs may be reluctant to bring up problems for fear of abandonment or rejection (as in the case of Paul and Jake) or to avoid being a burden to family members (Hays et al., 1990). Family members also differ in the ways that various problems are discussed or concealed, the level of conflict associated with problems, and the ways that conflict is expressed. These differences are related to family immigration history, cultural norms, and values. Indeed, two or three adult generations within one family may express highly divergent values and beliefs about AIDS, health care, care, and support.

In sum, families affected by HIV/AIDS can expect to face multiple problems related to illness and treatment, but the occurrence, timing, and severity of these problems are unpredictable. AIDS-related problems do not occur in isolation, as families are often called on to meet many different problems and crises. However, the presence of HIV/AIDS in the family member increases emotional distress, introduces additional barriers to support, and constrains options for coping. In light of multiple problems, daunting obstacles, and unclear choices, we decided that families could clearly benefit from a program that provided them with flexible tools that would help them respond to changing demands and arrive at the best possible solutions. The social problem-solving paradigm offered this kind of training model.

Problem-Solving Approach

The problem-solving approach is an empowerment model, in the sense that families gain tools and develop skills that they can apply to problem situations as they see fit. This model does not presuppose individual or family deficits. Rather, the focus is on helping family members develop and use existing competencies to cope with even the most difficult problems. The goal is to help family members develop and enhance skills that they can use in the problem-solving approach whenever problems occur. This flexibility is especially important because of the many obstacles to problem solving that families affected by HIV/AIDS may encounter. Once they have learned the approach, families should be able to apply their problem-solving skills to new situations, making it feasible to offer a time-limited program. The problem-solving approach also makes sense given the diversity of families because every family can arrive at solutions that fit their own unique circumstances, values, and beliefs.

THEORY AND RESEARCH
UNDERLYING THE FAMILY
PROBLEM-SOLVING MODEL

The Social Problem-Solving Approach

Our program for families affected by HIV/AIDS is based on one of the oldest and most widely used approaches in cognitive behavior therapy. Over the past 30 years, a core set of interpersonal cognitive problem-solving skills has been identified, and methods for assessing and enhancing these skills have been developed in work with numerous populations. Social problem-solving interventions focused on individuals attempt to enhance a range of cognitive skills that can be used to analyze and solve any variety of problems. These skills include (a) sensitivity to interpersonal problems, (b) causal thinking, (c) alternative thinking, (d) consequential thinking, (e) means-ends thinking, and (f) perspective taking. Many versions of the general problem-solving approach have been developed. One of the most comprehensive is D'Zurilla's (1986) transactional problem-solving model of stress, which integrates cognitive interpersonal problem-solving models with Folkman and Lazarus's (1984) work on coping with stress. This expanded conception of problem solving emphasizes that problem-solving skills can be used to cope with emotional distress as well as tangible problems.

Evidence That Problem-Solving
Training Benefits Patients

A number of studies have demonstrated the benefits of problem-solving skills enhancement for individual patients. Worden and Weisman (1984) found that identification of current problems and exploration of possible coping strategies significantly reduced the emotional distress of newly diagnosed cancer patients. Cain, Kohorn, Quinlan, Latimer, and Schwartz (1986) found that low- and middle-income gynecological cancer patients became less depressed and less anxious following a group program that helped them to identify problems, set goals, and obtain needed social support. Telch and Telch (1986) contrasted the benefits of a problem-solving training curriculum with supportive group therapy for cancer patients. They found that the more structured problem-solving program led to significantly lower levels of mood disturbance and higher levels of vigor. Similarly, Fawzy et al. (1990) found that active problem-solving training increased cancer patients' sense of efficacy in coping with a wide variety of illness-related stressors.

Extending the Social Problem-Solving
Model to the Family Level

These studies demonstrate that training in problem-solving skills can help individuals to identify problems and arrive at solutions that suit their personal values and circumstances. Clearly, PWAs could benefit greatly from a program to enhance their skills as individual problem solvers. However, we believed that there would be even greater advantages in viewing the family, rather than the individual, as the "problem-solving" unit. Table 10.1 summarizes ways in which family process enters into different social problem-solving steps. It also suggests how family members working together have the potential to recognize one another's problems earlier, generate alternative solutions from different perspectives, weigh pros and cons of solutions more fully, and cooperate in implementing plans and overcoming obstacles.

As the son in the Victor family amply demonstrated, individuals understand themselves as being part of a family and naturally think of their own needs and problems in this context. The son's own coping strategies very much hinged on the well-being and availability of his parents, which in turn depended on how well they coped with the demands of their extended family and their tenuous health status. The advantage of a family problem-solving approach is especially evident in situations such as the Victor family, who must cope with multiple problems simultaneously.

If successful, FPS training should benefit both individual family members and the family as a whole. Individuals should be better able to anticipate and avert problems and to mobilize formal and informal supports. In terms of outcomes for the family, problem-solving training should decrease burdens related to support and caregiving (including care *for* PWAs and care *given* by PWAs). Training should also help to improve family communication about problems, reduce conflicts, and lead to more stable living situations. FPS may be understood as a *prevention* program, allowing families to reduce or avoid negative mental health and social consequences associated with HIV/AIDS. By helping individuals and families attain desired goals, the FPS approach should help to improve quality of life for all concerned.

FAMILY PROBLEM-SOLVING
TRAINING PROGRAM

Program Overview

The FPS program that we developed is designed to help families affected by HIV and AIDS increase their ability to use the problem-solving concepts and skills summarized in Table 10.1. To explain this program, we will trace how we work with families from recruitment through termination. At each juncture, we

TABLE 10.1 Interpersonal Problem-Solving Skills at the Individual and Family Levels

Problem-Solving Skill	Definition of Problem-Solving Ability	Effective Family Problem-Solving	Relevance to HIV-Affected Families
Problem identification/ goal setting	To recognize problems; establish priorities; set attainable goals	To openly discuss concerns, ask about feelings and needs; recognize others' goals and needs, resolve conflicting priorities	Some families feel resigned to their fate; others deny problems; still others are too weary to address new concerns; multiple challenges, novel situations make goals uncertain.
Preparing for problem solving	To use emotion-focused coping to minimize or manage stress; to cue problem solving	To help one another to relax; create an atmosphere for problem solving; recognize affect as cue	Families may be overwhelmed; conflicts among family members may interfere with coping.
Alternative thinking	To generate alternative solutions to problems	To brainstorm together, share ideas, encourage suggestions	Families face new challenges, need to try out new strategies to find what works for them. Families and PWAs who have lost some capacity to function need new approaches.
Consequential thinking/decision making	To evaluate alternatives, maximize positive outcomes for self, others	To give and accept critiques of strategies, reach consensus, compromise if need be	Sense of crisis encourages indecision or impulsiveness; long-term consequences of decisions may be difficult to know or accept.
Means-ends planning/ enactment	To think through implementation of solutions, account for others' actions, anticipate obstacles and needs; to implement a plan	To plan together, base strategy on cooperation; to provide tangible support; to coordinate efforts to carry out plans	Plans help families track progress toward goals; some families feel reluctant to initiate action, especially if outcomes are uncertain or there is potential for failure or conflict.
Reevaluation/persistence	To maintain motivation, follow through with plans; appraise solution outcomes, reinitiate problem solving if needed	To encourage others when obstacles are encountered	Low-income families' motivation to pursue goals can be sapped by fatigue, poverty-related stress, prior frustration, or a sense of hopelessness.

will highlight special provisions necessary to meet the needs and circumstances of families affected by HIV/AIDS. Our work with Paul and Jake and the Victor family will serve to illustrate the ways this program can be used with different families. Briefly, it is useful to consider the FPS program in three distinct phases: (a) outreach/intake, during which we inform PWAs about this program, determine eligibility, and identify which family members will participate in the program; (b) curriculum, during which family members come to three psychoeducational sessions for an introduction to problem-solving concepts; and (c) consolidation/termination, during which families receive periodic telephone calls from problem-solving advisers who help families to incorporate program concepts and techniques to address new problems in their everyday lives.

Outreach/Intake

The goal of this phase of the program is to inform families affected by HIV/AIDS about the FPS program and encourage them to participate. The FPS program is designed to benefit a wide range of families affected by HIV and AIDS. Families learn about our program through our direct outreach to patients and through our networking with staff at designated AIDS care centers and AIDS service organizations throughout the New York City metropolitan area. Note that we do not restrict our program to families with specific deficits or needs. Rather, as a competency-based model, our program attempts to help families make use of and enhance their problem solving. Even families without overt complaints can use the FPS approach to anticipate potential future problems and obtain positive goals. FPS was developed for the following:

- There must be at least one other adult family member or close friend with whom the PWA is willing to discuss HIV-related problems. These individuals may or may not be seropositive. If a particular family member does not want to participate, the PWA may select another.

- Family membership is determined by PWAs and families; if all parties concerned perceive themselves as "family," then they are family.

- Family members need not live together, although they must live in close enough proximity to attend sessions.

- PWAs and family members must be mentally and physically able to attend three prevention programs.

Due to the curricular format and frank nature of problem discussions, this prevention program is offered to adult family members only. In the case of Paul and Jake, it was Jake who first found out about the program at an AIDS service organization where he had been an active volunteer. However, it turned out that Paul was experiencing worse health than Jake and that Paul's blood kin were more centrally involved in this couple's current problems.

Furthermore, intake staff are trained to avoid sharing information offered by one family member in interviews with others. In a case such as the Victor family, the intake worker would necessarily avoid telling either parent that the son was primarily seeking help for their burdens and health problems. In general, it is essential that family members control how and when their concerns are revealed to one another. Thus, intakes are conducted with individual family members. Information from intakes is *not* introduced into curricular sessions where families meet together.

Clearly, we check carefully with the PWAs to ensure that they give us permission to contact family members to whom they have already disclosed their serostatus. In some instances, nondisclosure of HIV status has severely restricted the number of family members who can participate.

Typically, two or three members from a given family participate in our program. In some instances, we have extended invitations to additional members. We have found that it is sometimes necessary to involve additional family members in the program after the initial intake (and after curriculum training sessions have begun), as the composition of the family and the nature of their problems become clearer. In such instances, we conduct special intakes with these newcomers to orient them to the program and answer their questions.

Unfortunately, identified family members may not always be able to attend. In the case of the Victor family, the index PWA approached his two younger brothers and asked them if they would like to participate in this program. When they refused, he took it as another indication of how too many burdens fell onto his parents alone. In contrast, in our intake, neither Paul nor Jake considered inviting Paul's brother to sessions. Only after they were able to articulate what was wrong in their household did they tell him about this program and invite him to participate. Although Paul's brother was unable to attend our scheduled sessions, he ultimately became involved in his family's efforts to solve problems in their household. As these instances demonstrate, our approach has been to work with all adult family members who are able to take part in our program and to help them engage other relevant family members in the problem-solving process when possible. In this sense, the need for outreach to family members and intake/orientation to the FPS program can arise at any time during our work with families.

As part of our evaluation process, we ask each family member to complete several questionnaires to assess his or her problem-solving skills, recent problems the family has encountered, social support, quality of life, and family adjustment. We also ask family members to engage in two brief family interaction tasks to observe their problem-solving communication. This information permits us to better tailor this program to different families.

The Family Problem-Solving Curriculum

The goal of the curricular phase of the FPS program is to introduce families to the language and concepts of problem solving and to show them how the FPS approach can be used to address the problems and challenges that they face. Families come to the program with many types of problems, some directly related to AIDS and some not. There are also great differences within and between families, in terms of communication skills and the ability to grasp FPS concepts. Thus, it was necessary to design our curriculum with sufficient flexibility to address families' different concerns and different problem-solving styles and competencies.

Many problem-solving training programs use hypothetical examples and vignettes to help participants understand what problem solving entails. However, we found that this format was not effective with families affected by HIV/AIDS. Some families even stated that stories about other families' problems seemed irrelevant. Rather, we have found that families participating in the FPS program are often highly motivated to address the problems of greatest current concern. Given the urgency families tend to feel about these problems, we ultimately decided to focus the curriculum around problems provided by the family.

Similarly, problem-solving curricula are generally organized around specific skills (such as those summarized in Table 10.1). However, actual problem situations often change rapidly. We found that it is usually not possible or desirable to limit discussion of "real-life" situations to a single problem-solving skill. Rather, we settled on an approach to problem-solving training that allowed families to identify, analyze, and make provisional decisions about a focal problem in a relatively constrained timeframe. Indeed, the watchwords for our problem-solving training sessions are, "In with a problem, out with a plan."

One major difficulty that we encountered in working with families affected by HIV/AIDS involves scheduling of sessions. In addition to illness, families are often juggling multiple demands that compete for members' time and attention. After experimenting with several different formats, we found that it was most feasible to limit the number of face-to-face training sessions to three 3- to 4-hour meetings. Families find it easier to come in fewer times but for longer appointments. Longer meetings also give families time to discuss problems in sufficient depth to arrive at provisional plans. Of course, maintaining comfort of families and staff is a key concern in this format. Depending on the time of day, we provide families with a light meal or snack midway through each session. Given the length of meetings, family members could also take breaks as needed.

In general, we try to schedule curriculum sessions once per week over 3 weeks, but we have exercised considerable flexibility to accommodate families' needs. To encourage families' attendance and use of the FPS approach, staff routinely call families one or more times between sessions.

Weekly curriculum sessions are conducted by a clinician (psychologist or social worker) and a FPS peer adviser. The role of the clinician is to serve as a teacher and problem-solving resource for the family. Clinicians are responsible for the timing of the session and for ensuring all topics are covered, according to program fidelity criteria. The role of the peer adviser is to host the family, to "join" the family as needed to model effective problem solving. Advisers may take part in role-plays, model FPS behavior for family members, or make suggestions when the family seems stuck. As we shall discuss below, FPS advisers continue playing this role with the families throughout the consolidation phase. Peer and clinician teams are assigned to each family after intake and remain with the family through the completion of the program.

All three sessions have the same general format, although there are also session-specific goals and milestones that we try to achieve with each family. In general, each session starts with a preparatory exercise such as guided relaxation, deep breathing, meditation, or prayer. This is followed by identification of a "focal" problem for that session. Focal problems are discussed using a FPS workbook. This workbook was designed to help families develop problem-solving plans and to monitor outcomes as they carry out plans outside of sessions during the coming week. Figure 10.1 shows the six steps of the problem-solving model that families follow in discussing their problems. Following the problem-solving discussion, the team asks questions to ensure that family members understand and feel comfortable with the curriculum and offer feedback about the FPS approach. Family members are also invited to ask questions, provide suggestions, and share what they have learned about problem solving during the session. Working from this general framework, session-specific goals and activities are summarized as follows.

Session 1. In this session, the team uses an active and directive approach in working through the focal problem with the family to explicitly demonstrate to family members each step of the FPS approach. Family members are presented an audiotape and slideshow to explain program components and ground rules (see below). The team demonstrates how the FPS workbook is used to analyze and plan a solution to a focal problem selected by the family.

Session 2. During this session, a family member is selected to lead the discussion of the focal problem. The peer adviser and clinician prompt, answer questions, clarify points about the FPS workbook, and help the family overcome any impasses. In preparation for the consolidation phase of this program, families

Six Steps of the Family
Problem-Solving Model

- Recognizing a Problem
- Getting the Family Together
- Finding a Solution
- Planning Your Solution
- Carrying Out Your Solution
- Reviewing the Results

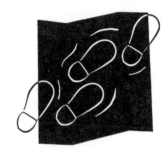

Figure 10.1.

also spend some time at the beginning of this session generating a list of problems they would like to work on and discussing their priority.

Session 3. In this session, the team encourages the family to discuss the focal problem independently, using the FPS workbook. The team tries not to participate in the family's discussion of the problem but does provide feedback to the family members when they have completed their plans. This session ends with planning for the consolidation phase, including a review of priorities and a discussion of using FPS at home.

Ground Rules

We established a number of FPS program ground rules (see Figure 10.2) to provide a setting where all family members could feel safe enough to participate. These include (a) being an active participant, (b) listening to others, (c) respecting others' rights to an opinion, (d) attending on time, (e) coming to sessions alert and sober, and (f) keeping what is said in sessions private. We also explicitly remind families about the stipulation that we must report child abuse and neglect, as well as plans to hurt oneself or others.

Our major source is the FPS workbook. The workbook table of contents is reproduced in Table 10.2. The workbook is organized into six different-colored sections, according to the six major FPS steps. Each section includes several pages that prompt families to use certain FPS skills. An instructor's version of

Ground Rules

- **Be an active member**
- **Be on time**
- **Respect yourselves and the rest of us too**
- **Be alert, attentive and aware during sessions**
- **Keep what is said in the sessions in the sessions**
- **Focus on the problem**

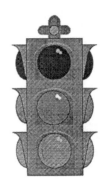

Figure 10.2.

the workbook also was created, which includes prompts for facilitating discussion of each workbook page.

The FPS workbook was designed to be used for any kind of problem by individuals, dyads, or larger groups of family members. The workbook encourages a thorough, in-depth discussion and analysis of an identified problem. To make the workbook useful to the widest range of participants, we have included cartoon images that reinforce the text and color-coded reminders of the main problem-solving steps. To keep track of decisions while using the workbook, family members keep records using "FPS worksheets" that correspond to the workbook.

It will be useful to draw on the Victor family's experience to demonstrate how families learn the FPS model during the curricular phase. We have included figures depicting several sample workbook pages to show the kinds of questions that guided the Victor family's discussion. Following the FPS workbook in Session 2, we identified one of this family's key focal problems—taking care of ourselves as well as others (Figure 10.3 depicts FPS workbook questions on problem identification).

Even after the problem was labeled, members of the Victor family differed markedly in how distant they felt from the solution. The stepfather gave it a 3 (*not too distant*), consistent with his pattern of denying his own needs. The son thought that the distance was an 8 (*far from solution*). He said that he felt even further away than before his family started our program. The mother acknowledged

TABLE 10.2 Family Problem-Solving Workbook Table of Contents

Recognizing a Problem
  1. How Do You Know There Is a Problem?
  2. Identifying Examples
  3. Labeling the Problem
  4. Putting the Problem in Focus
  5. Check Your Distance

Getting Together to Solve the Problem
  1. Who Else Should Be Involved as a Problem Solver?
  2. How to Tell the Ones You Have Chosen About This Problem
  3. Finding the Right Times and Places to Discuss This Problem
  4. Setting the Mood for Solving This Problem

Finding a Solution
  1. Understanding This Problem Better
  2. What Has to Change?
  3. Are These Changes Within Reach?
  4. Problem-Solving Ideas
  5. Deciding on Your Best Ideas

Planning Your Solution
  1. Setting Up the Plan
  2. Support Needs
  3. Getting Support
  4. Putting Your Plans Into Action
  5. Barriers to Problem Solving
  6. Talking Through Your Plans
  7. Reviewing Your Plans

Carrying Out Your Solution
  1. Checking Up on Your Plans
  2. Checking Your Progress
  3. Supporting One Another

Reviewing the Results
  1. Reviewing the Results of the Plan

Your Thoughts and Reflections

her husband's perspective but rated the problem a 7, to echo the son's concern about family burden. In reviewing the family's history with this problem, both parents had been called on to take responsibility for other family members because they were much younger. (See Figure 10.4 for workbook questions to help families explore a problem's history.) Part of their strong bond seemed based on the recog-

How do you know there's a problem?

You can tell there is a problem because of...

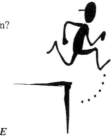

- *FEELINGS*
  - What feelings point to this problem?
- *NEEDS & WANTS*
  - What do you need or want?
- *UNPLEASANT EVENTS*
  - What happened?
- *OTHERS' BEHAVIOR*
  - What did they say or do?
- *CONCERNS ABOUT THE FUTURE*
  - What might happen?

Figure 10.3.

nition of how much each cared for others, and they often supported one another in these efforts (e.g., they each would do many things for the other's mother).

As we discussed goals, the mother and stepfather in the Victor family recognized that it was necessary for them to set limits. This was especially difficult for the stepfather to do. Indeed, he had a very difficult time saying no, especially to his brothers. At times, he would control the demands on him by staying away from home and not returning telephone calls. These obstacles were a source of conflict with his wife, who felt caught in the middle because her husband would not face his brothers or others, to refuse their requests. (The workbook page used to prompt discussion of obstacles is included in Figure 10.5.) The Victor family's plan encompassed several complementary alternative solutions, including saying no to others, asking their own children for help that they needed, and exploring a few new ways to relax. (These plans were discussed according to the workbook questions represented in Figure 10.6.)

Although the workbook provides a valuable tool for learning the FPS curriculum, we were concerned that this kind of written modality would be unfamiliar and difficult for many participants to use. In fact, our debriefing of program families suggests that this is not usually the case. The workbook approach has been very well received. Many family members use it spontaneously, and some have asked for extra copies to give to friends and relatives not involved in our program. Based on a suggestion made by the father in the Victor family, we also offer the workbook in audiotape format to participants who have difficulty with reading or who are visually impaired.

The FPS workbook provides a detailed, step-by-step approach to problem solving. The workbook raises questions that must be asked to fully understand a

Understanding This ProblemBetter

- Has your family had a problem like this before?
- Has anyone else you know?
- What did you/they do?
- Would you handle it the same way?
- What would you do differently?

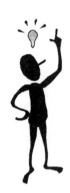

Figure 10.4.

problem and to stimulate discussion of the widest possible range of solutions. Clearly, families do not need to approach every problem in this way. Families receive suggestions about situations in which the workbook might be most helpful (see Figure 10.7). We suggest that they follow the workbook when they are learning the FPS approach, when they are having trouble getting started, when the problem is complicated, when other solutions have not worked, when there is conflict among family members, and whenever they feel like using it. In less demanding situations, family members have told us that they have used one page or one section to help them think about an impasse. Families have also found the language of the workbook helpful, even when they do not follow its linear structure.

Given the limited time available, we found that it is often difficult to fully discuss more than one focal problem in any given curricular session. However, there are many instances when families raise issues or request services that warrant referrals to outside agencies. Of course, it would be most inconsistent with the FPS approach to simply tell families what help they needed and where to go to find it. Rather, we developed a "referral module" to incorporate such referrals into the curriculum as a special opportunity to demonstrate the problem-solving model in action. This module prompts the clinician or peer adviser to walk the family through the steps in the FPS workbook, analyze the problem, and arrive at a plan for seeking, using, and monitoring formal services. Designed to take 10 to 15 minutes, this module reinforces use of the FPS approach, rather than simply telling families where to seek help.

Barriers to Problem Solving

- List the possible barriers you may face.
- What is the way around each barrier?
- Is it necessary to change your plan, in order to avoid or overcome barriers?

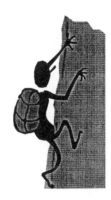

Figure 10.5.

Similarly, there are instances in work with families affected by HIV/AIDS when staff become aware of urgent problem situations or when one or more family members are so distressed that it would be difficult to proceed with the session as planned. We have developed a "crisis module" to use in such situations. Like the referral module, the crisis module also draws on the FPS workbook. However, in the crisis module, program staff may take a more direct and active role in the problem-solving process than they would in other situations, including suggesting problem labels, offering alternatives, and pointing out consequences. Unlike the referral module, staff take as much time as needed to complete the crisis module, even if it is necessary to preempt the discussion of any other focal problem within a given session. Note that the crisis module would not be used in case of an emergency requiring immediate outside assistance.

We found it necessary to use the crisis module in our work with Paul and Jake. In our first session, these men discussed arguments that they were having and initially framed the focal problem in general terms of wanting a more "cooperative and collaborative household," without specific discussion of the baby. Despite their focus, the FPS team was highly concerned about the baby's well-being. This concern became heightened when the couple casually mentioned that the baby recently "needed to go to the emergency room for stitches." At this point, the clinician decided to switch gears and to refocus discussion on care of the baby. Although the baby received stitches after a minor accident, the couple went on to report difficulty getting him follow-up medical attention because neither parent was available to take the baby to the doctor. Paul and Jake were afraid

Setting Up the Plan

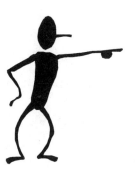

- What are the steps that make up your plan?
- Who should do what?
- When should you begin?
- When will each step happen?
- Where will each person be at each step?
- Don't begin a step until earlier steps are complete.
- Think about what else might conflict with this schedule.

Figure 10.6.

to take the baby to the doctor because neither had permission to serve as the baby's legal guardian.

Using the workbook in "crisis" mode, the team helped Paul and Jake frame a specific problem: getting the baby regular medical care. Plans included trying to get one or both of the baby's parents to take the baby, obtaining a letter from the parents, and getting help from Jake's case manager. Although the solution took several weeks to enact, this "crisis" actually became the first instance in which Paul confronted his brother about taking more responsibility for the baby. Ultimately, Paul persuaded his brother to take the baby to a clinic. Paul accompanied them to their first appointment so that he could be introduced to the clinic staff as the baby-sitter, in case he needed to get him care in the future. Monitoring the well-being of the baby became a routine part of our work with Paul and Jake, extending into the consolidation phase.

Consolidation/Termination

The goal of the consolidation phase is to help families use the FPS approach for an extended period of time and find ways to draw on these skills independently as they confront new and unfamiliar problems. Many cognitive problem-solving programs focus on the process of solution generation and means-ends planning. However, given the multiple serious problems affecting families in our program, we also felt it necessary to emphasize skills related to actual imple-

Use the Workbook When ...

- You're learning the Family Problem-Solving Approach.
- You're having trouble getting started.
- The problem is complicated.
- Other solutions haven't worked.
- There is conflict among the family.
- You feel like using it.

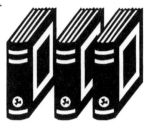

Figure 10.7.

mentation of plans in real life. To accomplish this, we decided to work with families over the telephone for a 6-month period following completion of the curricular phase. Telephone contacts between the team and the family focus on troubleshooting the family's problem-solving efforts and encouraging the family to use the FPS approach on new problems that arise. Calls decrease in frequency from weekly to biweekly to monthly, ending after 6 months. The peer adviser makes most of the calls, with clinicians checking in every fourth call and as needed. FPS staff members contact a different family member participating in the program with each call, if possible. Families may also call to request problem-solving assistance if needed.

During the telephone calls, peer advisers routinely check with families about solutions on which they have been working, as well as new problems or concerns. Often, families request help revising solutions and plans. Discussion focuses on the steps that families have tried to take to carry out plans and obstacles they have encountered along the way. When necessary, they also encourage families to use the FPS workbook at home (see Figure 10.8). The workbook includes calendars and rating scales for families to monitor their progress and keep them focused as they implement plans (see workbook distance rating that families use in Figure 10.9). Staff may use role-plays on the telephone to rehearse conversations and practice assertiveness. Families also are prompted to use stress management techniques to help them deal with obstacles and persist in problem solving (following questions from the workbook in Figure 10.10). Peer advisers are trained to use the referral and crisis modules with family members during

Finding the Right Times and Places
to Discuss This Problem

- What discussions are needed?
- When can you get together?
- Where do you want to get together?
- How long do you want to talk?
- What other arrangements are needed?
- Did you speak with everyone who will be involved as a problem solver?

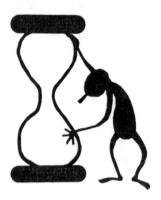

Figure 10.8.

telephone contacts. Peers are trained to contact the clinician by pager whenever they need to initiate a crisis module and at any time they feel they need backup during or after a call.

Often, the consolidation phase continues themes identified during the curricular sessions and allows families to refine and expand their solutions.

Throughout our calls with Paul and Jake, we discussed ways to make their household situation more stable and supportive for the baby and more satisfactory for the two of them. During these calls, the complementary problem-solving style of these two men became apparent. Jake was always able to generate a lengthy list of strategies. With the assistance of his peer adviser, Jake created a plan that included bringing the brother into the problem-solving process, getting his help dealing with the girlfriend, and moving to a bigger apartment near to Paul's aunt, who could then also help with child care. Paul and Jake discussed this plan at home and agreed to give it a try. It seemed that Paul was much more involved with taking care of the baby, leaving Jake with more of the responsibility for implementing the plan. Paul's declining health made it more difficult to take a larger role. Jake tacitly acknowledged this difference and seemed satisfied taking the lead role in solving the problem.

The couple worked on this plan throughout the consolidation phase, although there were some definite obstacles along the way. One ideal apartment fell through, and another was too expensive. The peer adviser helped Jake to continue

Checking Your Progress

- How close are you to solving the problem?
- Are you headed in the right direction?
- What changes are necessary to reach the goal?

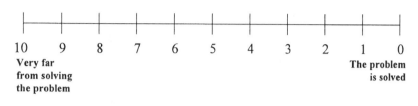

10	9	8	7	6	5	4	3	2	1	0

**Very far
from solving
the problem**

**The problem
is solved**

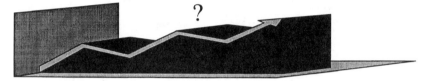

Figure 10.9.

looking for an affordable place and to negotiate with Paul's brother to pay a larger share of the rent. For a time, the girlfriend and the brother broke up, and the baby went to live with the girlfriend's mother (the baby's grandmother). This was not satisfactory to Paul and Jake because the grandmother was already caring for a large number of other grandchildren. (It turned out that the accident that required the baby to get stitches had actually happened at this grandmother's house.) Using the workbook section that focuses on identifying family members involved in the problem (see Figure 10.11), it became clear that Paul and Jake had never spoken with the grandmother about the baby's care. Jake made plans to visit the grandmother and discuss the best child care arrangements. This proved to be a productive conversation because it brought in yet another adult to help with the baby's care. By bringing the grandmother into the discussion, it became possible to ensure that there was someone who was responsible for the baby's well-being while the baby was visiting his mother. At the same time, the grandmother agreed that the baby should stay with Paul, Jake, and his father. As of our last contact with this family, the three men—Paul, Jake, and Paul's brother—and the baby had moved into a new apartment near Paul's aunt. The plans they had developed seemed to be working out (see Figure 10.12 for follow-up probes used to help families reflect on problem outcomes).

◇ ◇ ◇

Supporting One Another
As obstacles come up, how do you want to
cope with stress and show support?

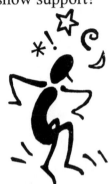

- Identify where the
  stress comes from
- Think of ways to cope:
  - Take a break, Relax
  - Take a walk, Exercise
  - Sports, Music, Hobbies
  - Other ideas?
- What can you do to
  show appreciation for
  one another's efforts?

Figure 10.10.

To be sure, many families encounter difficulties in implementing solutions, which must be addressed during our consolidation telephone contacts. Family members sometimes do not carry out problem-solving activities between calls. Often, new problems arise between calls that demand the family's attention and interfere with carrying out plans. To address these issues, we developed a FPS troubleshooting guide to help peer advisers respond to these problems in a consistent manner.

In general, when a family member reports a problem using the FPS approach, peer advisers engage the family member in a problem-solving process to identify and define the problem and arrive at a solution. For example, at one point, the father in the Victor family did not follow through on steps to tell one of his brothers he was unable to help repaint his house. This made his wife quite angry, especially because we had discussed this particular problem in our sessions. The peer adviser engaged the family at several levels. Discussions with the mother focused on her frustration with her husband's failure to follow through with plans. However, rather than following their pattern of engaging the father in a head-to-head battle (which usually did not resolve the situation and led to him going off for several days), the mother and peer arrived at a different tact. She decided to take an "at-home vacation," both to reduce her own sense of feeling overwhelmed and to show her husband how to take it easy. She liked this so

Who Else Should Be Involved
as a Problem Solver?
Decide who else will work
with you to solve this problem.

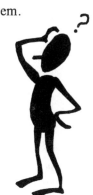

- Do you want others to take part in solving the problem?
- Who else? Family members? Others?
- What are your reasons for asking others to work with you to solve this problem?
- Are there reasons not to ask others to help solve this problem?
- Decide who you will ask to work with you on this problem.

Figure 10.11.

much that she actually put everyone else out of the house and spent a couple of days just taking care of herself. After that, it was easier for her to discuss the problems she was having without "blowing her stack." Since then, she has taken several briefer vacations at home when she has needed them, at times joined by her husband. Although the father did not say no to his brother about painting the house, he was subsequently able to tell his family members that he could not meet their demands in other situations. Helping oneself as well as others remains an ongoing challenge to the Victor family, but they were able to find new ways to address this problem and the feelings it engenders in their relationship.

In many ways, concerns about termination enter into the entire FPS program. Our goal is to help families become autonomous and effective problem solvers. The workbook provides families with a flexible set of tools that they can use independently. Over each of our three curricular sessions, families are called on to take a more active role in leading discussions of problems. The FPS referral module provides families with an example of how they can locate new services and supports when needed. Consolidation contacts focus on the family's efforts and are faded out over 6 months. Throughout the program, we explain to families that our goal is to help them solve problems independently to achieve the outcomes that they desire.

Reviewing the Results of the Plan

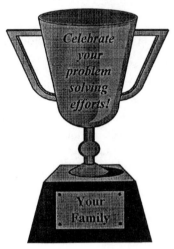

- **Is the problem solved?**
  - Does everyone in the family agree?
- **If the problem wasn't solved:**
  - Look over your plan.
  - Which steps were successful and which were not?
  - Start the Workbook again, using what you have learned.
- **If the problem is solved to everyone's satisfaction:**
  - Are there any new problems?
  - What problem would you like to work on next?

Celebrate your problem solving efforts!

Your Family

Figure 10.12.

Our formal consolidation phase ends with a termination/booster session. This final meeting provides an opportunity to review what the family has learned and accomplished in our program and to set the stage for independent problem solving. Families also have the opportunity to provide feedback to our team about the program. These final sessions are conducted jointly by the clinician and peer adviser.

Of course, completion of the program does not mean that all (or any) of a family's problems are resolved. Toward the end of our program, the son in the Victor family began to complain of conflicts he was having with his seronegative lover of 3 years. The son reported a combination of frustration that he had to abstain from certain sexual activities and fear that he would transmit the virus to his partner. During the process of breaking up with this partner, the son became sexually involved with another man. Many members of the Victor family, including the parents, felt that the son was making a mistake breaking up with his longtime partner and getting involved with this other man. At our final session, the son identified several strategies he wanted the family to try so that they could communicate with him about the situation in a nonjudgmental way. However, the son himself was clearly having his own conflicted feelings about this situation, and any resolution was still uncertain at our final session. Even so, the Victor family stated that they were communicating about problems more often and more effectively as a result of the FPS program.

CONSIDERATIONS IN FPS
PROGRAM IMPLEMENTATION

Staff Training and Supervision

One of the most important features of our program involves the role of peer FPS advisers working in tandem with clinicians. FPS advisers are themselves people infected or affected by HIV. They are selected to serve as paraprofessionals on this project by virtue of past work experience as a buddy, peer counselor, or support group leader. Peer advisers have been involved in developing our program from the beginning. Clinicians include faculty, fellows, and consultants trained in clinical psychology, psychiatry, and social work with prior background working with people living with HIV/AIDS. Several of the FPS advisers and clinicians are bilingual, in Spanish and English.

We view training of clinicians and peer advisers as an ongoing process in this program and an integral part of supervision. We have devised the program to be straightforward, and we provide many supporting documents, including an academic discussion of problem-solving guidelines, session checklists and scripts, an instructors' version of the workbook, the FPS troubleshooting guide for telephone contacts, and forms for charting sessions and telephone contacts.

We orient new staff to this program and, to the use of these materials, during weekend training sessions. New staff members also take part in role-plays to gain an understanding of how the program works. After orientation, new staff members observe peer and clinician teams working with families and take part in supervision discussions. Then, new staff are teamed with a more experienced staff member and observed in working with a case.

We have found that ongoing training is necessary because each family brings new issues and requires staff to consider the best way to implement the FPS approach. Indeed, the ultimate goal of training is to help staff learn to think in terms of the FPS model and respond to families accordingly.

To stay on top of the changing needs of the families, the peer advisers' ongoing telephone relationship during the consolidation phase, and the advisers' needs for support, we have implemented a multitiered supervision system. First, clinicians provide guidance and supervision to the peer advisers in all work with families. Charting forms are used before and after sessions, to assist teams in reviewing cases and addressing supervision issues. During the consolidation phase, clinicians also review tapes and notes of the peer adviser's telephone contacts with families and make occasional telephone contacts to independently assess the family's status. Second, the clinicians have weekly individual telephone contacts and monthly group supervision with the project's clinical director. The clinical director also reviews session tapes and notes to ensure that sessions are carried out with fidelity to the prevention program. Third, the clinical director holds weekly meetings with the peer advisers, for ongoing training and support. These meetings are often more like a mutual help group and afford the peer advisers the opportunity to assist one another in dealing with difficult issues in their work with families.

Peer Adviser Role

The most difficult aspect of the peer adviser role involves work with the families by telephone during the consolidation phase. It is demanding for our staff to accommodate families' schedules by calling in the evening or on the weekend. At times, peer advisers could not free up the time or did not want work to intrude into things they were doing at home. As people affected by HIV, peers' own issues also affect their ability to engage families. On several occasions, peers were reluctant to make calls when they felt the family's problems were too close to ones they had experienced. Peers also became frustrated when they were not sure how to help the family within the FPS model. We took a number of steps to address these issues, including the following:

- working individually with each peer adviser to help him or her plan the best time and place to make calls and to take this into account when scheduling;
- keeping the clinician involved with the case throughout the consolidation phase, to help the adviser when difficult issues arose, and to serve as a backup for the peer;
- preparing a guide for telephone contacts called "Troubleshooting Family Problem Solving," which provides peers with explicit examples of problems and ways to respond; and
- tracking all telephone calls in supervision on a weekly basis.

Holding Sessions at a Community Site

In planning this program, we felt that it would be best to hold our sessions away from a hospital environment, where the focus is on "treating the patient." Rather, we wanted to create a setting in which families would feel comfortable coming in together to discuss the problems and needs facing all of the family members.

Use of the FPS Program With Culturally Diverse Families

Given the disproportionate impact of HIV/AIDS on communities of color, it was vital to take cultural issues into account in developing and implementing the FPS program (Boyd-Franklin, 1989). One common criticism of the social problem-solving approach is that it emphasizes a rational, linear way of thinking, without taking into account more intuitive, affective, or spiritual approaches. In our program, we have tried to leave open opportunities for affective, intuitive, and spiritual facets of problem solving to come into play. In particular, sections on problem recognition, perceived distance from solutions, setting the tone for problem solving, supporting family members' problem-solving efforts, and review of outcomes encourage expression of affect and creative leaps. We encourage families to select their own ways to create an atmosphere for problem solving, including relaxation, meditation, prayer, song, reminiscence, or other rituals. Problem exploration and finding solutions encourage families to look to their own histories and to models that they respect. At several points in the FPS process, family members are asked to consider whether rationally derived problem-solving plans feel comfortable and realistic to them. Although our program has been well received by families of many different ethnic and cultural backgrounds, it remains to be seen whether all families benefit equally from this approach. Future refinements may lead us to modify program activities, materials, and procedures to better suit the needs of specific ethnic and cultural groups.

The Place of the FPS Program in the Continuum of Care

Often, PWAs in New York and other major epicenters face a vast and fragmented service system. Medical care, substance use treatment, housing assistance, nutritional assistance, and social activities are provided by different agencies. Family members must seek health care and social services within substantially different systems. Families may have multiple "case managers," each charged with overseeing a different, narrow aspect of their care. As our discussion of preceding examples indicates, the FPS program is designed to help families make best use of any variety of resources and services available to them. In a sense, our program helps family members become their own "case managers." Ideally, families will carry the FPS approach into their relationships with providers, to arrive at better decisions about care.

It is important to note that the FPS program may be useful for families affected by HIV/AIDS outside of the dense service environment of New York City. Families living in communities that are not AIDS epicenters may encounter different problems in locating care than those in our program. The FPS approach can still help them to arrive at the most optimal solutions given the resources at hand.

ISSUES AND FUTURE DIRECTIONS IN PROBLEM SOLVING FOR FAMILIES AFFECTED BY HIV/AIDS

As these case studies demonstrate, families have been able to use the FPS program to discuss important problems, to develop solutions that draw on the strengths of different family members, and to overcome difficult obstacles to carry out these solutions. The program is still being evaluated to determine whether it has long-term benefits for families. Ideally, families will be able to make use of the FPS approach whenever problems arise long after this program ends.

Before adapting this FPS model, the following issues should be considered.

Number of Curricular Sessions. We chose to limit the number of sessions to three sessions (a total of 9-10 hours) to foster attendance and completion of the program. However, this has proven to be a relatively brief time to introduce the program and define the families' priorities. It may be that families would benefit from more sessions, perhaps spread over a longer period of time, interspersed with consolidation telephone calls. The program could be readily adapted to this format.

Selection of Peer Advisers. As noted above, the peer advisers have played a significant role in the development and implementation of this program. However, the role of advising families can be very demanding, and we had a relatively high rate of turnover of advisers, especially in the first year of the project. Despite close supervision and monitoring, the peer adviser role requires people to work autonomously in a systematic and organized manner. It also requires the ability to discuss families' problems in a nonjudgmental fashion, even when they disagree with the family's decisions (e.g., to go off medications). Although it would be possible to conduct the sessions and telephone calls using staff other than peer advisers, this would sacrifice an important dimension of the training: the availability of a role model who can show families how to really make use of the problem-solving model. The individuals who have proven to be most effective as peer advisers have been people who are employed or in school, have a track record as volunteers or peer counselors, and who have a personal and political commitment to supporting families affected by AIDS. Individuals who have had more difficulty as peers are those who have had less work experience or who are facing their own health problems.

Implementation of the FPS Program. Of course, any intervention must be implemented in a way that fits local conditions. It would be possible to implement this program as part of an ongoing service or clinic. For example, the program might be mounted in day treatment programs or clinics where PWAs must spend a considerable amount of time. Although families do not routinely attend these programs with PWAs, provisions might be made to bring families in. The FPS approach might also be a useful basis for conducting psychoeducational programs for multifamily groups. More generally, the FPS might be a useful adjunct to AIDS case management by providing an approach for the family, the PWA, and the case manager to work together as a problem-solving team.

LESSONS LEARNED

In sum, perhaps four main lessons have been learned so far from our experiences developing and implementing a program for families affected by HIV/AIDS. First, programs must anticipate and accommodate the inherent diversity of families. One size does not fit all when it comes to responding to family needs. Even families coping with exactly the same problem may differ in the members that they choose to involve, the goals that they set, the solutions they pursue, and the outcomes that they accept. Second, families of people living with HIV/AIDS must be defined in an open and flexible fashion. The lives of our program participants were intertwined with extended nontraditional family members (such as "my partner's brother's girlfriend's baby's grandmother"!). Programs can anticipate and capitalize on this ecology. Third, people understand problems in a family context. Even problems that "belong" to an individual PWA such as pain or adherence have direct ramifications for the family. Families are indeed a natural problem-solving unit. Fourth and perhaps most important, families affected by HIV/AIDS have multiple strengths and competencies that they can and do bring to bear to address the problems that affect their lives. Like the Victor family and Paul and Jake, the families in our program have been highly motivated to take care of one another and improve their quality of life. Our role has been to help them to spend time focusing on problems, to ask some necessary questions, and to find ways to keep working together when solutions prove to be elusive.

REFERENCES

Bor, R., Miller, R., & Goldman, E. (1993). HIV/AIDS and the family: A review of research in the first decade. *Journal of Family Therapy, 15*(2), 187-204.

Boyd-Franklin, N. (1989). *Black families in therapy: A multisystems approach.* New York: Guilford.

Cain, E. N., Kohorn, E. I., Quinlan, D. M., Latimer, K., & Schwartz, P. E. (1986). Psychosocial benefits of a cancer support group. *Cancer, 57,* 183-189.

Carl, D. (1986). Acquired immune deficiency syndrome: A preliminary examination of the effects on gay couples and coupling. *Journal of Marital and Family Therapy, 12*(3), 241-247.

Dunkel-Schetter, C. A., and Wortman, C. B. (1982). The interpersonal dynamics of cancer: Problems in social relationships and their impact on the patient. In H. S. Friedman & M. R. DiMateo (Eds.), *Interpersonal issues in health care* (pp. 69-100). New York: Academic Press.

D'Zurilla, T. J. (1986). *Problem-solving therapy: A social competence approach to clinical intervention.* New York: Springer.

Fawzy, F. I., Cousins, N., Fawzy, N. W., Kennedy, M. E., Elashoff, R., & Morton, D. (1990). A structured psychiatric intervention for cancer patients: I. Changes over time in methods of coping and affective disturbance. *Archives of General Psychiatry, 47,* 720-725.

Fiore, J., Becker, J., & Coppel, P. B. (1983). Social network interactions: A buffer or stress? *American Journal of Community Psychology, 11,* 423-439.

Flaskerud, J. H. (1987). AIDS: Psychosocial aspects. *Journal of Psycho-social Nursing, 25,* 9-16.

Fobair, P., Hoppe, R. T., Bloom, J., Cox, R., Varghese, A., & Spiegel, D. (1986). Psychosocial problems among survivors of Hodgkin's disease. *Journal of Clinical Oncology, 4*(5), 805-814.

Folkman, S., & Lazarus, R. S. (Eds.). (1984). *Stress, appraisal and coping.* New York: Springer.

Good, M. D., Good, B. J., Schaffer, C., & Lind, S. E. (1990). American oncology and the discourse on hope. *Culture, Medicine, and Psychiatry, 12,* 59-79.

Hays, R. B., Chauncey, S., & Tobey, L. A. (1990). The social support networks of gay men with AIDS. *Journal of Community Psychology, 18,* 374-385.

Namir, S., Alumbaugh, M. J., Fawzy, F. I., & Wolcott, D. L. (1989). The relationship of social support to physical and psychological aspects of AIDS. *Psychology and Health, 3,* 87-92.

Peters-Golden, H. (1982). Breast cancer: Varied perceptions of social support in the illness experience. *Social Science and Medicine, 16,* 483-491.

Shinn, M., Lehmann, S., & Wong, N. W. (1984). Social interaction and social support. *Journal of Social Issues, 40*(4), 5-76.

Smith, M. Y., & Rapkin, B. D. (1995). Unmet support needs of persons with AIDS. *AIDS Care, 7*(3), 353-363.

Starrett, R. A., Bresler, C., Decker, J. T., Waters, G. T., & Rogers, D. (1990). The role of environmental awareness and support networks in Hispanic elderly persons' use of formal social services. *Journal of Community Psychology, 18,* 218-227.

Stoller, E. P., & Pugliesi, K. L. (1989). Other roles of caregivers: Competing responsibilities or supportive resources? *Journal of Gerontology, 44,* 31-38.

Telch, C. F., & Telch, M. J. (1986). Group coping skills instruction and supportive group therapy for the cancer patients: A comparison of strategies. *Journal of Consulting and Clinical Psychology, 54*(6), 802-808.

Weissman, J., & Epstein, A. M. (1989). Case mix and resource utilization by uninsured hospital patients in the Boston metropolitan area. *Journal of the American Medical Association, 261*(24), 3572-3576.

Worden, J. W., & Weisman, A. D. (1984). Preventive psychosocial intervention with newly diagnosed cancer patients. *General Hospital Psychiatry, 6,* 243-249.

Chapter 11

Structural Ecosystems Therapy With HIV+ African American Women

Victoria Behar Mitrani   José Szapocznik
Carleen Robinson Batista

University of Miami

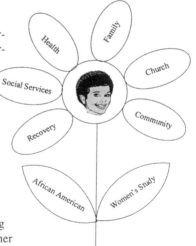

Diane is a 33-year-old African American woman who suffered a miscar-
riage and was diagnosed with HIV infection 2 years ago, leading her to
assess her many years of street
life and enter drug treatment. She
completed residential treatment 8
months ago and remains drug free. She
lives with her parents and her two
daughters and is committed to rees-
tablishing herself as a mother. Her
parents have done a fine job raising the
girls, one of whom has neurological
problems associated with Diane's drug
use during pregnancy. Although her mother

AUTHORS' NOTE: This work was funded by Grant 1 R37 MH 55796 to José Szapocznik, principal investigator, from the Center for Mental Health Research on AIDS, National Institute of Mental Health. For further information about the intervention, please contact José Szapocznik, Center for Family Studies, Department of Psychiatry and Behavioral Sciences, University of Miami School of Medicine, 1425 NW 10th Avenue, Miami, FL 33136; e-mail: jszapocz@med.miami.edu. We grate-fully acknowledge Debra Greenwood, Ph.D., our clinical team and all project staff, and our families with HIV.

anxiously watches Diane for signs of impending relapse, Diane, who appreciates the concern, finds this vigilance suffocating. The family is well established in their community, with ties to the church and a network of neighbors. Diane, however, spends most of her time at home or attending group meetings because she fears the temptation of running into old places and old faces from her street days.

This was Diane's life situation when she enrolled in Structural Ecosystems Therapy (SET), an intervention designed to help HIV+ African American women improve their psychosocial functioning (c.f. Jackson-Gilfort, Mitrani, & Szapocznik, in press; Nelson, Mitrani, & Szapocznik, in press). The focus of SET is on assessing and improving the woman's relationships within her entire social *ecosystem,* that is, with family, extended family, friends, social service providers, health care workers, and other relevant persons in her life. The goal of SET is to empower the woman to increase the extent to which her emotional, material, health, and social needs are achieved, and, in turn, her psychological adjustment is improved. SET helps the woman (a) transform problematic interactions that create and maintain stress and distress, (b) promote supportive interactions in existing relationships, and (c) develop new supportive relationships. The SET therapist helped Diane negotiate with her mother for more personal space and for cooperatively transferring parenting tasks, assisted the parents in linking Diane to their church, and facilitated the difficult family task of ejecting Diane's drug-abusing brother from their home in collaboration with the legal system.

Because relationships are such an important part of a woman's definition of self (Amaro, 1995; Miller, 1986), helping a woman to improve her condition requires an assessment and improvement in the social relationships that are central to her life. Among HIV+ African American women, key relationships often have been strained by HIV risk behaviors such as drug use and association with drug-abusing men. The tensions in these relationships become more burdensome when a woman must face the challenges of living with HIV, including the stigma that HIV still carries in many African American communities.

SET's ecosystemic perspective is ideally suited for the complex environment of HIV+ African American women and their families, who live in the extremely adverse social conditions found in the inner city. It is designed to help inner-city families challenged by HIV to skillfully and strategically interact with service systems and to capitalize on and enhance the tradition of strong social supports in African American families and communities. As such, SET is part of a movement in mental health toward approaches that attend to social ecological contexts (Aponte, 1976; Aponte & Van Deusen, 1981; Auerswald, 1968; Bronfenbrenner, 1977, 1979, 1986; Szapocznik & Kurtines, 1993; Szapocznik & Williams, in press). One of the most unique features of the SET approach is that we seek to network the various support systems in the woman's life (e.g., family, friends, health care), so that they can collaborate more effectively in supporting her. The goal is to develop a "small-town" context of support in which a person's family, friends, neighbors, and service providers know each other.

> SET therapists emphasize strengths, adapt their treatment to match each woman's particular life situation, and respect the woman's wishes regarding how many people are "in her business." For these reasons, women who are not comfortable participating in traditional psychotherapy can be engaged in SET.

This chapter describes the SET intervention as it was implemented with 65 women like Diane in a study conducted by the Center for Family Studies, in the University of Miami's Department of Psychiatry and Behavioral Sciences. Subsequent sections describe (a) the women, (b) program characteristics, (c) the SET model, (d) clinical findings, and (e) therapist characteristics, supervision, and training. Case examples such as that of Diane and other women from the project are presented throughout the text. All client names and some case details have been changed to protect confidentiality.

THE WOMEN

Like the other women in our project, Diane is an HIV+ African American woman who has given birth to at least one child, reports some family problem, and did not report drug dependence or a pattern of drug abuse at the time of enrollment. Recruitment takes place largely in HIV/AIDS health care facilities that serve the inner city. Because the women do not seek us, but rather we seek them, in general, they are not in the midst of a major personal crisis when they enroll.

The women vary widely in their knowledge, attitudes, and adherence regarding available medical treatments for HIV/AIDS. The vast majority are very poor and on welfare. Also, because of the prevalent routes of HIV infection in the past decade for inner-city women, most of the women have a history of drug addiction.

The women often have had more than one child, with the youngest and the oldest children having different fathers. Contrary to the usual lore, more than 80% of the women have a mate, who is frequently the father of the youngest child or children and who has a central role in the nuclear family. The women often have children in more than one household who have been formally or informally adopted by older female relatives. Because of the eligibility requirement for the project of "some family problems," the women's personal relationships with mates, children, and family members are frequently sources of stress and distress. For that reason, much of our emphasis in SET has been in improving these relationships.

The women's extrafamilial social supports often include neighbors, church, and self-help support groups. A few women are remarkably isolated, and treatment focuses on identifying potential social supports and the barriers that keep the women from accessing them. The women typically enter the intervention with a complex service network in place (e.g., health care, social services). This may be a function of our having recruited mainly from HIV/AIDS health clinics, which often offer or refer women to ancillary services.

PROJECT CHARACTERISTICS

This section describes the general framework of the SET intervention. Specific SET techniques will be presented in a later section.

The SET intervention lasts approximately 9 months, a time frame that was selected to provide some standard amount of contact and to allow sufficient time to meet treatment goals. There is considerable variability within and between cases regarding the frequency of therapy, with an average of 2 hours per week of contact. These include face-to-face or telephone contacts with the woman alone and/or with relevant persons from her ecosystem.

Pacing of treatment in this population is quite different from one that presents in crisis. The treatment course often has the pattern of moderate contact followed by a relatively inactive period (often due to a life disruption such as moving or illness), followed by a period of intensive contact around a crisis. In some cases, therapy starts out quite slowly because the woman is not in the midst of a major problem. Early contacts in such cases are typically short and informal and are aimed at building rapport until a problem occurs and the woman views the therapist as a relevant figure. Even in the midst of a crisis, the women are rarely receptive to meeting with the therapist more frequently than once per week.

Most sessions take place in the woman's home and are videotaped for clinical supervision and review. Contacts may also take place in other settings, such as a relative's home, a clinic, or a community center, wherever the therapist can gain access to the woman and the people whose relationships are being targeted in treatment. A few women, particularly those who are concerned with disclosure or domestic violence, prefer to have their sessions in the office. The therapist listens carefully for clues regarding the woman's unstated preferences and accommodates to maximize the chances of engagement into treatment, including foregoing videotaping if necessary.

> The primary principle regarding the location of therapy is that under no circumstances should this issue become a barrier to treatment. After considering therapist and client safety, the therapist goes wherever the woman and her support persons are available.

The Initiation of Treatment

Within 48 hours of being enrolled in SET, the woman is contacted by her therapist, who immediately begins building rapport and schedules the first meeting. In the initial sessions, the therapist most likely meets with the woman alone or sometimes with the woman and other members of the household and conversationally gathers the woman's life story, with an emphasis on the status of important relationships. This story gathering provides information for understanding the woman's relationships and opportunities for developing a therapeutic alliance and for linking past to present interactions (e.g., "I see how it came to be that you and your brother don't talk"). In the first sessions, the therapist also guides the woman in defining her treatment goals.

Next, the therapist plans the initial set of interventions, which are likely to involve family or familylike members who are potentially available for support. In cases in which there is a moderate or high degree of conflict between family members, it is useful to contact individual family members to develop trust and a working alliance. A working alliance is built by listening supportively to the family member's "side of the story" and looking for signs that the family member cares about the woman and is interested in an improved connection.

Once the therapist has obtained the collaboration of the key family members, she begins to orchestrate opportunities for new interactions that reflect increased emotional or instrumental support for the woman.

In the case of Shanequa, for example, her father, in whose home she was living, agreed to participate in the second session. The father was initially highly negative about Shanequa, offering a laundry list of her shortcomings and misdeeds. The therapist noted that the father made repeated references to scripture and learned that he was a church elder. Shanequa had disconnected from the church following her mother's death but indicated that she was interested in returning. The therapist then guided a discussion between father and daughter that resulted in his inviting Shanequa to attend a church gathering. Hence, the father's negativity about Shanequa was redirected to his reaching out to her for a joint activity.

◇ ◇ ◇

For the most part, the remainder of therapy involves continued reinforcement and solidification of the newly acquired interactions within different content areas.

> Shanequa's father went on to help her work out a financial plan (one of his primary complaints was her irresponsible spending), which helped Shanequa to realize her goal of moving into her own apartment. The desired interaction was to establish direct and productive communication between Shanequa and her father, and this was practiced and reinforced around various contents (e.g., church, financial planning) until the direct line of communication was firmly established and no longer required intervention by the therapist.

Depending on the case, extrafamilial interventions may precede, follow, or be a part of family sessions. On occasion, there are immediate needs, such as medical or legal crises that may require urgent attention from the therapist. However, because SET is an empowerment model, the family work often precedes extrafamilial interventions in the hope of assisting the family to develop the skills to conduct the needed interactions with other systems.

WORKING IN THE WOMAN'S HOME
AND OTHER NATURAL SETTINGS

Most therapists are taught that to facilitate emotional processing, sessions must take place in a private and sacrosanct space. Home sessions, in contrast, are frequently interrupted by telephone calls, unexpected visits, household members entering and leaving the room, and noise from the street or from television sets that are left on (Shanequa's first session took place while a manicurist worked on her nails). To be effective in home-based therapy, the therapist must be able to structure a therapeutic environment, yet blend in and respect the authority of the client in her own home.

Spontaneity is essential in home-based work. The therapist must not only sustain therapeutic contact in the context of a disrupted environment but must also respond to these disruptions as opportunities for carrying out interventions. Unexpected visits or phone calls may provide opportunities to engage members of social support or service systems into the therapeutic system. With the woman's permission, a visiting neighbor could be invited to join the session and be engaged as a resource for the woman. Household members who are reluctant to become involved in a session often pass through the room where the session is taking place. This is an opportunity for the therapist to engage the family member in some light conversation, gradually building a bond (see Figure 11.1).

Home-based therapy provides an opportunity for the therapist to
* *access* persons otherwise unavailable,
* *assess* and *intervene* in interactions that would not occur in the office, and
* become *integrated* in family events.

Figure 11.1. Opportunity Knocks

In the woman's natural environment, the therapist has an opportunity to gain a better understanding of relationships and to transform interactions as they naturally occur. In addition, interactional changes that are made in the natural environment may be more likely to generalize outside of therapy. Contacts at events that are part of the woman's life, such as family funerals or graduation ceremonies, allow the therapist to become acquainted with important persons and gain insight regarding the woman's position within her ecosystem.

Termination

When the family interactions are more positive and the woman has established better connections within her ecosystem, it is time to move toward termination of therapy. Termination is typically determined in terms of behavioral objectives, including symptoms (such as substance abuse or depression) and the targeted relationships, as well as project parameters for the duration of treatment. One indicator of readiness for termination is how the woman and her ecosystem respond to crises, that is, whether they spontaneously respond to challenges in a more functional manner.

Shanequa's treatment was coming to an end as she was solidly connected with a drug support group, preparing to obtain a high school equivalency degree, attending church, and adhering to her medical regimen. Shanequa's relationship with family members had become closer, and she had gained status in the family by opening a bank account and saving money for the first time in her life. A week before the final session was to be held, Shanequa was hospitalized for an infection. This crisis provided an opportunity to observe the new family patterns in action. Without any therapist intervention, the family mobilized to provide physical, emotional, and financial support. Shanequa experienced a new level of nurturance and respect from her family. She left the hospital feeling physically recuperated, confident in her family's future support, and truly ready for termination.

Termination is a process that begins in the first session. Every intervention is directed at developing interactions that will continue beyond the duration of the therapy. The therapist's job is to work herself out of a job, and the SET therapist's competence is judged by her effectiveness in helping the woman and her family to build competence in relating to each other and outside supports.

THE SET MODEL

This section presents the more technical aspects of the intervention, including SET theory and techniques.

SET Theory

SET is derived from a combination of two theoretical approaches: (a) the structural/systemic approach and (b) the ecosystemic approach. The structural/systemic approach provides the "rules" for making sense of interactions, and the ecosystemic approach provides an organizing framework for the "field" in which these interactions occur. We will now describe each of these theoretical roots and the manner in which they are integrated to form SET.

The Structural/Systemic Approach

Structural/systemic theory (Kurtines & Szapocznik, 1996; Minuchin, 1974; Minuchin, Montalvo, Guerney, Rosman, & Schumer, 1967; Szapocznik & COSSMHO, 1994; Szapocznik & Kurtines, 1989) explains that the nature of the interdependence among and within systems can be understood in terms of patterns of interactions. The central principles of this approach are systems, structure, and strategy.

Systems. A system is composed of parts that are interdependent or interrelated. Human systems are made up of persons who are responsive to each other's behaviors. Two major aspects of systems that are important to our work are that (a) the woman's problems are identified as occurring not in isolation but in the context of the systems in which she finds herself, and (b) the behaviors of members within systems are viewed as interactive and interdependent. That is, each individual's behavior is quite different from what it would be if it were possible for the individual to act in isolation. The family is one type of system in which individual members of the system are interdependent and interrelated. When a woman is irritable due to the side effects from her medications, for example, she is less able to come to agreement with her mate about their parenting functions, resulting in the woman's children being exposed to inconsistent parenting.

Structure. The interactions that occur in established systems tend to be repetitive and predictable and define the system's structure. When these repetitive interactions are unsuccessful in achieving the goals of the system or its individual members, then they are considered maladaptive and become an important focus of treatment.

Changing structures is the challenge of systemic therapies such as SET because natural forces within the individual and system conspire to maintain the status quo.

An example is the case of Jackie, who as a result of our interventions began to spend some time out of the home and with friends and began to rely on her mate's cousin next door to do occasional parenting. This led Jackie's mother to make disparaging remarks about Jackie's resolve as a mother. Without further intervention, Jackie would have reverted to her prior behavior, having been pulled back by the forces of the system. The therapist elicited the mother's support of this structural change by suggesting to the mother that the new behavior would make Jackie a better mother because it would give her an opportunity to "recharge her batteries." The mother's support was solidified when she agreed to be available on the telephone in the event that the children wanted their mother or grandmother while Jackie was out.

If new behaviors are rewarding (e.g., Jackie being able to "recharge"), they tend to recur, and the system is forced to recalibrate to accommodate the new behavior, albeit with therapist interventions. In the new arrangements, other members of the system (Jackie's mother and children) change their behaviors to complement the new behaviors of the person (Jackie) who initiated the change.

Strategy. Strategy refers to treatment interventions that are practical and planned. To be "practical" means that we implement an intervention because it helps to achieve therapeutic objectives. A common strategic intervention is for the therapist to highlight a convenient piece of reality, a frame or perspective, that helps to move the intervention in the desired direction. For instance, in a case in which a woman's mother is berating her for being a "pothead," if the therapist is most concerned with lowering the negativity of the interaction, she may choose to focus on the mother's concern for the well-being of her daughter as a way of building a bridge between them while minimizing the hostility. Conversely, if the therapist is most interested in having the mother set limits to dangerous behavior, she might select to exacerbate the sense of crisis surrounding the drug abuse, validating and magnifying the mother's concerns by emphasizing that her daughter's way of life will lead her to lose custody of her baby or worsen her medical condition.

Structural/systemic interventions are "planned" in that the therapist assesses interactions, determines which of these might be targeted or used in treatment, and establishes a plan to transform interactions. This approach involves (a) developing a clear understanding of the nature of supportive and problematic interactions, (b) understanding how these interactions are related to the woman's current level of psychosocial functioning, and (c) intervening in a very deliberate fashion to enhance supportive and reduce maladaptive interactions. In the example given earlier, once the therapist has determined that there is a caring bond between the woman and her mother, a planned set of interventions might include (a) strengthening their alliance by having them talk together about a common concern (e.g., the woman's health), (b) having them work together on practical problem solving regarding how the woman might better manage her stress (an outcome of which might include a plan for the mother to watch the baby so that the woman can attend an HIV support group), (c) prompting a facilitator or member of an existing support group to reach out to the woman, and (d) meeting individually with the woman to enhance her motivation to stop using drugs, break off drug-using relationships, or enter drug treatment.

Process Over Content

The purpose of SET is to transform interactional process so that the woman is able to attain her immediate content goals (e.g., negotiating so there is agreement about who takes out the trash) and is able to go beyond them to achieve a more effective and rewarding interaction with her ecosystem (applying these negotiation skills to other contents and other people).

Process. The most important implication of the structural/systemic approach is its emphasis on process over content. Process comprises the behaviors of system members and of the interplay between behaviors. Content, on the other hand, is the manifest aspect of the communication. For example, when a couple is arguing about who takes out the trash, the content is the trash. The process is how they argue (e.g., they attack each other) or the meta-communication in the message (e.g., "I want you to be my partner, but I don't experience you as doing your fair share," or "You are not good for anything, not even to take out the trash.").

Our typical client is convinced that content is the basis of her unhappiness (i.e., it is the trash that is the problem). In contrast, SET aims to transform the

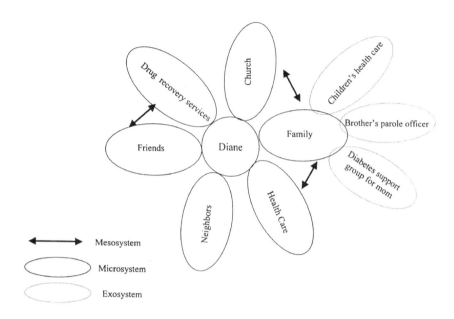

Figure 11.2.   Diane's Ecosystem Template

processes that block the resolution of content concerns (the attacking manner in which they argue about the trash). Attacking one another over who takes out the trash is merely one instance of the couple's inability to resolve conflicts.

The Ecosystemic Approach

The second theoretical foundation of SET is the ecosystemic approach. This perspective provides a systemic template through which to organize the relationships that define the woman's context (i.e., her ecosystem). The ecosystem is organized in terms of (a) microsystems, (b) mesosystems, and (c) exosystems (Bronfenbrenner, 1979). To illustrate these terms, we have drawn an ecosystemic template for Diane (see Figure 11.2), who was introduced at the beginning of the chapter.

Microsystems. Microsystems refer to systems in which the woman is a member in direct interaction with other members of these systems. The microsystems are represented by the petals of the "flower" in Figure 11.2. The most common microsystems for our women include family (nuclear and extended); social support systems such friends, church, and neighbors; and service systems such as social services, drug abuse treatment, and health care. Diane's microsystems include family, health care, neighbors, friends, drug recovery services, and church.

Mesosystems. Mesosystems consist of the connections between persons from the woman's microsystems. In Figure 11.2, these are represented by the arrows between the petals. Mesosystems do not necessarily include the woman directly, yet their presence and quality play an important role in defining the quality of her supportive context. For example, a mesosystem may involve a collaborative relationship between the woman's parents (family microsystem) and a close friend (friend microsystem) in which responsibilities for caring for the woman and her children in the event of a hospitalization may be distributed. The absence of mesosystems may indicate risk because persons from different systems cannot compare notes or collaborate on what is happening with the woman (e.g., in the case of a woman who is not attending prenatal visits, the absence of a connection between a health care worker and a family member limits the health worker's options for intervening). Mesosystems in Diane's case include the relationship between her friends and the drug recovery system (she was beginning to socialize with peers that she had met in drug treatment), between family and church (the family was well connected to the church), and between the family and Diane's health care system (Diane's younger brother had accompanied her to a clinic appointment and wanted to learn more about HIV).

> We believe that it is SET's emphasis on targeting mesosystems (i.e., the relationships between support systems in the woman's life) that critically distinguishes it from other psychosocial interventions. By targeting mesosystems, SET provides a wide field in which to create new interactions (i.e., supportive networks) throughout the ecosystem. Mesosystems have great potential for impact while placing little demand on the woman.

Exosystems. Exosystems do not directly involve the woman. They are those relationships between a member of one of the woman's microsystems and a system that does not directly contain the woman. These exosystems, through their impact on persons in the woman's life, have an impact on the woman. In Figure

11.2, exosystems are represented by the dotted ovals that touch on a petal. In the case of Diane, exosystems include Diane's children's health care, her mother's diabetes support group, and her brother's parole officer. Exosystemic interventions are not a specific target in SET but are attended to in cases in which a family member or other support to the woman is in need of improvements in support system functioning. In the case of Diane, an exosystemic intervention involved having the family work with Diane's older brother's parole officer to help set limits on the brother's access to the home and pressure him to enter drug treatment (because the parole officer is a relationship of the brother that does not directly include Diane, we consider it an exosystem).

On the Treatment of Natural Ecosystems. The primary emphasis in SET is in restoring the functioning of the woman's natural social support network (e.g., family, friends, and neighbors) rather than the prevalent approach among psychosocial services of giving families surrogate support systems (e.g., support groups and other services) while disregarding natural supports, which are more enduring. Although SET therapists work to connect women and their families with services, they emphasize naturally occurring supports because these are the most likely to have ongoing and enduring influences on the woman. Also, as we have argued elsewhere (Szapocznik & Mancilla, 1995), we are concerned that the overreliance on surrogate supports may be contributing to the breakdown of natural support systems.

In addition, SET emphasizes the *treatment* of maladaptive interactional patterns at all levels of the ecosystem. If a woman's family and friends are disconnected or she is not attending clinic appointments, we assume that underlying processes interfere with connectedness (such as a history of negativity or power struggles between the health system and the woman or a deliberate fracturing of connections on the woman's part that may indicate an underlying problem such as depression, drug abuse, or domestic violence). Rather than just linking family with friends or women with doctors, we transform the interactions between them to overcome barriers that preclude ongoing communication and collaboration.

An example is the case of Angela, who wanted to be better informed about her condition and whose primary care nurse was focused on Angela's failure to adhere to her medical regimen. Although both clearly had the common goal of improving Angela's health, they were locked in conflict because each viewed the other as uncooperative or insensitive. The therapist engaged Angela and her nurse in a collaboration by highlighting their common goal.

◇ ◇ ◇

Integrating the Structural/Systemic
and Ecosystemic Approaches

SET merges the structural/systemic and ecosystemic approaches by applying the concepts of system, structure, and strategy to interactions that occur at every level of the woman's ecosystem (microsystem, mesosystem, and exosystem).

The issue of Diane's brother's substance abuse provides an example for the integration of these concepts. The *interdependence* of the family *system* is illustrated by the fact that the brother's substance abuse had an impact on each member of the family: providing cues that triggered Diane's cravings for drugs, pulling at the mother's competing desires to nurture her son and protect other family members, exposing the children to drugs and paraphernalia, and creating tension between the mother and stepfather. The family *structure* (before intervention) was one of making few demands on this oldest son, leading him to expect special treatment and Diane to be resentful of the "double standard." In addition, delicate problems in this family were rarely managed head on and often were avoided until a crisis emerged. The pattern of interaction between the family and the legal system (*exosystem*) was governed by fear; the family kept their distance because they did not view the legal system as helpful. The therapist employed a *planned* set of interventions: (a) helping the family confront the tensions and problems that the drug abuse caused within the family, (b) guiding Diane's mother and stepfather in their contact with the parole officer (an intervention that *strategically* excluded Diane to minimize her burden), and (c) helping the family to confront Diane's brother with the limits they were setting. Concurrently, the therapist assessed the *ecosystem* for potential sources of support and the family's patterns of interactions with these support systems. She encouraged the family to reach out to those systems with which they already had positive bonds: their church (for Diane and her parents) and drug abuse peer counselors (for Diane).

The structural/systemic approach also provides the techniques used in SET and applies them as needed throughout the ecosystem.

SET Techniques

The following section describes the SET techniques, which are divided into three categories: (a) *joining,* or building and strengthening therapeutic alliances; (b) *pattern diagnosis,* or mapping and assessing the ecosystem; and (c) *restructuring,* or shaping new interactions (Kurtines & Szapocznik, 1996; Minuchin & Fishman, 1981; Szapocznik & COSSMHO, 1994; Szapocznik & Kurtines, 1989). These three elements of therapy, although somewhat sequential (the earliest phases of treatment emphasize joining and diagnosis, whereas restructuring is predominant later in treatment) all take place throughout treatment and are used strategically as needed. For example, with every restructuring intervention, the therapist is straining the therapeutic alliance and therefore needs to do some joining, and the therapist must assess (diagnose) how the system responds to the emerging patterns of interactions that result from the restructuring.

Joining

The first category of techniques is joining. In this chapter, we will emphasize joining over the other techniques because we believe that this is where many other interventions fail. Because women are making important life changes as part of this intervention, we concentrate on building and nurturing the therapeutic relationship between the therapist, the woman, her family, and other members of her ecosystem.

In the process of joining, the therapist becomes a leader of the therapeutic system by earning the trust of persons in the system, particularly its most powerful members.[1] The therapist enters a system by matching its style, tempo, and mood and accepting its rules of interaction. For example, if the therapist recognizes that one person serves as the central pathway through which communication is routed, she joins with the system by talking directly to this person and allowing this central person to mediate her communications to other system members.

Even after a therapeutic alliance is established, the therapist continues to join by matching some aspects of the system's structure while challenging others.

In the case of Shirley, for example, the therapist noted that Shirley held a lower status than her husband, James. Moreover, when it came to mother-child conflicts, James would render a decision as if Shirley and the children were all equal in status. The therapist matched this structure by employing the metaphor of James as "judge" of the family court but simultaneously challenged the structure by designating Shirley as "the state prosecutor" and the children as "the defendants." Thus, Shirley remained below her husband but was elevated to a higher level than the children. The family accepted this metaphor and spontaneously held "family court" several times during the week. At the next session, Shirley, who usually looked disheveled and dispirited, was well dressed and groomed and sat proudly in the chair next to James, who stated that Shirley had not even needed to present her case; he knew that the children were in the wrong.

As this case illustrates, a critical aspect of joining is that it requires the therapist to muster genuine feelings of acceptance for all members of the system, regardless of whether she likes and agrees with them. In fact, sometimes the person with whom it is most critical to establish an alliance (the most powerful member of the system) may be the person who is liked least. Establishing alliances and a therapeutic system, then, is the art of politics.

The therapist establishes alliances around goals. She learns what each individual in the system wants to achieve, identifies systemwide goals that will benefit the woman, and offers help in attaining these goals. By identifying the goals of the various family members, the therapist weaves together a coalition in which different members strive to achieve their individual goals, all of which contribute to the common goals that ameliorate problems the HIV+ woman is experiencing.

Although in most cases it is possible to identify common goals that benefit the woman and every member of the system, occasions require that some members of a system be left out of the therapeutic coalition. In particular, drug-abusing individuals will typically have to be excluded from the coalition because their drug use threatens the coalition's stability, as was evident in the case of Diane, whose drug-using brother was threatening her recovery. In some cases, then, a strategic aspect of the intervention is to create more solid boundaries between the woman and individuals jeopardizing her well-being.

Disclosure: An Important Consideration in Joining. When approaching any member of the ecosystem to participate in treatment, the therapist must be aware of whether this person has been told about therapy, the woman's HIV/AIDS diagnosis, and/or the woman's personal history. The woman's decision on disclosure in any issue is always respected (to the limits of the law) and is a critical factor in determining whether or how a person should be included in treatment. HIV/AIDS and other sensitive issues do not necessarily have to be mentioned in sessions, making it possible to include persons to whom the woman has not disclosed.

HIV disclosure issues may become central in treatment, however. Many women become estranged from important sources of support due to their anxieties related to HIV disclosure. The woman may want to disclose to her friends and family but may fear rejection and abandonment. The therapist works with the woman in assessing the advantages and disadvantages of each disclosure decision. Although disclosure may not be advisable in every instance, treatment can be a "safe" place for the woman to develop skills in managing her fears and disclose to friends and family.

Working through disclosure of HIV was an important theme in the case of Andrea, who was engaged to her live-in partner, Kevin. Andrea wanted to begin married life with a "clean slate" and disclose her HIV status to Kevin. She suspected that Kevin already knew, but when she had tried to broach the subject in the past, Kevin stated that he did not want to know about it and left the house for 2 days.

This was the manner in which the couple managed other difficult problems, including Kevin's drug abuse, the intrusiveness of Andrea's family, and Kevin's mother's terminal illness. Kevin's avoidance of difficult issues frustrated Andrea, who would respond by persisting or berating Kevin, leading to an escalation of conflict until Kevin would leave home or they would enter long periods of tense silence. The couple worked in therapy on this pattern, using the "safest" of the difficult issues (the matter of Andrea's sister's meddling) as content. At an individual session about 4 months into therapy, after the couple had overcome their troublesome pattern of managing conflict and problems around the "safer" issue, Andrea announced that she was ready to present Kevin with the truth about her HIV. Andrea and the therapist rehearsed how Andrea would present the information, how she would manage Kevin's response, and how to judge if she should back off and give Kevin "space" if he seemed on the verge of an explosion or of walking out. The therapist also guided Andrea in securing support from Kevin's brother's wife, who would send her husband to look for Kevin should he leave home again. Andrea decided that it was best to tell Kevin in private. The following week, she called the therapist to say that she had told Kevin, that he had stated that he knew all along, but that he was not yet prepared to discuss the topic in treatment. The opportunity to process the disclosure in therapy occurred 1 month later when Kevin brought up his concerns regarding Andrea catching his cold. At that time, the therapist observed that Kevin and Andrea were able to speak openly about her health, about their mutual fears, and about Andrea's fears of rejection.

In some cases, relationships that have been damaged in the course of disclosure may need to be repaired in the process of therapy.

In the case of Doreen, for example, she had disclosed to her favorite aunt and not to other members of her family. The aunt revealed this information to Doreen's mother, who was extremely hurt by Doreen's apparent lack of confidence in their relationship. The therapist conducted a session with Doreen, her mother, and her aunt in which the secretiveness was presented as an attempt by Doreen to spare her mother the anguish of knowing about the HIV diagnosis.

Joining in the Family Context. Families have deeply ingrained patterns of interaction and therefore require especially skilled joining. The therapist must enter the family system but avoid becoming inducted into the family's maladaptive patterns. In some families, for example, the therapist may be viewed as the ultimate arbiter of arguments, whose expertise can be used to judge "rights" and "wrongs" within the family. The therapist must avoid getting caught in these family processes, or his or her effectiveness will be compromised.

In our work, the HIV+ woman is the initial contact through whom the therapist enters the family. Other family members may be difficult to engage because they view the therapist as being the woman's ally rather than theirs, they have negative attitudes toward therapy, or they do not have the time to be bothered with the woman's problems. For whatever reason family members state (which is content) that they will not participate in therapy, resistance to participation is always viewed from an interactional perspective (i.e., as process). Resistance is a function of therapist-system interactions, and when therapists change their response to disengaged behaviors, they can be enormously successful in increasing engagement into treatment (Szapocznik & Kurtines, 1989).

Some people, although they care about the woman and want a better relationship, may be difficult to engage because they expect to be devalued, blamed, or criticized in therapy. This is often the case with the women's male mates, who have historically been overlooked or identified as negative influences by social service agencies. The therapist approaches these family members in a highly supportive and validating manner and illustrates for them how therapy may be instrumental in achieving their goals and improving their relationship with the woman.

In the case of Michelle, for example, her partner Greg had been living with Michelle and her children for 2 years. Greg played the role of surrogate father to Michelle's two young sons and baby-sat when Michelle attended her medical appointments. Because Greg never accompanied Michelle to her appointments, her health care workers did not know Greg and the important role he played in assisting Michelle with many of her practical daily life tasks. In meeting with Michelle and Greg, the SET therapist discovered that although Greg knew of Michelle's HIV diagnosis, he was uneducated about HIV/AIDS and unaware of some of the health-related problems Michelle was experiencing. In addition, the therapist was concerned that the couple was not practicing safe sex. The therapist punctuated the positive aspects of Michelle and Greg's relationship (i.e., love, supportiveness, concern) and acknowledged the key role that Greg played in building a solid relationship with Michelle based on open communication about an array of interpersonal and intimate issues. By emphasizing Greg's care for Michelle, the therapist was able to engage Greg in the process of becoming more involved in and knowledgeable about Michelle's health. With the therapist's guidance, the couple planned to have Greg attend a clinic with Michelle to begin the process of his learning more about HIV and meet the health care workers.

Often, it is the woman herself who blocks the therapist's access to family members. This process is particularly important in cases in which there is a history of conflict and the woman feels that the relationship is tenuously balanced. The woman may tell the therapist directly that she wants to keep family members out of the therapy, or she may offer repeated excuses for them being unable to participate. It is important that the therapist work directly with the woman to explore her concerns about bringing these individuals into therapy and assuage her fears that the therapist will stress fragile relationships.

Sherry and her three children lived with Sherry's mother. Sherry was reluctant to include her mother in treatment because they were finally on speaking terms after years of estrangement, and Sherry feared her mother's disapproval if she learned of Sherry's HIV diagnosis and other personal issues. Sherry described her mother as a devout Christian who had expressed strong sentiments about HIV/ AIDS as "God's punishment." Sherry also did not want the children to hear her mother say anything negative about her, for fear that this would damage their relationship with herself and her mother. The therapist began the first session by talking about general family life and how she could assist the family with important issues such as parenting, coparenting (between Sherry and her mother), household management, communication, privacy issues, and so on. Sherry warmed up to this approach because these issues were very real concerns in her everyday experience. For the second session, Sherry asked her mother to attend. The mother shared her concerns and desire to get closer to Sherry. The issue of HIV was raised much later in the therapy and in a very natural and nonthreatening way for both the mother and daughter.

The importance of joining does not imply that the therapist presses for engagement of all family members. In cases in which the woman is involved in an abusive relationship, safety considerations are paramount in deciding whom to include in therapy and how they should be approached. Pressuring the woman to include the abuser prematurely may result in her terminating treatment. If there is an indication that approaching a person may result in abuse, the therapist must explore alternative strategies to rectify this relationship.

Joining in Extrafamilial Systems. The woman is often hesitant to allow the therapist to engage persons from outside of the family due to her concerns about having others know her "business." This privacy concern is often due to cultural values against "airing one's dirty laundry" as well as the stigma attached to HIV/ AIDS. The therapist can usually allay the woman's concerns by demonstrating that she is sensitive to the woman's need to maintain appropriate boundaries and by working with her to identify a rationale and goals for involving these persons in the treatment in a circumscribed manner. The therapist gains access to persons from extrafamilial systems by identifying the barriers to access and creating conditions that make it acceptable for such a person to become part of the treatment process.

Joining with persons from social support systems often takes place in informal circumstances and requires the therapist to have a flexible and spontaneous approach. It is often the case that the therapist meets members of these systems when they arrive unexpectedly, as she is escorted to her car or on social occasions such as funerals or hospital visits. As the therapist meets persons from social support systems, she discretely explores where these people fit in the woman's life and their potential as sources of support. This process must be accomplished with utmost sensitivity to the woman's privacy and requires that the therapist be able to tactfully evade questions that threaten confidentiality. Once important individuals have been identified, the therapist gains the woman's permission to bring them more formally into the therapeutic process.

Joining with persons from service systems carries its own special set of considerations because these systems often have complex political structures. Therefore, the therapist must be adept at identifying the unwritten rules of the system and not threaten its territoriality regarding "ownership" of the woman's (or her child's) case. Our therapists spend considerable energy in establishing collegial relationships with agency personnel to proactively identify and counteract system barriers. Effective tools in counteracting resistance from service systems include validating the good work and intentions of the system, identifying common goals, and inviting system members to attend team meetings. Case "ownership" is never a struggle because the SET therapist remains aware that SET is time limited, and her goal is to help establish a strong connection between the woman and the agency. Meetings that include the woman and members of service systems require the therapist to maintain an alliance with both parties, recognizing the service provider's expertise while supporting the woman in meeting her goals.

An example is the case of Cassandra, whose primary goal in treatment was to regain custody of her adolescent daughter following an episode of sexual abuse by Cassandra's former boyfriend. The therapist invested a great deal of effort in establishing working relationships with the guardian ad litem and the state protective services worker. Both of these workers held a negative view of Cassandra and were members of complex, turf-sensitive systems. The therapist recognized the seniority of these workers in Cassandra's case and asked them to bring her up to date. She also affirmed their accomplishments in helping Cassandra to improve her situation (she had cut off contact with the boyfriend and relocated to better housing), which served to have the workers invested in Cassandra's success. These relationships proved pivotal in helping Cassandra to fulfill all of the requirements for regaining custody while maintaining a cooperative relationship with the workers, who became important resources for Cassandra and her daughter during the transitional period of custody.

Table 11.1 (p. 264) presents some additional examples of joining interventions in the family, social support, and service systems.

Pattern Diagnosis

The second category of SET technique is pattern diagnosis, whereby the full complement of a woman's ecosystem is mapped and assessed. The *mapping* of the woman's ecosystem generally proceeds from those relationships with which she is most involved to those that are more peripheral. The genogram is a map of the woman's relationship with individuals in her immediate and extended family. The ecogram is a map of the woman's ecosystem, which shows the quality of the relationships between the woman, her immediate family, and the other systems with which they are involved. Figures 11.3 and 11.4 show Diane's (case presented at the beginning of the chapter) genogram and ecogram, respectively.

Diane's genogram (Figure 11.3) shows three generations of family and extended family, as well as significant relationships between them, and indicates who are the members of the household. Genograms are an invaluable guide for determining which relationships might be targeted in therapy and how they can be strategically approached. For example, Diane's genogram indicates that she is in conflict with Hazel, the grandmother of one of her children. This is a stressor for Diane as well as a possible barrier to her effectively parenting this child (because of the potential for Diane's parenting to be undermined by her conflict with Hazel), indicating that this relationship might be a target for intervention. It also shows that Diane has a close relationship with Juanita (Hazel's daughter), which alerts the therapist to the possibility that Juanita might provide a bridge between Diane and Hazel.

The ecogram (Figure 11.4) shows the relationships between Diane, her parents, and the various extrafamilial systems that are relevant in their lives. Among other things, it indicates that Diane's sole close connection with an extrafamilial system is with her drug recovery system. As with the genogram, the ecogram is an important tool for illustrating relationships that can be targeted in treatment. For example, the parents' strong church ties were targeted as providing a link between Diane and the church. In addition, extrafamilial interventions are often intertwined with within-family interventions. For example, an important strategy used to help Diane and her mother successfully negotiate Diane's increased parenting role was to have the mother serve as Diane's mentor. One intervention used in this realm was to have the mother introduce Diane to her children's teachers.

In the process of mapping, the therapist begins to systematically assess the various systems to determine their potential for conflict and support. Assessment takes place along the following dimensions: (a) system organization, (b) resonance, (c) developmental stage, and (d) conflict management.

TABLE 11.1 Examples of Joining Interventions

	Example 1	Example 2
Family microsystem	The stepmother of our client, who is in drug recovery, is reluctant to participate in family therapy sessions. She is a successful business owner. The therapist appeals to the stepmother's business expertise and enlists her advice and guidance on how her stepdaughter can become financially independent.	Our client has decided to reach out to her estranged sister. The sister is considered the "good and competent" one by the family and is often the one everyone depends on. The sister is ambivalent about getting pulled into the client's complex problems. The therapist explains the importance of family getting closer to one another and that being strong is not always an easy place to be in, especially when you may have to look for support. She also explains that in family therapy, it is good to hear more than one side of the story. The sister agrees that there are times she would like to have someone to talk to and that it might be a good thing to share some of her feelings with her sister every now and then. She likes the idea of telling her side of things and begins to regularly participate in therapy.
Social support system	A friend of our client drops by to ask if she needs anything from the store. The friend introduces her to someone who is "always helping" her (i.e., the therapist). Without disclosing her role or any information about the client, the therapist talks to the friend and learns that she is aware of the client's health status (HIV+) and that she is available to lend support. The friend is also involved in a church that has an AIDS ministry. The therapist suggests that the friend stay for the session if she is comfortable discussing ministry activities. The friend replies that she does not want to impose on the client's "territory" or embarrass her in any way. The client quickly tells her that would not be the case. The therapist encourages them to talk about what it would be like for the client to join the HIV support group at the church.	Our client wants to have a Narcotics Anonymous (NA) support group member visit her at the home that she shares with her mother. The mother fears that this person will be a negative influence on the client. The therapist suggests inviting the NA member over for a session to discuss her role as a support person for the client. A session is held that includes client, NA member, and mother. The therapist creates an atmosphere of comfort in which the client and NA member explain their similar experiences in recovery and how their relationship would be helpful for the client's sobriety and her need to be around positive people. The mother is wary at first but then decides that she likes the NA member and explains that she was just being protective of her daughter.

	Example 1	Example 2
Service systems	Our client has a 10-year-old son who is acting out in school. She is at her "wit's end," and although she has tried to be involved with the school, she has found it difficult to communicate and maintain a consistent presence because she is often ill and overwhelmed by other hardships. She requests the involvement of the therapist in reaching out to the teacher, whom she feels probably considers her a "bad mom." The therapist suggests telephoning the teacher during the session and making arrangements to meet. The client contacts the teacher and explains she is going through some rough times but would like to meet with her and that her family therapist would be happy to come along. The therapist introduces herself and expresses her belief that both mom and the teacher are obviously concerned about the child's education and future. A meeting is set up between client, teacher, and therapist for the following week.	Our client perceives her health care manager as somewhat hostile whenever the client asks questions and requests assistance. The therapist attends the clinic with the client and introduces herself to the manager and expresses her appreciation of how difficult her job must be and wonders if there are some ways to help the client be more prepared for clinic. The worker explains to the client that she would like her to come to clinic a little earlier so as not to be delayed in getting through the day. She apologizes that sometimes she is too busy to stop and listen to the client but that she does have some material she can pass along to her that may answer her questions. She also explains that although she cannot guarantee a quick exit, she will try to help make it easier to manage the long wait (e.g., by providing vouchers for lunch, having the chart ready). The client adjusts her perception of her manager's attitude and becomes more active in her health care.

265

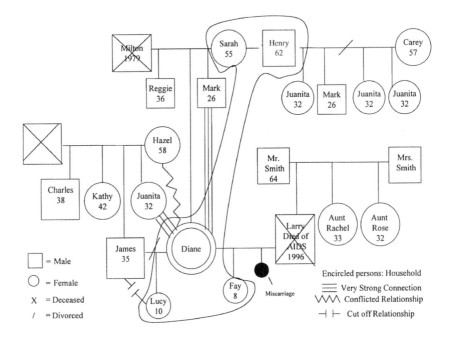

Figure 11.3. Diane's Genogram

System Organization. System organization considers the leadership functions of the system, such as who takes charge (especially in regard to the woman's concerns), whether there are power struggles, and the extent to which the woman is empowered within the system. System organization also is concerned with alliances, such as who supports whom and whether relationships are cooperative and supportive or highly competitive and adversarial, and the ability of system members to be direct and specific in their communications, which is essential for resolving conflicts and providing support.

Resonance. Resonance refers to the connectedness between and among persons in the system. At one extreme, boundaries can be highly rigid, resulting in emotional and psychological distance between people. Many women become alienated from important people in their lives due to the stigma of HIV/AIDS and problems associated with past HIV risk behaviors. Reconnecting women with these cutoff supports is one of the primary goals of SET.

Boundaries can also be far too tenuous, leading to a level of emotional and psychological closeness between people that is too great and intolerable for some. A strength of close systems is that members are very sensitive to each

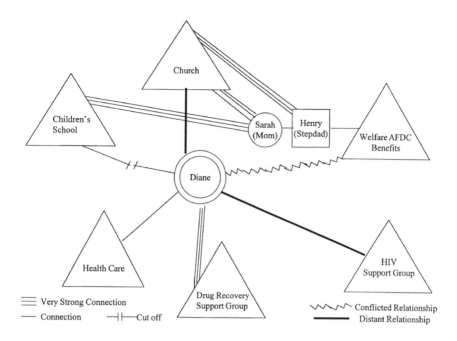

Figure 11.4. Diane's Ecogram

other's emotional states and are often available for support. A weakness is that they do not tolerate uniqueness and may engender dependency, and there is a tendency for members to make assumptions about each other's thoughts and feelings and therefore not communicate about important issues.

Developmental Stage. Systems, like individuals, go through a series of stages that require adjustment and the completion of stage-specific tasks. The women and families we treat experience multiple destabilizing disruptions of the life cycle. For example, many of these women had their first children during adolescence, when they were unprepared for the tasks of motherhood. When the women enter treatment, the family landscape has been influenced by the lack of synchronicity in the developmental stage of the woman, the couple, and the family.

Drug abuse recovery is an important milestone for many of the women in this intervention. The determination to end their drug abuse was often spurred by some life-shaking event such as their HIV diagnosis or a significant loss that was brought about by their drug use. As in the case of Diane, the recovery process requires numerous relationship adjustments such as reintegration into the family and other prosocial community systems, as well as separation from drug-abusing peers.

The most dramatic developmental upheaval confronted by the families of our women is the nature of their illness and, occasionally, the untimely illness and death of some of their younger HIV-infected children. A person's adjustment to his or her own impending death or to the chronicity of the illness, in the context of untimely deaths and overburdened family supports, is a formidable developmental challenge. Some of this important work can take place in HIV support groups or in the reconnection with the church that occurs with spiritual awakenings.

Conflict Management. Disagreements and problems are natural, and a viable system needs ways of managing them. Healthy systems are flexible and use a variety of conflict management approaches depending on what the situation warrants, with the goal of eventually resolving conflicts or problems. We have identified three conflict management styles: (a) denial/avoidance, (b) diffusion, and (c) resolution, which are presented in ascending order of functionality. Some situations, however, call for temporarily using one of the lower forms of conflict management rather than a higher form. For example, when a system member is having an intense emotional reaction to a discussion, it is preferable to avoid the issue temporarily until the person is able to face the issue more calmly.

• Denial/avoidance occurs when conflict is not allowed to emerge or begins to emerge but is stopped or inhibited in some way. Sometimes this is done by adopting the attitude that "everything is fine," instant agreement when one opinion is expressed, or attempts to squelch disagreement or the discussion of sensitive topics. Sometimes denial/avoidance even takes the form of exaggerating a problem such as, "I feel like I'm going to lose my mind if I have to think about this anymore." A pattern of conflict avoidance was illustrated in the case of Andrea and Kevin, which was presented earlier, in that when Andrea insisted on discussing a sensitive topic, an argument would ensue, leading to Kevin leaving home or periods of tense silence. Denial/avoidance of conflict also takes place when situations are arranged to bypass the reemergence of a conflict or sensitive issue. In the case of Laurel, whose stepfather had sexually abused her and two younger sisters, the sisters rarely got together due to their fear that this shared trauma would be mentioned.

• Diffusion refers to situations in which systems do not resolve a problem or conflict because clear emergence and confrontation are undermined by bringing up one issue after another, never letting any issue emerge fully. Diffusion can also take the form of making personal attacks that do not contribute to resolving the conflict issue. In the case of Betty, the problem of her not receiving help with housing could not be resolved because in addressing the housing issue, Betty and her case manager would begin to argue about other issues such as the long waiting period on clinic days, Betty's diet, and parenting practices.

- Resolution takes place when system members give different opinions, discuss them fully, and reach a reasonable decision. System members are able to negotiate their conflicts, generating solutions that are appropriate and in the best interests of the system and its members. Conflict resolution requires effective communication and negotiation skills.

Diagnostic Dimensions

System organization—system leadership, alliances, and communication patterns

Resonance—system boundaries and connectedness among members

Developmental stage—system adjustment to life cycle stages and events

Conflict management—system response to conflict and problems, including denial/avoidance, diffusion, and resolutions

---

Table 11.2 shows examples of problematic interactions across different systems.

Restructuring

As discussed, SET relies on three categories of techniques. Two of these, joining and pattern diagnosis, already have been discussed. The last category of SET techniques is restructuring. Restructuring involves orchestrating opportunities for system members to interact in new ways. The following section describes the two restructuring techniques in SET: (a) working in the present, and (b) reframing.

Working in the Present. The active ingredient of SET is changing interactional processes in the here and now. Working in the present thus refers to the process of transforming problematic interaction patterns by directing and creating opportunities for new interactions. To change interactions, therapists are expected to facilitate direct contact between members of the system, preferably in session or via coaching.

TABLE 11.2 SET Diagnostic Dimensions and Examples of Interactions

		Diagnostic Dimensions		
Domains	Structure	Resonance	Development Stage	Conflict Management
Family microsystem	**Examples:** Leadership—Woman lives with parents and children and is not involved in parenting. Spousal alliance—Couple constantly argues about how to manage household tasks. Communication flow—Woman and daughter use grandmother to speak to each other.	**Examples:** Closeness—Woman's family does not allow her to have private time because of fears related to former drug use. Distance—Woman does not want to participate in family activities.	**Examples:** • Woman's 12-year-old daughter is overwhelmed from parenting younger siblings. • Woman and mate in conflict over children from previous marriage.	**Examples:** Denial/avoidance—Woman does not respond to criticism from stepfather, which leads her to explode later on. Resolution—Woman and husband design a schedule for preparing meals.
Social support systems	**Examples:** Leadership—Power struggles among support group members (support group microsystem). Communication flow—Woman's friends do not speak to family to arrange schedule for hospital visits (family/friends mesosystem).	**Example:** Woman's friends are not allowed to visit the home by the woman's mother, who thinks they are a negative influence on her daughter (family/friends mesosystem).	**Example:** • Church in turmoil due to loss of pastor (church microsystem).	**Example:** Diffusion—Woman and friend unable to develop a schedule for transportation because they argue about failed promises in the past (friend/microsystem).

Diagnostic Dimensions

Service systems	**Examples:** Leadership—Case worker imposes rules for woman's children without first consulting woman (children's social service exosystem). Communication—Woman refuses to tell physician that she is not taking her medication regularly because of side effects (medical microsystem).	**Examples:** Closeness—Field-worker drops by woman's home unannounced (social service microsystem). Distance—Woman's primary doctor is not aware that she is being treated by a psychiatrist (medical microsystem).	**Example:** • Health care worker expects woman to keep track of her medications without training or providing tools to help her accomplish this (medical microsystem).	**Examples:** Denial/avoidance—Case manager and woman make appointments to meet but never do (social service microsystem). Resolution—Woman meets with case worker for pregnancy planning (social service microsystem).

extent necessary by the therapist. The goal is for these new interactions to eventually take place without therapist involvement. To that end, the therapist must gradually become decentralized from the interaction between system members.

In some instances, the therapist may have direct access to only one party of a targeted interaction, most likely the woman. In these cases, changing interactions involves coaching the woman to change her behavior to bring about a change in her interactions with another person, which is likely to lead to changes in the other person's behavior (Szapocznik & Kurtines, 1989). Coaching interventions are less powerful than enactment but can be used when the therapist determines that the woman has the necessary skills to carry out the plan and the power to influence the other person's behavior.

Working in the present can be costly in terms of rapport and therefore must be accompanied by joining interventions. It is crucial that the therapist appreciate the difficulty of changing highly ingrained patterns. As the therapist encourages these changes, system members experience the frustration and pain of abandoning the familiar. The therapist needs to offer encouragement and support and, whenever possible, build changes on strengths that already exist in the system. It is crucial that the therapist appreciate the difficulty of changing highly ingrained patterns.

An experienced therapist is always equipped with some standard reframes that he or she can access in various situations: anger as pain or loss (underlying the anger), highly conflictive relationships as close or passionate, crises as opportunities (to pull the family closer, to become a stronger person, etc.), feeling overwhelmed as a signal that one must recharge one's batteries, impulsiveness as spontaneity, and insensitivity as "telling it as it is."

Reframing. Reframing is a powerful tool to facilitate changing interactions. A therapist uses a reframe when she feels that the affective tone of the session blocks the interactional change that the therapist is trying to induce. For example, a mother may believe that our client is criticizing her, thus preventing them from engaging in the more positive interaction that the therapist is trying to establish. The therapist may explain to the mother that her daughter fights with her as a way of connecting with her, thus jarring the mother's perceptions to allow for a different interaction. Reframes shake up the emotional valence in a relationship by offering a reinterpretation of the situation that allows for concomitant flexibility in interactions. Reframing is a restructuring technique that typically does not cost the therapist a loss of rapport and thus is preferred over confrontation as a tool for managing and modifying negativity in interactions.

> ## SET Techniques
>
> Joining—forming a therapeutic alliance with the woman and persons from her ecosystem (family, social supports, and service providers)
>
> Pattern diagnosis—mapping the ecosystem and assessing interactions along four dimensions (system organization, resonance, developmental stage, and conflict management) to identify interactions to target for change
>
> Restructuring—transforming interactions to render relationships more supportive and/or less of a burden to the woman. Specific techniques include working in the present and reframing.

CLINICAL FINDINGS

Findings in the Family System

When first approached, many of the women presented themselves as single. However, after an effective therapeutic alliance was established and the woman was convinced that the intervention would not place her welfare receipts in jeopardy or threaten her relationship with her mate, mates were often identified and brought into the therapeutic system. In fact, we found that the most frequently cited source of distress was couple relationships. Our couples therapy structured opportunities for couples to communicate more effectively, moving from vague and indirect communications to specific and direct communications. The case of Athelie, presented below, illustrates a typical couples therapy within SET.

Athelie and Jake were both HIV+ and in drug recovery. They had been married for 5 years and were raising three small children. Athelie and Jake's marriage had recently been shaken by the death of Athelie's sister, which had resulted in Athelie's emotional withdrawal from Jake and Jake's seeking other female companionship (although he denied infidelity). The therapist met alone with Athelie in the first session and established a therapeutic alliance around the goal of addressing the suspected infidelity and improving the marriage. In Session 2, the therapist met with Athelie and Jake, attentively joining with Jake and approaching the issue of their commitment to each other from a positive angle (an upcoming anniversary). The subject of infidelity was addressed more directly beginning with Session 3.

Athelie often made statements to Jake such as, "I can't trust you," which blamed and injured without providing information about what he did wrong and could do differently to improve the relationship. The therapist guided Athelie in making the more specific statement, "I don't like it when you don't answer your beeper because it makes me think you're with another woman," which is very direct (speaking directly to Jake) and specific (exactly what it is he does that Athelie does not like). This transformation opened opportunities to move from blaming and hurting to examinations of the nature of the behaviors that were problematic to the interaction, certainly to Athelie.

Next, attention was given to the negativity of Athelie and Jake's communications, which resulted in mutual defensiveness. These negative communications, although direct and specific, needed to be reframed by the therapist to open new opportunities for supportive and constructive discussions. Hence, when Athelie would tell Jake that she suspected him of disloyalty, the therapist first supported the openness of that communication and then created the opportunity for Jake to respond constructively by representing both the negative and the positive aspects of the communication. To Jake: "I hear Athelie telling you that she wants to hear from you and that she worries that you are with someone else." Hence, without distorting the directness and specificity of Athelie's communication, Jake was helped to hear that Athelie's communication had a caring side. Creating this kind of balance that expresses the positive side (I care) of a valid complaint permitted Jake to respond in a less defensive fashion. The therapist quickly moved to asking, "Did you know that Athelie cared this much for you? Did you know that she noticed what you do? And can you understand that if she cares so much, she would feel so angry—angry because she feels hurt—when you don't answer your beeper?"

As these discussions ensued, the therapist addressed Athelie and Jake's conflict diffusion. When Jake said he was not available to help Athelie search for a new apartment, Athelie responded by attacking Jake: "You only care about yourself. You never care about what's important to me and the children." Although Athelie may have had good reason to be angry at Jake's lack of involvement, in this case, her attack on Jake prevented a discussion on the specific issue of searching for housing. The therapist helped Athelie and Jake to express their needs and differing opinions in a constructive manner across this and other content areas.

Findings in Social Support Systems

Many of the women had adequate informal social support. In such cases, therapy with informal systems tended to involve fine-tuning and bolstering existing relationships via coaching and some direct therapist contact.

Although a few women presented as being highly isolated, most women's networks were star shaped, with the woman at the center and only herself connected with each of the members of her network (a lack of mesosystemic relationships). There are tremendous deficits to a star social network configuration because support system members cannot collaborate with each other to help the woman. For example, an HIV support group member alerting a family member that the woman has stopped attending group can lead to positive action. If there is no relationship between a group member and the family, this protective function cannot take place. This lack of interconnectedness is problematic for some women but not for others, and many of the women preferred the lack of connection between the different areas of her life. In all cases, however, interconnected-ness between systems is a useful protective and preventive mechanism that the therapist makes efforts to promote. Intervention plans for the isolated women typically involved a combination of strengthening the woman's relationship with supportive persons in different systems (i.e., helping to build a star) and then bridging the support systems (i.e., connecting the points on the star). An example of such a woman is Barbara, whose case will be presented below. Figure 11.5 shows Barbara's network before and after the therapist's intervention.

> Barbara was living alone in a sparely furnished room. She had no telephone, had only minimal contact with neighbors, and was in violent (including physical assaults) conflict with much of her family over the custody of her children. Barbara had recently been arrested and was also in conflict with her attorney. Barbara identified a friend of her deceased grandmother, whom she had known since childhood, as the only supportive person in her life. The therapist followed a three-step plan of action as follows: Step 1 was a session with Barbara and her friend, which resulted in a solidification of their alliance and an agreement by the friend to accompany Barbara to her court hearing. Step 2 was a session with Barbara and her attorney, which resulted in lessened negativity between them. These two steps prepared the ground for Step 3, the court hearing in which the therapist facilitated the first contact of the friend and attorney, thus bridging these two points of Barbara's star-shaped network and laying the groundwork for future support for Barbara via this relationship between her attorney and her friend.

Findings in Service Systems

The women typically entered the intervention with complex and very involved formal health and social service systems in place. Although many of the women were well served and good consumers, we did find some problems. In some cases, service providers seemed to overidentify with the women and compete for their loyalty. These service providers often highlighted the shortcomings of the women's informal supports and failed to see or pursue their potential as significant resources. In other cases, the involvement of multiple providers either overwhelmed the woman or led to the fracturing of services. Although we found little need to supplement what was already taking place in the formal support systems, in some cases it was necessary to alter the woman's interaction with these providers and among the providers to improve the woman's use of services and her quality of life.

> Judy was a 34-year-old mother of five children. She was grossly overweight and had numerous health problems for which she had been hospitalized several

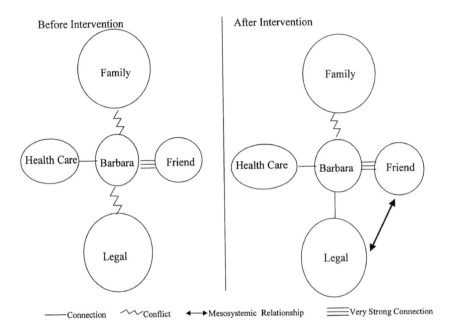

Figure 11.5.   Barbara's Network

times. Judy complained about a lack of energy and drive to accomplish even the smallest tasks, and she was often irritable. Judy was involved with numerous agencies and had approximately six case and health care workers from five different agencies. Due to her children's difficulties at school, she was frequently called for parent-teacher conferences. In addition, she had housing problems that required crisis-oriented interventions. Scheduling and managing to keep up with her various appointments had overwhelmed Judy. Furthermore, because she felt conflicted about her dependence on these agencies, she often expressed herself in an angry manner, which stressed her relationships with the various workers. Despite these feelings, Judy wanted to maintain a positive relationship with her workers.

It was clear to the therapist that she could be helpful by assisting Judy to coordinate her services, manage her time, and smooth these relationships. With Judy's permission, the therapist contacted some of the workers and asked them to cooperate with Judy in coordinating her commitments in a more efficient and productive manner. They were very willing do so because they were experiencing a sense of failure in how Judy was responding to their efforts. Sessions were conducted to get the workers and Judy to "iron out" some of the "wrinkles" in their relationship, with the therapist orchestrating the work on improving communication, accepting the limitations that agencies and individuals have in trying to access services, and working together in trying to assist Judy with her needs. The therapist reframed negative statements of blame and fault finding by pointing out that Judy would sometimes lose track of appointments and that the workers were concerned about her well-being, which served to shift the mood. The workers began to appreciate Judy's situation and became more effective at presenting helpful suggestions on how to provide follow-up (i.e., an appointment book, reminder telephone calls, and transportation). Within 4 months, Judy found new permanent housing, regularly attended medical appointments and health-related support groups, and had worked out child care assistance from the school.

THERAPIST CHARACTERISTICS, SUPERVISION, AND TRAINING

It is helpful to separate two aspects of skills required to conduct SET: (a) nonspecific clinical skills, which are common across therapies, and (b) skills specific to SET. The common clinical skills needed across therapies include empathy, timing, ability to provide support and validation, ability to establish working alliances with individuals, enthusiasm, and optimism (see Rotheram-Borus & Leonardo, 2000 [this volume]). Therapists who are selected for training in SET are carefully screened to ensure that they already have mastered clinical competence in these areas. Typically, this will require master's-level training in mental health, social work, or counseling and several years of supervised clinical experience. In addition, all of the therapists in the study are female. This is due to the complications inherent in having a male therapist conduct individual sessions in a woman's home.

Skills that are more specific to SET include competence in conducting therapy in environments other than the office, knowledge of the concepts underlying SET, and mastery of the SET techniques. SET training also requires reading, practice in mapping and diagnosis of systems in cases being seen by other therapists, and closely supervised experience with at least one practice case. SET training and practice also require frequent review of videotaped sessions by the therapist alone, with her colleagues, and with her supervisor.

Beyond training, it is crucial for the SET intervention to take place within a supervisory context. Support and guidance from the supervisor and treatment team are necessary even for highly experienced SET therapists because the woman's ecosystem will pull the therapist to look at only her and her immediate surroundings. The SET approach represents a radical departure from the usual way of viewing the problems of women and, as such, requires the counterbalancing effect of the supervisory/treatment team to keep the therapist true to the SET intervention.

The essential ingredients for treatment are the mapping and diagnosis of the ecosystem, interventions that are interactional, and a focus on process rather than content. In our work, all therapy sessions are videotaped, permitting frequent reviews of actual sessions. In addition, therapists complete clinical forms for each case that outline interactional diagnoses and treatment goals.

CONCLUSION

Our work with HIV+ African American women has confirmed our belief that these women, their families, and their community have untapped resources that, with careful and sensitive intervention, can be harnessed to improve the woman's psychosocial functioning. The elements of SET that are most crucial in bringing about positive interactional change are (a) meeting the woman and her ecosystem "where they're at," not only by offering sessions in their natural environment but also by respecting current interactional patterns while gradually helping them evolve; (b) the therapist's constant recognition that she is a temporary figure in the woman's life who must help to build relationships that will outlast the therapy; (c) a flexible, vigilant, and creative approach that capitalizes on opportunities for restructuring interactions; (d) a supportive context for the therapist in which supervisors and colleagues can help the therapist to overcome the isolation that might otherwise be inherent in doing home-based therapy and the powerful forces of the women's ecosystems that might otherwise pull the therapist to be overwhelmed by the multiple and complex problems that the women face; and (e) a theoretical model that guides the intervention.

NOTE

1. It is important to note that although the therapist starts out as the leader of the therapeutic system, it is the woman herself who is the central actor in her therapy. An important goal of SET is to help nurture the woman's emerging leadership of her treatment and every other aspect of her life.

REFERENCES

Amaro, H. (1995). Love, sex, and power. *American Psychologist, 50*(6), 437-447.

Aponte, H. (1976). The family-school interview: An ecostructural approach. *Family Process, 15*(3), 303-311.

Aponte, H., & Van Deusen, J. (1981). Structural family therapy. In A. Gurman & D. Kniskern (Eds.), *Handbook of family therapy* (pp. 310-360). New York: Brunner/Mazel.

Auerswald, E. (1968). Interdisciplinary versus ecological approach. *Family Process, 1*, 204.

Bronfenbrenner, U. (1977). Toward an experimental ecology of human development. *American Psychologist, 32*, 513-531.

Bronfenbrenner, U. (1979). *The ecology of human development.* Cambridge, MA: Harvard University Press.

Bronfenbrenner, U. (1986). The ecology of the family as a context for human development. *Developmental Psychology, 22,* 723-742.

Jackson-Gilfort, A., Milrani, V. B., & Szapocznik, J. (in press). Conjoint couple's therapy and preventing violence in low income, African American couples: A case report. *Journal of Family Psychotherapy.*

Kurtines, W. M., & Szapocznik, J. (1996). Family interaction patterns: Structural family therapy within contexts of cultural diversity. In E. D. Hibbs & P. S. Jensen (Eds.), *Psychosocial treatments for child and adolescent disorders: Empirically based strategies for clinical practice* (pp. 349-359). Washington, DC: American Psychological Association.

Miller, J. B. (1986). *Toward a new psychology of women.* Boston: Beacon.

Minuchin, S. (1974). *Families and family therapy.* Cambridge, MA: Harvard University Press.

Minuchin, S., & Fishman, H. C. (1981). *Family therapy techniques.* Cambridge, MA: Harvard University Press.

Minuchin, S., Montalvo, B., Guerney, B. G., Rosman, B. L., & Schumer, F. (1967). *Families of the slums.* New York: Basic Books.

Nelson, R. H., Mitrani, V. B., & Szapocznik, J. (under review). Applying a family-ecosystemic mode to reunite a family separated due to child abuse: A case study. *Contemporary Family Therapy.*

Rotheram-Borus, M. J., & Leonard, N. R. (2000). Training facilitators to deliver HIV manual-based interventions to families. In W. Pequegnat & J. Szapocznik (Eds.), *Working with families in the era of HIV/AIDS* (pp 45-64). Thousand Oaks, CA: Sage.

Szapocznik, J., & COSSMHO. (1994). Structural family therapy. In J. Szapocznik (Ed.), *A Hispanic family approach to substance abuse prevention* (pp. 41-74). Rockville, MD: Center for Substance Abuse Prevention.

Szapocznik, J., & Kurtines, W. M. (1989). *Breakthroughs in family therapy with drug abusing problem youth.* New York: Springer.

Szapocznik, J., & Kurtines, W. M. (1993). Family psychology and cultural diversity: Opportunities for theory, research and application. *American Psychologist, 48*(1), 400-407.

Szapocznik, J., & Mancilla, Y. (1995). Rainforests, families and communities: Ecological perspectives on exile, return and reconstruction. In W. J. O'Neill (Ed.), *Family: The first imperative: A symposium in search of root causes of family strength and family disintegration* (pp. 279-294). Cleveland, OH: The William J. and Dorothy K. O'Neill Foundation.

Szapocznik, J., & Williams, R. A. (in press). Brief strategic family therapy: A case study. *Contemporary Family Therapy.*

Chapter 12

The WiLLOW Program

Mobilizing Social Networks of Women Living With HIV to Enhance Coping and Reduce Sexual Risk Behaviors

Gina M. Wingood   Ralph J. DiClemente

Emory University

J ean illustrates how the WiLLOW program promotes healthy relationships, the adoption of low-risk sexual behaviors, and more effective coping. Jean (not her real name) is a 27-year-old African American woman who has been living with HIV for the past 6 years. Jean now lives at a shelter. However, until recently, she was living with her boyfriend, Jason. Jason has a history of abusing Jean. Jason is an injection drug user and he introduced Jean to using drugs. Jason and Jean have a 6-year-old child, Jerome, who is also living with HIV.

Jean is an articulate woman who has not disclosed her HIV status to her parents, both of whom she describes as extremely religious. Though she still maintains a relationship with Jason, he resists using condoms, continues to be abusive, and drains Jean's emotional and fiscal resources. Like many women who have entered

AUTHORS' NOTE: The writing of this chapter was supported by a grant from the Center for Mental Health Research on AIDS, National Institute of Mental Health (1R01 MH54412), to the second author. We would also like to express our thanks to the many staff members who have given tirelessly of themselves to implement this project. Finally, we would like to acknowledge all the women who have participated in the project. They have demonstrated a depth of courage that cannot be plumbed. To them we owe a great debt of gratitude. For more information about this prevention program, please contact Dr. Ralph DiClemente, Behavioral Sciences and Health Education and Emory/Atlanta Center for AIDS Research, Rollins School of Public Health, Emory University, Atlanta, GA 30322; e-mail: rdiclem@sph.emory.edu.

the WiLLOW program, Jean is a caretaker. She does not delegate care of her children to relatives or friends. In fact, when asked why she did not rely more on friends for support, Jean responded, "Friends are there so long as you have got no troubles. Soon as you need something and they find out you got HIV, they're gone."

When Jean was recruited, she stated explicitly that one reason she was willing to participate in the program was the monetary incentives. She was apprehensive about disclosing her HIV serostatus to strangers and blamed herself for having been infected with HIV. In fact, she had never previously participated in any group-based intervention.

Initially, during the first group session, Jean was uncomfortable talking. Many of the women were discussing how they became infected with HIV, many were sharing feelings of anger and self-deprecation, and many were talking about their struggles with addiction, with relationships, and with their families. However, when Jean started sharing about herself and her pains, upon disclosing her feelings, she felt a huge emotional release as the participants started to listen to her story and validate her pain. A week later, Jean was less anxious about sharing with the group and excited to join her newly formed peer group. When asked by health educators why she came back, she replied, "I wanted to learn more about myself. I wanted to know how I can live. I want to live with HIV. HIV is just something I have, but it's not me. I have a family, and I want to live a long life with my family." In subsequent group sessions, Jean was extremely active. She felt comfortable enough to disclose her sexual abuse history, something that evoked a great deal of emotion for her as well as for the other participants.

Jean is currently being followed through telephone and mail contact. She still loves Jason. Moreover, she has discussed condom use with him and recognizes the need to avoid high-risk sex. Equally as important, Jean has learned new coping strategies and has reached out to other group members for social support. Her social network still contains drug users, but the women in her group and the WiLLOW peer educators now provide a countervailing force, creating an atmosphere supportive of safer sex, caring, and support.

Women comprise an increasing proportion of persons with HIV. However, women living with HIV remain an understudied and underserved population. Because HIV infection is as much a social condition as it is a medical condition, living with HIV affects a woman's physical, social, psychological, and emotional aspects of living (Pergami et al., 1993). This may be particularly burdensome for those women whose lives are complicated by poverty, other chronic illnesses, discrimination, and unresponsive bureaucracies. These challenges are further compounded by the stigmatizing nature of HIV disease.

There are several compelling clinical and public health reasons to design a secondary prevention program for women living with HIV aimed at building supportive social networks, increasing coping skills, and reducing stress, risky sexual behaviors, and sexually transmitted diseases (STDs). First, an effective program could reduce the risk of disease progression among women living with HIV that may result from women's exposure to other strains of HIV or sexually transmitted diseases during unprotected sex. Second, an effective program could promote the quality of life among women living with HIV that may result from reducing stressors, enhancing coping skills, and building stronger social networks. Third, an effective program could reduce risk of HIV transmission to seronegative sexual partners. Finally, an effective program could reduce the risk of HIV transmission to their unborn children.

In this chapter, we present a program for women living with HIV. Women living with HIV, particularly in rural areas, are often isolated, and because of the stigma of HIV, they fear even disclosing their serostatus to their families and therefore often rely on networks that provide negative support, such as substance users. We therefore felt that building a network to provide social support to them was critical. The name of the program is WiLLOW, which stands for Women involved in Life Learning from Other Women. Currently, we are evaluating the WiLLOW program to test whether this social network intervention can enhance supportive social networks, reduce stress, increase coping skills, and reduce high-risk sexual practices and their adverse health consequences such as sexually transmitted diseases. WiLLOW is grounded in a social support networks framework as well as the transactional model of stress and coping.

Women Living With HIV Are Exposed to Many Stressors

Few studies have examined the unique stressors that affect women living with HIV. Semple et al. (1993) identified the major stressors among Caucasian women living with HIV. The main HIV-related stressors were (a) being informed of their HIV serostatus (27.8%), (b) having chronic financial strains (11.1%), (c) terminating an exclusive relationship as a result of learning their HIV serostatus (11.1%), (d) having a child develop behavioral problems subsequent to learning their serostatus (11.1%), and (e) having a friend die from AIDS (11.1%). Other studies report additional gender-specific stressors for women with HIV such as the caretaking responsibilities for an HIV+ child, the decision to continue or terminate a pregnancy, the shame and stigmatization of having HIV, the isolation of not knowing other women with HIV, the lack of physicians' knowledge about the medical and gynecological conditions that are common among women with HIV, and the lack of HIV support groups (Rehner, 1994; Selwyn et al., 1989). These burdens are made worse by the absence of a supportive kin network to assist women in effectively coping with these stresses.

Women Living With HIV Residing in Rural Areas

Although stressors are common among all women living with HIV, stressors such as stigma, secrecy, and confidentiality may be more pronounced for women residing in nonurban areas. Prior to developing the WiLLOW program, we conducted a series of qualitative interviews. One interview, typical of women's responses, was with a woman named Meg.

M eg is a 40-year-old White widowed woman living with HIV residing in rural Alabama. Her HIV infection was diagnosed 7 years ago following the death of her husband from AIDS. Meg has private medical insurance. Although she and her children visit a family physician for their routine medical care in their hometown, the local physician is unaware of her HIV diagnosis. Once a month, Meg drives 2 hours to see an infectious disease specialist in the urban medical center. She states, "I want to keep living until my children are grown up." She further reports that she has no one with whom she can talk about her disease and is mildly depressed and nervous.

Although the medical care provided by an urban HIV specialty clinic may be more comprehensive than the care provided in rural settings, it is not just the higher standard of care that motivates Meg's 2-hour journey. Meg is fearful of the stigma associated with HIV—not only for herself but, more important, for her family, her children, and grandchildren. Meg states,

They don't understand. No one would understand. They'd just condemn me and my family. One day we'd be part of the community, the next, we'd be social outcasts. It's not fair. But it's real.

Meg's assessment of the threat of stigmatization if local townspeople become aware of her condition probably is not much different from many other women with HIV living in rural areas.

Meg's experiences as an HIV+ woman seeking medical care are consistent with the findings from a recent survey conducted among rural residents living with HIV in Kentucky. In this study, 74% of the residents went outside their county for HIV-related ambulatory care, with 64% of the respondents traveling to an urban area. The primary reasons for traveling to urban areas included concerns regarding confidentiality and beliefs that their physician was not knowledgeable about HIV.

THEORETICAL APPROACHES

Relationship of Social Networks and Social Support to Health

There are a variety of ways through which social networks and social support affect an individual's physical, mental, and social health. Social networks and social support can improve health by (a) reducing stress, (b) enhancing organizational and community resources, (c) reducing behavioral risks and increasing preventive health practices, and (d) increasing an individual's coping resources (Berkman, 1984; O'Donnell & Haris, 1994). The WiLLOW program recognizes that all of these mechanisms are important in enhancing the physical, mental, and social health of women living with HIV. However, the WiLLOW program focuses primarily on building supportive social networks to enhance women's social support and coping resources and, as a consequence, reduce their stress. One stress and coping theoretical framework that is used to guide the WiLLOW program and has been effectively applied to people living with HIV is the transactional model of stress and coping.

Transactional Model of Stress and Coping

The transactional model of stress and coping provides a framework for evaluating the processes of coping with stressful events. Stressful events are defined as person-environment transactions in which a stressor is mediated by two processes: an individual's appraisal of the potential threat of the stressor (primary appraisal) and appraisal of personal resources and perceived ability cope to with the stressor (secondary appraisal; Lazarus & Folkman, 1984). For example, Meg has appraised the threat of disclosing her HIV serostatus to her neighbors as extremely stressful, but she has the personal resources to cope with it by keeping it private and driving to another community for her care.

Those strategies that Meg uses to handle the primary and secondary appraisals are referred to as coping efforts. According to this model, the two primary types of coping efforts are problem management and emotional regulation. Problem management strategies, also referred to as problem-focused coping, are directed at changing the stressful situation. Examples of problem-focused coping include problem solving, decision making, assertive communication, and information seeking. Emotional regulation strategies, also referred to as emotion-focused coping, are directed at changing the way an individual thinks or feels about the stressful situation. Examples of emotion-focused coping include seeking social support, using spiritual or religious resources to reframe a stressful situation, engaging in relaxation and meditation exercises, reappraising the situation positively, and learning adaptive strategies to avoid the stressful event, such as through exercise. Coping efforts aimed at problem management and emotional regulation influence the outcomes of the coping. Three main categories of outcomes are emotional well-being (quality of life), functional status (health status, disease progression), and health behaviors (practicing condom use, adherence to treatment recommendations, seeking social support).

Creating a Family of Supportive
Social Network Members

For the purpose of the WiLLOW program, we broadly define *family* as supportive social network members. These members include the participants, the program's peers, and the health educators. This network is evident in the bonds that develop between each of the members and with one another. The WiLLOW program is designed to use trained peers and health educators from the community to enhance women's existing social networks, develop new personal networks, and develop new linkages to community resources.

Identifying the peers and health educators is a critical step in developing WiLLOW. The WiLLOW program selected peers based on the evaluations of social workers, nurses, and community-based organizers working with women living with HIV. The peers complete a training program focusing on group dynamics, building social networks, enhancing coping skills, and using sexual risk reduction techniques. To identify health educators, WiLLOW built linkages with community-based programs, such as SISTALOVE, which provide social services and sex education for women living with HIV. Organizations such as SISTALOVE often have staff that have experience working with women living with HIV, have excellent group dynamics skills, understand the life challenges faced by many women living with HIV, are trained in providing referrals to community resources, and have training in stress reduction and safer sex education.

In the WiLLOW program, women participate in four 4-hour group sessions led by a health educator and HIV+ peers. Following completion of the four-session intervention, women are contacted bimonthly via telephone to reinforce prevention messages, support maintenance of newly adopted behaviors, and reduce feelings of social isolation. During the months that women are not contacted by telephone, they receive WiLLOW newsletters reinforcing the importance of adhering to newly adopted behaviors and maintaining a healthy social support network.

Structure of the Group Sessions

Following introductions by the health educators and greetings to the participants, women in WiLLOW begin each session with the peers leading a poetry reading. The poem, written by a female poet, is relevant for the content emphasized in that particular day's session. Following the poetry reading and discussion, the previous session is reviewed by the health educator prior to implementing the current session. Each session is interactive. The peers initiate each activity by discussing its purpose, and then the health educator and peers either provide didactic training or role model session activities (described in the section immediately below) to enhance the woman's understanding of the activity objectives. Subsequently, the participants role-play the modeled activities to reinforce learning and to encourage active participation. At the end of the role-play, the peers and health educator provide positive reinforcement and corrective feedback regarding the participants' performance. Throughout the session, to master the requisite skills and knowledge, role-play activities become successively more challenging, as participants are asked to act out scenarios that are either emotionally laden, more cognitively demanding, or require greater skill dexterity. Each session begins and ends by all participants reiterating the WiLLOW motto: "We are *W*omen *i*nvolved in *L*ife *L*earning from *O*ther *W*omen."

THE WiLLOW PROGRAM

Content of the WiLLOW Program

Women in the WiLLOW program receive information and training designed to enhance gender pride, social networks, emotion-focused coping skills, problem-focused coping skills, sexual risk reduction skills, condom use management skills, and healthy relationships. The content of the WiLLOW program is summarized in Table 12.1. Each session is more fully described below.

Session 1: Gender Pride and
Enhancing Our Social Networks

Subsequent to introductions and explaining the ground rules, participants are introduced to the WiLLOW program. They are taught that WiLLOW is an acronym that stands for Women involved in Life Learning from Other Women. The WiLLOW program originates from the belief that historically, women have learned about life and about how to cope with life's challenges by having relationships and friendships with other women. These interactions and friendships are important sources of inspiration for women and evolve into a sense of support, love, harmony, caring, and sisterhood that represent the essence of the WiLLOW program (see Figure 12.1).

Figuratively, the name WiLLOW represents a willow tree. The willow tree is associated with great beauty and splendor, but at the same time, the willow tree can be strong and flexible. It is this combination of attributes, exuded by many

TABLE 12.1 The Four-Session WiLLOW Program

Session	Session Title	Figures
Session 1	Fostering Gender Pride and Enhancing Our Social Networks	Figures 12.1 and 12.2
Session 2	Strengthening Our Emotion-Focused and Problem-Focused Coping Strategies	Figure 12.3
Session 3	Providing Sexual Risk Reduction Education and Condom Use Skills	
Session 4	Developing and Maintaining Healthy Relationships	Figure 12.4

women living with HIV, that has come to symbolize the WiLLOW program. The willow tree is used in multiple exercises during the sessions.

After providing an overview of the WiLLOW program, women engage in an activity that is meant to foster gender pride. There are several reasons for beginning the first session with a discussion of gender pride. First, participants voice their needs and concerns *prior to* our providing any information about healthy behaviors. This allows us to understand the participants' personal motivations for engaging in unhealthy behaviors. It also allows the women to voice positive qualities about themselves, and it provides the educators with an opportunity to validate participants' feelings. This creates an atmosphere that allows the program to start on a very positive note. Moreover, this activity sets a tone, one that is reflected throughout WiLLOW, that the health educators and peers want to hear the voices of the participants.

During the gender pride activity, women discuss what they enjoy about being a woman and the importance of taking pride in being a woman. Several of the women in WiLLOW mentioned that being a woman to them meant being "caring, supportive, nurturing, compassionate, flexible, proud, passionate, giving, sexy, intelligent, proud, and strong." Many of the WiLLOW participants stated that if they could strengthen something in women, "they would strengthen women's self-respect, sense of adventure, independence, and confidence" (see Figure 12.2). Participants then engage in an exercise titled "Personal Values," in which they identify those values that are most important. Participants are encouraged to prioritize their values when entering into a relationship. Women often mention that they value their children, their family, their sense of freedom, their faith and spirituality, and their health. Health educators emphasize that an individual's values can help serve as guidelines for setting personal goals. The theme of pride in oneself is emphasized throughout the entire program by using

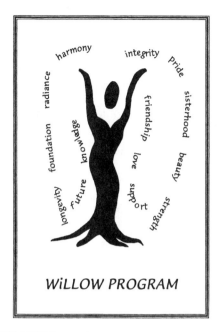

Figure 12.1.   The WiLLOW Program

poetry and film by female artists. The end of the first part of this session concludes by the entire group reciting, in unison, a poem written by Maya Angelou titled "Phenomenal Women." Afterward, participants discuss what they perceive is "phenomenal" about themselves. The activities in this session are also designed to provide affirmational support by validating the women's self-worth and their personal values.

The second part of Session 1 focuses on enhancing women's social support network. Women engage in an activity in which they identify people who constitute their social network. These individuals may be people such as their friends, family members, social workers, personnel at community-based organizations, neighbors, coworkers, pastor or priest, and nurses and doctors. To help women identify members of their social support network, we use the figure of the willow tree, the project's logo. Using their WiLLOW tree, women are asked to write along the roots of their tree those individuals in their life who constitute "root people"—individuals who may assist them with child care activities or help in purchasing groceries and people they can really talk with when they have had a bad day or who can provide financial support when they need a little extra money for rent. The health educator emphasizes that the number of individuals in one's social support system is not as important as the quality of the support received

---

1. Women in the WiLLOW program mentioned that being a woman to them meant being

caring	sensitive	beautiful	proud
supportive	compassionate	strong	giving
nurturing	flexible	passionate	loving

2. Women in the WiLLOW program mentioned that they enjoyed being a woman because

they are able to show their emotions,
they are able to care for others,
they are loyal to their friends,
they are fun-loving.

3. Women in the WiLLOW program mentioned that if they could strengthen something among women, they would strengthen women's

self-respect
adventure
independence
confidence

Figure 12.2.   Gender Pride Activity

from one's social support system. Subsequently, women are asked to write around the branches of their tree those individuals from whom they would like to receive more support. These may be people who are currently providing a small amount of support or people who are not providing any support. The health educator explains that the goal of the program is to move some of the individuals who are listed on the branches of the WiLLOW tree to "root people" so that these new "root people" may provide additional and diverse supportive roles and ease the burden on those who currently serve as "root people." The peers explain that maintaining a social support system (i.e., preventing burnout) is just as important as developing a social support system.

The health educators then briefly define and discuss different types of support—namely, informational, emotional, and practical social support. Using their WiLLOW tree, the participants place an "I, P, and/or E" next to each person listed, indicating the provision of informational, practical, and/or emotional support, respectively, to identify what type of social support is provided by each member of their support network. This activity allows the participants to identify who is in their existing social support network, who they would like to see in their social support network, what types of social support they are currently receiving, and what types of social support they need. The peers and health educators then discuss, model, and role-play activities designed to enhance women's social support networks; increase the amount of informational, practical, and emotional support they receive; and identify barriers to obtaining and maintaining their social support network.

Session 2: Emotion-Focused and Problem-Focused Coping

The first part of Session 2 emphasizes enhancing participants' emotion-focused and problem-focused coping skills. Initially, the health educators define stress and subsequently engage participants in an exercise titled "What Stresses You?" As part of this exercise, participants identify the three most prominent stressors in their lives. Among the WiLLOW participants, major sources of stress include relationships with their sexual partners, decisions regarding disclosing their HIV serostatus to their sexual partners and their family members, financial burdens, and health-related stressors. This activity allows participants to discuss how stress affects them emotionally (i.e., feeling depressed), behaviorally (i.e., using drugs), and physically (i.e., feeling sick).

The peers then engage in appraisal training designed to teach women how to distinguish between stressors that are changeable and stressors that are unchangeable or difficult to change. Women are taught to use emotion-focused coping strategies for reducing stressors that are unchangeable or difficult to change. Using the acronym RELAX, participants learn that each letter stands for a different emotion-focused coping strategy:

R = Relax
E = Express your emotions
L = Let others help
A = Allow positive thoughts
X = Exercise

Realizing that some strategies may be more appealing to some women than others, our intent is to teach women a range or "menu" of strategies, so that they may select the coping strategy that best fits their personal style and situation.

Relax. The first emotion-focused coping strategy that is discussed is relaxing. During this activity, women lay on gym mats for 10 minutes while listening to the soothing sounds of the ocean on meditation tapes to help them physically and mentally calm their mind and body. The women slowly rise to a sitting position and engage in deep breathing exercises. Women enjoy these meditational exercises and find these activities soothing, refreshing, and healing. At the end of the session, all women receive relaxation tapes.

Express Your Emotions. The health educators also discuss the importance of expressing emotions. The health educators instruct the women to express their feelings by talking with a friend, partner, or sibling; having a good laugh; crying to release emotional tension; and writing down the recurring thoughts and feelings that are emotionally draining or that are motivational and uplifting. At the end of the session, all women are provided with a WiLLOW journal to chronicle their thoughts and feelings.

Let Others Help. The peers also discuss the importance of letting others help when the participants are having trouble coping with a situation. During this activity, participants are asked to refer to their WiLLOW tree, identify those individuals who could provide them with particular types of social support, and let these people know that they can help—call them, write them, or just share their feelings with other people to assist in dealing with whatever situation that is challenging. At the end of the session, all women are provided WiLLOW stationery and encouraged to initiate contact with network members and express their need for support and their gratitude.

Allow Positive Thoughts. Because many women living with HIV have negative thoughts about themselves, women participate in an activity designed to allow women to act and think positively about themselves. Negative thoughts common among the WiLLOW participants include thinking everything about themselves is bad, thinking that they are unattractive, believing that nobody will ever want them, and thinking that they cannot enjoy life anymore. To counter these feelings, we engage in an esteem-enhancing activity. Each participant is provided 12 leaf-shaped stickers. On each leaf-shaped sticker, the participants write down two positive thoughts about each of the women in the group except for themselves. All of the leaf-shaped stickers for each individual are collected from all the participants. In round-robin fashion, each participant shares two of the positive thoughts that have been written about her and subsequently sticks her leaf stickers to her WiLLOW tree. Their WiLLOW tree is then "blooming" with brightly colored stickers, each with positive messages about themselves. This is one of the participants' favorite activities.

Each woman experiences this exercise slightly differently, although they all acknowledge its impact on enhancing their self-esteem and self-concept. It is sometimes difficult to imagine the power of positive feedback. Perhaps an illustration will help.

Sandra is a drug user. She readily acknowledged her "weakness," as she puts it, for drugs. She was not, in her words, "strong-willed enough" to avoid drugs. It was during the trimming of her WiLLOW tree that Sandra realized, perhaps for the first time in a long time, that people really appreciated her sense of humor, her compassion and caring, and her willingness to share her most intimate and frightening feelings about herself. As she read the accolades written by the other women—"beautiful," "loving," "supportive," and "sharing"—Sandra began to softly sob. Finally, the trickle of tears became a torrent as she burst out in tears. These were tears of joy because, as she said later, no one had ever told her so many "nice" things before.

Exercise. The final emotion-focused activity that is discussed and role-played is the importance of exercising. Women are taught that exercising not only means working out at a gym but also includes activities such as dancing as a way of relieving stress. To demonstrate, the health educators and peers ask the women to rise and move to a large open area in the room. Then they proceed to demonstrate the "Electric Slide" and the "Macarena," first without music and then with music. Soon, the room is "rocking and rolling," and women are not only dancing but singing as well. At the end of the session, all women receive a CD of the "Electric Slide."

The second part of Session 2 emphasizes enhancing participants' problem-focused coping skills. Initially, participants learn a decision-making model to assist in problem solving and subsequently apply the model to enhance their use of problem-focused coping strategies. Problem-focused coping strategies taught include learning to distinguish between passive, aggressive, and assertive communication styles. Subsequently, women verbally and nonverbally communicate being assertive, aggressive, and passive (see Figure 12.3). Women are taught to assertively communicate with their social workers regarding seeking informational and practical support. Women enjoy this activity because being assertive with their social workers is a practical skill that they can apply in their daily lives. In addition, women are taught to assertively communicate with their sexual partners their desire (a) to abstain from having sex, (b) to negotiate safer sex, and (c) to refuse an unsafe sexual encounter.

Session 3: Sexual Risk Reduction Education and Condom Use Skills

This session focuses on sexual risk reduction education. Using multimedia educational materials (e.g., videos) that are appropriate for women living with HIV, the health educator presents information to increase participants' knowledge of STD prevention strategies and to personalize the risk of HIV reinfection. The health educator discusses the effect of STDs on a compromised immune system and the potential for perinatal transmission of STDs and HIV. Because many of the participants have children, plan on becoming pregnant, or are pregnant, the theme of "Stay Safe for Yourself and Your Child" is reinforced. Subsequently, women engage in an STD/HIV "Jeopardy Game" to reinforce factual

---

Passive

  You are unable to tell someone how you really feel about a situation or what you want or need.

  You go with the crowd when you are unaware of a situation.

  You say yes when you really want to say no.

  You act this way to be nice to someone, to keep from hurting another person's feelings, or so you will be liked.

Aggressive

  You express yourself by standing up for yourself in a way that is punishing, demanding, or threatening to someone else.

  You try to get your way by putting someone else down.

  You talk or get what you want without considering the feelings and rights of other people.

  You threaten or force people to give you something.

Assertive

  You communicate your feelings and opinions in a direct and honest manner.

  You say no to things you do not want to do if they will put you in a situation that might threaten your well-being.

  You express yourself honestly while considering the needs and feelings of other people, without jeopardizing your own needs.

  You do not let others use you, and you do not use others.

Figure 12.3.   Communication Styles

information provided during the session. During this game, women are divided into two teams, with score kept by the health educator. The peers ask questions from one of the three categories titled the following: (a) Facts About STDs, (b) Rating Your STD Risk, and (c) Why Condoms? The first person to answer a question correctly is awarded points. The team with the most points wins.

After women are instructed about why using condoms is important, participants are taught the steps to using condoms properly, using the acronym OPRAH. This acronym stands for the following:

O = Open
P = Pinch
R = Roll
A = Action
H = Hold

The health educators discuss the importance of each step and model proper condom use. The participants then role-play using condoms first with the lights on and then with the lights dimmed to simulate using condoms in a darkened environment. This is always a fun activity, as women enjoy learning about and playing with the dildos, condoms, and lubricants. During the last activity of this session, the peers personally endorse why they either use condoms consistently or abstain from sex. These personal endorsements are designed to create an atmosphere supportive of safer norms, including abstaining from sex.

By the end of the third session, participants have a greater sense of comfort about being in the group. Therefore, at this time, subsequent to the peers' personal endorsements about condom use, women are invited to share their thoughts about how living with HIV has affected their lives and how they are coping with HIV. Women are initially reticent about engaging in this dialogue. However, one by one, women often tearfully talk of the challenges and their newfound strengths in living with HIV. The room fills with tears, powerful convictions of living with the disease, hope, and recognition of the need to maintain the familial ties provided by WiLLOW as women exchange their names and phone numbers with one another.

Session 4: Developing and Maintaining
Healthy Relationships

The first part of the fourth session addresses how sexuality occurs within the context of a larger social relationship. Specifically, health educators emphasize that it is easier to receive support from a partner, to negotiate condom use, and to use condoms in a healthy relationship. In this session, women engage in an activity in which they identify healthy and unhealthy characteristics of relationships. During this activity, the health educator emphasizes that healthy relationships are relationships in which "power is balanced, communication is good, respect is real, trust is strong, and honesty is valued." Unhealthy relationships are characterized as relationships in which many of these qualities are lacking (see Figure 12.4). Subsequently, the health educators define emotional, physical, and sexual abuse. Health educators discuss different forms of emotional abuse (i.e., being humiliated, threatened, or kept from doing things that you want to do), physical abuse (i.e., being hit, shaken, choked), and sexual abuse (i.e., being pressured into having sex with threats or guilt or force). Then participants discuss how being in an abusive relationship can make it difficult to receive support and practice safer sex. Because abuse is not uncommon among these women, many of the participants share stories of their abuse histories. For many of the participants, it is the first time that they have disclosed their abuse histories.

The second part of Session 4 focuses on role reversal. This allows participants to reverse roles and serve as the health educators and peers while the health educators and peers become the participants. The participants enjoy this activity

In a *healthy* relationship:
> Power is balanced. No one has an unfair advantage over the other.
> Communication is good. Both partners talk and listen to one another.
> Respect is real for oneself and one another.
> Trust is strong. You feel safe both physically and emotionally with one another.
> Honesty is valued. Both partners talk with one another truthfully and have a faithful relationship.

In an *unhealthy* relationship:
> Power is not balanced. One partner has an unfair advantage over the other.
> Communication is not good. Both partners do not talk and listen to each other.
> Respect is not real for oneself and one another.
> Trust is not strong. You do not feel safe both physically and emotionally with one another.
> Honesty is not valued. One or both partners are not truthful or faithful to the relationship.

Figure 12.4.   Healthy and Unhealthy Relationships

because it provides them the opportunity to role-play being the group leader and sharing the knowledge that they have learned from the program. At the end of this session, women again recite the poem "Phenomenal Women" by Maya Angelou and receive certificates of empowerment for completing the program.

This is a very powerful and moving last session. Women exchange hugs, reinforce the need to stay in touch with one another, and begin solidifying their relationships with one another. Indeed, clinical staff have commented that they see marked changes in participants' attitudes, their sense of self, and their willingness to interact with each other.

As one nurse commented,

> Before they would come into the waiting room and sit quietly in a corner. They wouldn't talk to anyone. They'd just sit there. Not reading anything, just sitting and mostly staring blankly into space. After they go through WiLLOW, you can see them starting to talk with other women, carrying their head up high, asking questions about where to get one service or another. It's as though they had come out of a cocoon.

In essence, WiLLOW fosters the development of friendships and social support networks among the group members and enhances pride in oneself. Of the 800 group sessions that could have been completed by these women (200 women attending 4 sessions), only 7 sessions have been missed, yielding a participation rate of 99%. Among women who have missed a group session, the following two examples are indicative of how participation in WiLLOW has become a family system.

Agnes had been hospitalized for cervical cancer surgery, and she called the project director from the hospital while she was awaiting surgery. Selma found out that her father had died, and on the way to his funeral she called the project director. Both women wanted their group to know how much they would miss them and that they would keep the group spirit in their hearts through these tough moments. They also wanted the group to know that they were looking forward to rejoining them as soon as possible.

However, the fourth session is not the last time that the peer educators interact with the participants.

Personal Contacts Are Critical for Maintaining Program Effects

Subsequent to completing the four group sessions, for the next 12 months, every month peer educators alternate providing either a scheduled telephone call or a WiLLOW newsletter containing role model stories to each group participant. This strategy is designed to amplify the program effects by reinforcing prevention messages, supporting maintenance of newly adopted behaviors, and reducing feelings of social isolation. The telephone contacts also allow the intervention to be tailored to the clients' particular needs, continue to foster rapport established during the four-session intervention, and can reduce relapse to high-risk practices. Women enjoy the individualized attention that they receive from talking with and learning from the peer educators and each other.

TRAINING TO CONDUCT THIS PREVENTION PROGRAM

To engender this commitment to the program, clinicians interested in implementing a sexual risk reduction and coping program for women living with HIV need to carefully consider training issues. The health educators and peers should receive additional training in techniques for establishing group rapport, understanding group dynamics and cultural sensitivity, learning stress management, referring women to social services, and maintaining confidentiality. This training is essential in enhancing the quality of the program and being sure that the facilitators feel comfortable with the dual topics of HIV and sex.

IMPLICATION FOR PREVENTION
OF CONSEQUENCES OF HIV/AIDS

The WiLLOW program has as its overarching goal the improvement in women's ability to build supportive social networks that may increase their coping skills and reduce risky sexual practices and, as a consequence, their risk for STDs. Building supportive social networks is viewed as creating a "family" for women living with HIV—such as Jean, Meg, Agnes, and Selma. Unfortunately, there are few secondary prevention programs for women living with HIV. Given the potential adverse health consequences associated with unprotected sexual intercourse among women living with HIV, both for the women and their sex partners, such interventions could make a significant impact in reducing the spread of HIV as well as promoting the mental and social health of women living with HIV. Moreover, the integration of social support and sexual risk reduction program efforts with clinical services may strengthen the social networks of women living with HIV.

REFERENCES

Berkman, L. (1984). Assessing the physical health effects of social networks and social support. *Annual Review of Public Health, 5,* 413-432.

Lazarus, R. S., & Folkman, S. (1984). *Stress, appraisal, and coping.* New York: Springer.

O'Donnell, M. P., & Haris, J. S. (Eds.). (1994). *Health promotion in the workplace* (2nd ed.). Albany, NY: Delmar.

Pergami, A., Gala, C., Burgess, A., Durbano, F., Zanello, D., Riccio, M., Invernizzi, G., & Catalan, J. (1993). The psychosocial impact of HIV infection in women. *Journal of Psychosomatic Research, 37,* 687-696.

Rehner, T. A. (1994). *Depression in Alabama women with HIV.* Ph.D. dissertation, School of Social Work in the Graduate School, University of Alabama.

Selwyn, P. A., Carter, R. J., Schoenbaum, E. E., Robertson, V. J., Klein, R. S., & Rogers, M. F. (1989). Knowledge of HIV antibody status and decisions to continue or terminate pregnancy among intravenous drug users. *JAMA, 261,* 3567-3571.

Semple, S. J., Patterson, T. L., Temoshok, L. R., McCutchan, J. A., Straits-Troster, K. A., Chandler, J. L., & Grant, I. (1993). Identification of psychobiological stressors among HIV-positive women. *Women & Health, 20,* 15-36.

Epilogue

A Letter to Family Service Providers From Family Prevention Researchers

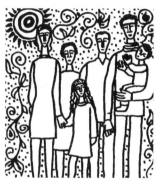

Dear Family Service Providers:

Although there is increased attention on families and HIV/AIDS in developing services and conducting research, there is a critical need for programs that can be easily delivered and are effective.

The work presented here has been conducted by academics working within the scientific rigor required of research funded by the National Institute of Mental Health. Often the resources that are available to researchers to carry out the interventions are greater than what is available at the practice level. We set up a paradox here. We may have developed programs that work but that are more resource intensive than providers are used to having. We suggest, however, that if providers measure their efforts not by the number of persons they include in their programs but rather by the number of persons with whom they are successful, you, the provider, will conclude that using some of the models proposed here yield for you a better outcome. That is, because the services are resource intensive, you might not have been able to work with as many persons and their families. However, because the programs are likely to be effective, you are likely to have a larger number of successes—even by working with a smaller number of families—than using less resource-intensive programs that may have very low success rates.

At the policy level, this kind of thinking is captured in the following question: "If I have enough antibiotics for 50 persons, but I have 200 persons to treat, shall

I have a better ultimate outcome (i.e., save more lives) by giving everyone one fourth of the dosage or by selecting carefully 50 persons in whom a full dosage could make a great impact?" Most likely, the latter would be a better model of public health: Provide an intervention that has the desired impact because less than adequate dosage might not be a good solution.

As the provider is likely to have noticed from our presentation of the work and the cases, our work has been far from the ivory tower. Our work has taken place in community settings not unlike the ones in which you provide services. We have worked with the same populations that you are likely to provide services. In fact, in these chapters, we have shown work with some of the neediest populations.

We now invite you to collaborate with us in the next step of the work. The next step is to bring this work to the front lines, to providers like yourselves. If you are interested in any of the models that you have seen presented here, we invite you to contact the team that developed the prevention programs. Every developer of these prevention programs is interested in helping providers implement these prevention programs throughout communities in the United States and abroad, assisting in the adaptation of this intervention to the unique terrain of your community, agency, and the clients that you serve.

In many cases, these programs have already been adapted for incorporation in service settings. For example, the work of Bauman and Rotheram-Borus actually grew out of requests for help from a community-based organization in the New York area. For this reason, their work has been intimately interwoven with the work of that practice agency. In Miami, the work of Mitrani, Szapocznik, and Robinson Batista has already been implemented in a comprehensive health and social services program at Miami-Dade County's main indigent hospital. Social service providers have been trained by clinicians who participated in the research, and the family work is now a part of the package of services that are provided to HIV+ women with the Special Immunology Obstetrics/Gynecology Clinic, in which these women are followed routinely for their primary health care. In this fashion, doctors, social service and family therapy providers, case managers, and family members collaborate in the care of the HIV+ women and their families.

The National Institute on Mental Health has a public health mission. It is our mission to develop services that improve the mental health of the public. We have completed development of the interventions using sound scientific principles and are now in the stage of completing evaluations to determine if these interventions work. Once these two steps are completed, for us to fulfill our mission of improving the mental health of the public, we must make these interventions available to front-line providers who ultimately will have the greatest impact by touching large numbers of lives. As presented here, these prevention programs represent the architectural blueprints for the work to be done.

However, only by having providers take these architectural blueprints and adapting them to the realities of their communities will these interventions ever reach their potential.

Without you, the providers, we cannot fulfill our mission. We stand ready to collaborate with you, the providers, in the next step in the work needed to improve the mental and physical health of the nation's families.

Sincerely yours,
Family Prevention Researchers

Willo Pequegnat, Chair   *Roberta Paikoff*
José Szpocznik   *James H. Bray*
Ralph J. DiClemente   *Colleen DiIorio*
Loretta Sweet Jemmott   *Bruce D. Rapkin*
Laurie J. Bauman   *Mary Jane Rotheram-Borus*
Beatrice J. Krauss

Index

Achenbach, T., 20, 158
Active listening, 204
Adolescents:
  African American, 135
  as caregivers, 183-184
  condom use, 6, 114
  high-risk behaviors, 11, 137
  role reversals, 200
  sexual behavior initiation, 11
  See also Adolescents, HIV positive
Adolescents, HIV positive, ix, 5, 114
  African American, 6, 135
  Hispanic, 6
  prevalence, 6
Adrian, C., 20, 158, 167
Africa, HIV/AIDS in, 4
African Americans:
  at-risk for HIV/AIDs, 12
  beliefs in HIV/AIDS conspiracy theory, 69
  denial of HIV/AIDS epidemic, 69
  See also Adolescents, HIV positive; African Americans, HIV positive; African American women, HIV positive; Women, HIV positive; Young adults of color, HIV positive
African Americans, HIV positive, ix, 5, 135, 170, 210
  prevalence among males, 6
  See also Adolescents, HIV positive; African American women, HIV positive; Women, HIV positive

African American women, HIV positive, 243-246, 278. *See also* African Americans, HIV positive; Structural Ecosystems Therapy (SET); Women, HIV positive
Age, HIV/AIDS and, 4, 6. *See also* Adolescents, HIV positive
AIDS. *See* HIV/AIDS
AIDS Serviceline, 171
Albert Einstein College of Medicine, 155
Aleman, J., 68
Aleman, J.-G., 5
Almeyda, L., 5, 13
Alumbaugh, M. J., 216
Alvy, K. T., 167
Amaro, H., 7, 244
Anderson, R., 3
Ankrah, E. M., 4
Aponte, H., 86, 244
Arena, V. C., 138
Armistead, L., xiii, 193
Ary, D., 12, 121
Assessment. *See* Family assessment
Audio taping interventions, 57
Auerswald, E., 244
Azjen, I., 106, 138, 139

Baca, L., 19, 190, 191
Baer, P. E., 34
Balk, D., 190
Balk, D. E., 19

303

About the Editors

Willo Pequegnat is Associate Director for Primary Prevention, Translational, and International Research in the Center for Mental Health Research on AIDS, National Institute of Mental Health (NIMH), National Institutes of Health (NIH). She provides scientific leadership for the largest national and international HIV/STD prevention and translational research program at NIH. She develops research program initiatives, sets priorities, and develops policies and initiatives. She serves as the senior scientist on a five-country (China, India, Peru, Russia, China) international behavioral prevention trial. In 1992, she initiated the NIMH Consortium on Families and HIV/AIDS and the annual research conference on the role of families in preventing and adapting to HIV/AIDS. Currently, she is coordinating the development of a mathematical program that can project the dynamics of HIV/STDs based on current prevalence and risky behavior patterns in a population and can also factor in the impact of specific prevention programs on the trajectories of the epidemic. Dr. Pequegnat serves on both national and international committees that address behavioral prevention issues. She was the coeditor of *How to Write a Successful Research Grant Application: A Guide for Social and Behavioral Scientists,* which is the most definitive guide on how to prepare a federal research grant proposal. In addition, she has prepared many articles on different aspects of HIV/STD behavioral prevention issues. She earned a Ph.D. in clinical psychology from the State University of New York at Stony Brook.

José Szapocznik, Ph.D., is Professor of Psychiatry and Behavioral Sciences, Psychology, and Counseling Psychology at the University of Miami. He is Director of the Center for Family Studies and the Spanish Family Guidance Center at the University of Miami School of Medicine. The Center for Family Studies is considered the nation's major systematic program of minority family therapy research. Dr. Szapocznik has served on the National Institute on Drug Abuse (NIDA) Extramural Science Advisory Board, the National Institute of Mental Health (NIMH) Advisory Council, the National Institutes of Health Office of AIDS Research Advisory Council, and the U.S. Center for Substance Abuse Prevention National Advisory Council. For his groundbreaking contributions in the development and testing of family interventions for poor urban minority families, he has received national recognition awards from the American Psychological Association, the American Family Therapy Academy, the American Association for Marriage and Family Therapy, the Association of Hispanic Mental Health Professionals, the Latino Behavioral Health Institute, the National Coalition of Hispanic Health and Human Services Organization, and the National Institute of Mental Health. Internationally, his work led to the designation of the Spanish Family Guidance Center as a World Health Organization Collaborating Center. Dr. Szapocznik has more than 140 professional publications, including a seminal book, *Breakthroughs in Family Therapy With Drug-Abusing and Problem Youth.* He is a frequent guest lecturer and plenary speaker on Hispanic or minority families, families and HIV, family therapy and family-based prevention, and mental health and drug abuse policy at universities, grassroots agencies, and national and international forums.

About the Contributors

Luis Almeyda, B.A., is Consultant for the Cornell Cooperative Extension, Cornell University, Ithaca, New York.

Donna Baptiste, Ed.D., is Research Assistant Professor and Psychology Supervisor at the University of Illinois at Chicago, Department of Psychiatry, Institute for Juvenile Research. She has coordinated the joint training of community parents and mental health interns for the past 5 years of the CHAMP Project. She also has conducted research related to parental monitoring of youth in high risk neighborhoods.

Carleen Robinson Batista, M.S.W., is Senior Research Associate with the Department of Psychiatry and Behavioral Sciences at the University of Miami School of Medicine. As a research associate with the University of Miami's Center for Family Studies, she has been a family therapist on clinical research projects funded by the National Institutes of Health. These studies have included adolescent conduct problems and substance abuse and adjustment to HIV.

Laurie J. Bauman, Ph.D., recently began a study of children as caregivers to their parents ill with AIDS, with Barbara Draimin in New York and Geoff Foster in Zimbabwe. She also obtained funding from the National Institute of Mental Health to evaluate Project Safe, a program designed to prevent HIV infection in sexually active teenagers. In addition, she has received an Investigator Award in Health Care Policy Research from Robert Wood Johnson Foundation to develop strategies to predict which children will have high health care costs and utilization using an algorithm that combines medical and social risk factors.

Jo Anne Bennett, RN, Ph.D., CS, ACRN, is a consultant public health nurse in the Office of Research, New York City Department of Health. She also has an appointment as Adjunct Assistant Professor of Nursing at New York University. She has over 15 years of experience in community-based AIDS services and education, including clinical trials of pharmaceutical and psychosocial interventions.

Nancy Boyd-Franklin, Ph.D., is an African American family therapist and Professor at Rutgers University in the Graduate School of Applied and Professional Psychology. She is the author of *Black Families in Therapy: A Multisystems Approach* (1989) and an editor of *Children, Families and HIV/AIDS: Psychosocial and Therapeutic Issues* (1995). Her latest books are *Reaching Out in Family Therapy: Home-Based, School and Community Interventions,* with Dr. Brenna Bry (2000), and *Boys Into Men: Raising Our African American Teenage Sons,* with A. J. Franklin and Pamela Toussaint (2000).

James H. Bray, Ph.D., is Director of the Baylor Family Counseling Clinic and Associate Professor in the Department of Family and Community Medicine, Baylor College of Medicine in Houston, Texas. He has received numerous awards, including the Karl F. Heiser APA Presidential Award for Advocacy on Behalf of Professional Psychology and the 1992 Federal Advocacy Award from the APA Practice Directorate. He has published and presented numerous works in the areas of divorce, remarriage, adolescent substance use, intergenerational family relationships, and collaboration between physicians and psychologists.

Emma J. Brown, Ph.D., RN, CS, is Associate Professor and Chatlos Endowed Chair in the School of Nursing at the College of Health and Public Affairs, University of Central Florida. Her research interests include STD/HIV prevention intervention among adolescents, women of color, and individuals who use illicit drugs (especially crack cocaine); drug use prevention and intervention; exploring the drug use cultures of small communities and rural areas; and developing and evaluating Faith-based HIV/AIDS and drug use prevention intervention models designed specifically for African Americans and other Blacks. She has received university and foundation awards to investigate these issues. She has recently submitted applications to the National Institute of Mental Health and the National Institute on Drug Abuse to study the impact of drug use on HIV risk behavior of rural Black women who use crack cocaine.

Edna Bula is Field Site Supervisor for the National Development & Research Institutes, New York.

Doris Coleman, LCSW, is a CHAMP Family Program Supervisor. She oversees all the social work interns placed on the CHAMP project, as well as, providing direction to CHAMP group facilitators. She is also conducting research related to the impact of CHAMP group factors on family outcome.

Teasha Daniels is Executive Assistant for the National Development & Research Institutes, New York.

W. Rees Davis, Ph.D., is Project Director for the National Development & Research Institutes, New York.

Jesse DeJesus is Research Assistant for the National Development & Research Institutes, New York.

Pamela Denzmore, M.P.H. is Research Project Coordinator, Senior at the Rollins School of Public Health at Emory University. She has worked as a research field interviewer on numerous research projects, volunteered with various HIV/AIDS organizations, and presented at several public health conferences including the1999 National HIV Prevention Conference and the American Public Health Association 127th Annual Meeting. Her interests include recruitment issues of African Americans into clinical research studies.

Ralph J. DiClemente, Ph.D., is Charles Howard Candler Professor of Public Health and Chair, Department of Behavioral Sciences and Health Education at the Rollins School of Public Health, and Professor of Medicine (Infectious Diseases) and Pediatrics in the School of Medicine, Emory University. He has focused much of his research on the development and evaluation of HIV prevention programs tailored to adolescents and women.

Colleen DiIorio, PhD, RN, FAAN, is Professor in the Department of Behavioral Sciences and Health Education of the Rollins School of Public Health at Emory University. She holds an affiliate faculty appointment at the Nell Hodgson Woodruff School of Nursing at Emory University and serves as Director of the Behavioral Core for the Center for AIDS Research at Emory University. She is a Fellow of the American Academy of Nursing and has received awards for her research, teaching, and service to the community. Her research includes the development and testing of HIV prevention programs for adolescents and the study of HIV risk factors among young adults.

Barbara Draimin, DSW, is Executive Director of The Family Center, a community-based agency providing custody planning services to seriously ill parents throughout New York City. She has worked with families with AIDS since 1988 focusing on the needs of well, orphaned children.

William N. Dudley, Ph.D., is Research Assistant Professor in the Department of Behavioral Sciences and Health Education, Rollins School of Public Health, Emory University. He also serves as statistician on a number of federally funded research projects that focus on HIV prevention, exercise and nutrition, and medication compliance in chronic disease such as HIV and epilepsy. His research interests also include the study of pain in those undergoing cancer therapy and quality of life in cancer survivors.

Ernest Frugé is Assistant Professor of Pediatrics and Family and Community Medicine at Baylor College of Medicine. He is also Director of Psychosocial Programs at the Texas Children's Cancer Center and Hematology Service. He holds adjunct appointments in the Department of Psychiatry and Behavioral Sciences, The University of Texas Health Science Center and the Department of Psychology at the University of Houston. His clinical and research interests focus on family and institutional factors that affect health care delivery, coping, and quality of life in chronic and life-threatening illnesses.

Evelyn Garcia is Research Assistant for the National Development & Research Institutes, New York.

Christopher Godfrey, M.A., is Principal Research Associate for the National Development & Research Institutes, New York.

Lloyd Goldsamt, Ph.D., is Coinvestigator for the National Development & Research Institutes, New York.

Brenda Howard Hopkins, MPA, is Project Director of the Mother-Son Health Promotion Project and Manager of the Center for Urban Health Research at the University of Pennsylvania School of Nursing. She has served as a project director on several NIMH funded HIV risk-reduction programs that target African American and Latino populations.

Monique Howard is a doctoral candidate at the University of Pennsylvania, Graduate School of Education. She has spent the past 8 years designing human sexuality education curriculum and has focused attention on reducing risk of sexually transmitted HIV and unplanned pregnancy. Presently, she is a consultant with YRM Consulting Unlimited where she develops culturally sensitive workshops that address human sexuality topics within communities of color in hopes of increasing positive attitudes and behaviors regarding human sexuality.

She has also co-edited an HIV risk reduction curriculum for domestic violence shelters.

Jan Hudis, MPA/MPH, is Director of Research for The Family Center in New York City, where she has worked with families with AIDS in the provision and evaluation of services for more than 10 years.

John B. Jemmott III, Ph.D., is the Kenneth B. Clark Professor of Communication and Director of the Center for Health Behavior and Communication at the Annenberg School for Communication of the University of Pennsylvania. He is a Fellow of the American Psychological Association and the Society for Behavioral Medicine and has served on the Behavioral Medicine Study Section and the AIDS and Immunology Research Review Committee. He currently is a member of the Office of AIDS Research Advisory Council of the National Institutes Health. He has been the recipient of numerous grants from the National Institutes of Health to conduct research designed to develop and test HIV risk reduction interventions for adolescents.

Loretta Sweet Jemmott, Ph.D., R.N., F.A.A.N., is Associate Professor and Director of the Center for Urban Health Research at the University of Pennsylvania School of Nursing and holds a secondary appointment in the Graduate School of Education. She received her M.S.N. in nursing, specializing in psychiatric mental health nursing, and her Ph.D. in education, specializing in human sexuality education, from the University of Pennsylvania. Her research has focused on designing and testing theory-based, culturally sensitive, and developmentally appropriate strategies to reduce HIV risk-associated sexual behaviors among African American and Latino populations.

Yolanda Jones is Junior Research Assistant for the National Development & Research Institutes, New York.

Beatrice J. Krauss, Ph.D., is Deputy Director of the Institute for AIDS Research and the Center for Drug Use and HIV Research at the National Development and Research Institutes in New York City. Her work has focused on HIV-affected communities and family adjustment to the HIV epidemic. She has been involved with more than 15 state or nationally funded HIV-related researches, and she has published and presented extensively on HIV prevention and adjustment to HIV in highly affected communities. In 1998, she received the Kurt Lewin Award for her social contribution in the area of HIV/AIDS.

Noelle R. Leonard, M.S., M.Ed., is Program Director at the Family Studies Unit, where she has worked since 1996 on the longitudinal study of adolescents living with HIV-infected parents as well as the replication of an HIV prevention program for runaway and homeless youth. She is currently a doctoral candidate at the University of Massachusetts at Amherst. She is writing her dissertation on the role of attachment in the adolescent bereavement process.

Carol Levine is Director, Families and Health Care Project, United Hospital Fund Director, The Orphan Project in New York City. She founded The Orphan Project in 1991 and was awarded a MacArthur Foundation Fellowship in 1993 for her work in AIDS policy and ethics.

Marguerita Lightfoot is Assistant Research Psychologist at the University of California, Los Angeles (UCLA), where she has been an integral part of a number of NIMH- and NIDA-funded grants, primarily intervention studies with adult and adolescent populations at high risk. She is published and has presented nationally and internationally on HIV issues. She is currently coinvestigator for a secondary prevention program with adults. In a randomized controlled design, the study delivers a computer-assisted risk assessment and intervention to seropositive adults in health care clinics.

Jenny Lipana, M.P.H., C.H.E.S., is Director, Educational Program Development for the Arthritis Foundation, National Office. Her interests include adolescent health as well as the use of the Internet for promoting self-management.

Sybil Madison, Ph.D., is Research Assistant Professor and Psychology Supervisor at the University of Illinois at Chicago, Department of Psychiatry, Institute for Juvenile Research. She has developed and supported the CHAMP Collaborative Board, consisting of community parents, teachers, representatives of community-based organizations and university-based researchers. She also is conducting research related to factors contributing to the resilience of urban youth.

Mary McKernan McKay, Ph.D., LCSW, is Associate Professor at Columbia University School of Social Work. She directs a program of research, including the CHAMP Family Program, geared toward testing innovative prevention and intervention programs to meet the health and mental health needs of urban youth and their families. She has a strong history of collaborating with community members and researchers to develop culturally and contextually sensitive programming.

Victoria Behar Mitrani, Ph.D., is Research Assistant Professor of Psychiatry and Behavioral Sciences at the University of Miami School of Medicine. As a faculty member of the University of Miami's Center for Family Studies, she has been a family therapist, family therapy supervisor, and investigator on numerous clinical research projects funded by the National Institutes of Health. She has been at the forefront of adapting structural ecosystems therapy, a family-based intervention model developed at the Center for Family Studies for ethnically and clinically diverse populations. She is also the coauthor of the *Structural Family Systems Ratings,* an observational measure of family interactions.

Michele Muñoz, Ph.D. is Research Project Director with the Department of Psychiatry and Behavioral Sciences at Memorial Sloan-Kettering Cancer Center. She has provided psychotherapy and psychosocial interventions to patients and families affected by chronic illness. Her interest lies in how Hispanic/Latin families cope with illness and their access to services. She has also studied language differences in the representation of biographical experiences among bilingual Latinos.

Paulette Murphy, Psy.D., is Clinical Research Director with the Department of Psychiatry and Behavioral Sciences at Memorial Sloan-Kettering Cancer Center. She has extensive experience in working with HIV/AIDS patients and with substance abusers. She has also completed training with the American Psychological Association HIV Office of Psychological Education.

Joanne O'Day is a Research Assistant for the National Development & Research Institutes, New York.

Freida H. Outlaw, DNSc, RN, CS., is Assistant Professor of Nursing and Program Director of the Psychiatric Mental Health Graduate Program at the University of Pennsylvania School of Nursing. Her research and clinical practice are focused on developing culturally competent evidence-based mental health interventions with poor minorities in urban communities.

Roberta Paikoff, Ph.D., is Associate Professor at the University of Illinois at Chicago, Department of Psychiatry, Institute for Juvenile Research. She is a developmental psychologist who directs a program of research, including the CHAMP Family Study and the CHAMP Family Program, which identifies child, family, and community level factors that influence the risk and health behaviors of urban youth. She is particularly committed to the translation of basic research findings into family-based prevention programming.

Michael Pierre-Louis, B.A., is Research Assistant for the National Development & Research Institutes, New York.

James Pride is Junior Research Assistant for the National Development & Research Institutes, New York.

Bruce D. Rapkin, Ph.D., is Associate Professor of Psychology in the Department of Psychiatry and Behavioral Sciences at Memorial Sloan-Kettering Cancer Center. He is a community psychologist with background in the development and evaluation of programs to address access to care, quality of care, and quality of life among the medically undeserved. He also has an interest in developing research methods to better understand health behavior and health outcomes in diverse communities. His work has been supported from NIMH, AHCPR, NIDA and the New York State Department of Health.

Dennis Reardon, M.S.W., C.S.W., is Field Site Supervisor for the National Development & Research Institutes, New York.

Ken Resnicow is Professor in the Department of Behavioral Sciences and Health Education, Rollins School of Public Health, Emory University. His research interests include: the design and evaluation of health promotion programs for special populations, particularly cardiovascular and cancer prevention interventions for African Americans; understanding the relationship between ethnicity and health behaviors; substance use prevention and harm reduction; motivational interviewing for chronic disease prevention; and comprehensive school health programs. He also serves as a co-investigator on the following: an NIMH funded HIV prevention intervention being conducted with African American adolescents and their mothers through the Boys and Girls clubs of Atlanta; an NIMH study to improve father-son communication regarding safer sex practices; an NIAAA-funded study to reduce substance use and problem behaviors in juvenile offenders; and an NCI study testing the efficacy of Zyban as a smoking cessation treatment for African American smokers.

Celestino Rivera is Research Assistant for the National Development & Research Institutes, New York.

Giesla Rogers-Tillman , BS, is a Senior Interviewer at the Rollins School of Public Health at Emory University. She has worked as an interviewer on a number of research projects including a multisite HIV prevention project to enhance risk reduction practices among adults at high risk for contracting HIV. She has expertise in interviewer training as well as developing and implementing strategies for retention of participants in research studies.

Mary Jane Rotheram-Borus is Professor of Psychiatry and the Director of the Center for HIV Identification, Prevention, and Treatment Services and the Center for Community Health in the Neuropsychiatric Institute, University of California, Los Angeles. Her research interests include HIV/AIDS prevention with adolescents, suicide among adolescents, homeless youth, assessment and modification of children's social skills, ethnic identity, group processes, and cross-ethnic interactions. She has received grants from the National Institute of Mental Health to study HIV prevention with adolescents and persons with sexually transmitted diseases.

Richard Scott, M.A., combines a strong business background with a degree in social work to support the infrastructure necessary to deliver the CHAMP Family Program at multiple community-based sites. He has been responsible for overseeing all financial and organizational issues related to CHAMP.

Jennifer Tiffany, R.N., is a Consultant for the Cornell Cooperative Extension, Cornell University, Ithaca, New York.

Elba Troche is Research Assistant for the National Development & Research Institutes, New York.

Deborah Fisher Van Marter, M.P.H., is a Data Information Specialist at Rollins School of Public Health, Emory University. Her research interests include HIV prevention among adolescents and health policy. She has been a contributing author on articles published in the *Journal of Health Communication* and *Research in Nursing and Health* and has presented at various industry conferences, including the American Public Health Association 127th Annual Meeting and the 1999 National HIV Prevention Conference.

Richard Velez is Junior Research Assistant for the National Development & Research Institutes, New York.

Dongqing T. Wang, M.S.P.H., is a Data Analyst at the Rollins School of Public Health, Emory University. She currently serves as the data manager on a number of federally funded research projects that focus on HIV prevention, exercise and nutrition, and adherence to HIV medications. Her research interests include research design and implementation, development and maintenance of research databases as well as statistical analyses.

Gina M. Wingood is Assistant Professor in the Department of Behavioral Sciences and Health Education at the Rollins School of Public Health, Emory University. She is the principal architect of the theory of gender and power. Her research focuses on designing, implementing, and evaluating culturally tailored HIV prevention programs for young African American women. She also conducts research on the influence of sexual and physical abuses and television viewing habits as HIV risk factors for young African American women.

Dorline Yee, B.A., is Senior Research Associate, the National Development & Research Institutes, New York.